The Art of Paediatric Medicine Beyond the Evidence Base

Catherine F Lynch • Sarah Arachchi
Sharmayne Brady • Ar Kar Aung
Ralph Junckerstorff
Editors

The Art of Paediatric Medicine Beyond the Evidence Base

Clinical Pearls from Experienced Clinicians

Springer

Editors
Catherine F Lynch
Alfred Health
Melbourne, VIC, Australia

Sharmayne Brady
Arthritis and Rheumatology Centre
Endeavour Hills, VIC, Australia

Ralph Junckerstorff
Monash Health
Melbourne, VIC, Australia

Sarah Arachchi
Department of Paediatric Emergency Medicine
Monash Health
Melbourne, VIC, Australia

Ar Kar Aung
Department of General Medicine
Alfred Health
Melbourne, VIC, Australia

ISBN 978-981-96-7233-2 ISBN 978-981-96-7234-9 (eBook)
https://doi.org/10.1007/978-981-96-7234-9

This Springer imprint is published by the registered company Springer Nature Singapore Pte Ltd.
The registered company address is: 152 Beach Road, #21-01/04 Gateway East, Singapore 189721, Singapore

Prologue

Storytelling is a fundamental part of being human. Stories let us share information in a way that creates an emotional connection and may enhance our ability to remember information clearly. Our patients bring their stories and teach us every day. Our colleagues also teach us every day.

The Art of Paediatric Medicine Beyond the Evidence Base: Clinical Pearls from Experienced Clinicians is not a traditional textbook with the usual comprehensive specialty-based coverage of all aspects of the fascinating field of paediatrics. This book is based on cases or stories, distilled into a "pearl of wisdom", and then refined by experienced clinicians who have cared for children. The delight of practising in paediatrics often comes from providing care for all ages and stages of children with differences in size, physiology, capabilities and charms. Most clinicians caring for children will deal with this wide range whether they are generalists or subspecialists. We asked a wide variety of colleagues working in diverse clinical settings to "send us a pearl". In Australia, primary care for children is provided by general practitioners in the community. Consultant paediatricians provide specialised outpatient and inpatient hospital care. Clinicians from all around the world, from every field of paediatrics, responded with insight and passion. We were humbled by their response and enthusiasm. The responses were as varied as the vast range of paediatric practice: from the neonatologist to the developmental paediatrician; from the tertiary paediatric hospital specialist to rural paediatricians. All were kind enough to share a nugget of wisdom. However, although diverse, at their core was a desire to share information that would improve the lives of our patients by helping those who care for them.

The book is organised by "Ages and Stages" rather than organ systems, reflecting the developmental nature of paediatric practices. However, there are pearls of wisdom applicable to all ages and stages. Each chapter begins with a clinical case that demonstrates how the pearl can be applied in clinical practice. This is followed by a discussion of the topic with relevant evidence-based references. The "Other Gems" section allows authors to share other practice points relevant to, but not directly related to, the clinical pearl. We hope this book will be useful for later-year medical students, medical educators, doctors in training, general practitioners and consultant paediatricians alike.

We sincerely thank all our contributors. As Editors we hope these pearls make you think, bring you hope, encourage the art of medicine and create a safer place for our patients and our practice. If this collection gives you an extra tool, or makes you think differently about a patient you see tomorrow, it will have achieved its purpose.

Melbourne, VIC, Australia Catherine F Lynch
Melbourne, VIC, Australia Sarah Arachchi
Endeavour Hills, VIC, Australia Sharmayne Brady
Melbourne, VIC, Australia Ar Kar Aung
Melbourne, VIC, Australia Ralph Junckerstorff

Contents

Part II Children (5–12 Years)

About the Editors

Catherine F Lynch, BMedSci, MBBS, M. Bioethics, FRACP, is a Consultant Paediatrician. She studied undergraduate medicine at University of Tasmania graduating in 1985. She trained in Sydney, Toronto and Melbourne, attaining her Fellowship in Paediatrics from the Royal Australasian College of Physicians (FRACP) in 2002. She also holds a Master of Bioethics (2000) from Monash University. She was founding director of Bayside Childrens Clinic (a private paediatric clinic. She worked as an Adolescent Medicine physician at Monash Childrens Hospital and was Head of Unit, Paediatrics at Alfred Health. She is the inaugural Clinical Advisor for Paediatrics and Adolescent Medicine for Alfred Health (2016–present). She has been involved in undergraduate and postgraduate teaching and has interests in quality and safety issues, disability, and transition for children into adult health services. She has three adult children, too many pets and loves bubbles and sparkles.

Sarah Arachchi, MBBS (Hons), FRACP, Dip.C.H is a General Paediatrician in the Emergency Department at Monash Children's Hospital in Melbourne, Victoria, and works in a private paediatric clinic at Victorian Children's Clinic and Clynden Ave Specialist Clinic in Malvern. She studied undergraduate medicine at Monash University in 2009 and finished her degree with honours. She became a fellow of the Royal Australasian College of Physicians in 2017. She has organised multiple medical conferences in Australia. She co-convenes educational sessions (Vic Feat) for the Royal Australasian College of Physicians (RACP) for paediatricians and advanced trainees and is also an active member of the Women in Medicine committee of AMA Victoria. She also recently published her memoir, *Brown. Female. Doctor.*, by Monash University Publishing, and in her spare time, enjoys writing media articles centred around healthcare and leadership. Some of her work has been published in Women's Agenda, the ABC and Guardian newspapers.

Sharmayne Brady, MBBS (Hons), BMedSc (Hons), FRACP, PhD is an adult rheumatologist working in private practice in Melbourne, Australia, and is a senior staff specialist at The Alfred Hospital. She studied undergraduate medicine at

Monash University in Melbourne and finished her degree with first-class honours. She completed her PhD in 2021 through Monash University, working with internationally renowned osteoarthritis experts. During her PhD, she was supported by a prestigious National Health and Medical Research Council (NHMRC) Clinical Postgraduate Research scholarship. She has published 16 papers in leading peer-reviewed journals and presented her research in several leading international and national conferences over the past 10 years. She has also co-edited medical textbooks for doctors *Clinical Integration: Medicine*, published in 2021, and *Beyond Evidence-Based Medicine: Clinical Pearls from Experienced Physicians* in 2023.

Ar Kar Aung, BMedSci, MBBS, FRACP, MPHTM is an adult General and Infectious Diseases physician, a researcher, a medical editor, an educator and an exhausted but proud parent to a cheeky toddler. He is a consultant physician at Alfred Health in Melbourne, Australia, and holds an adjunct clinical associate professor position at Monash University. He plays several leadership roles in the Internal Medicine Society of Australia and New Zealand. He has published more than 70 peer-reviewed articles, numerous clinical guidelines and book chapters, and co-edited two medical textbooks *Clinical Integration: Medicine* and *Beyond Evidence-Based Medicine: Clinical Pearls from Experienced Physicians.*

Ralph Junckerstorff, MBBS, FRACP, DTM&H is an adult General (Internal) Medicine and Infectious Diseases physician at Monash Health in Melbourne, Victoria. He graduated from undergraduate medicine from the University of Western Australia in 2000 and became a fellow of the Royal Australasian College of Physicians in 2010. He also holds a Diploma of Tropical Medicine from the University of Liverpool (UK). He is a co-editor of the medical textbooks *Beyond Evidence-Based Medicine: Clinical Pearls from Experienced Physicians* and *Leadership Pearls in Healthcare*. He has two children.

Part I
Babies, Toddlers, Preschoolers (0–4 Years)

If You Only See One Hole, It's the Wrong One

Carl Kuschel

1 Clinical Pearl

Neonatal intubation is a difficult skill to acquire and maintain. Consider all available resources that can support you if a baby requires intubation.

2 Clinical Case

A female infant, Rowena, weighing 3105 g was born at 41 weeks gestation after an unremarkable pregnancy and spontaneous labour. Thick meconium was noted when the membranes were ruptured just prior to birth. She took some initial gasps and was assigned a 1-min Apgar score of 7. However, she developed marked respiratory distress and bradycardia. An emergency call was made, with neonatal staff attending soon afterwards. Mask ventilation with 100% oxygen and cardiac compressions were commenced for bradycardia (heart rate <60 bpm) and thick meconium was noted in the oropharynx. Pulse oximetry showed a reliable heart rate trace with bradycardia and oxygen saturations of only 50%. The 5-min Apgar score was 6 with persistent bradycardia despite resuscitation efforts. Laryngoscopy was performed but there was difficulty seeing the vocal cords clearly despite suctioning, due to copious thick meconium-stained secretions. Following placement of an endotracheal tube, the heart rate and oxygen saturations did not improve and there was no colour change on carbon dioxide colorimetric testing. A laryngeal mask was inserted whilst preparations were made for a further intubation attempt. On the second

C. Kuschel (✉)
Neonatal Services, The Royal Women's Hospital, Parkville, VIC, Australia

The University of Melbourne, Parkville, VIC, Australia

C. F. Lynch et al. (eds.), *The Art of Paediatric Medicine Beyond the Evidence Base*,
https://doi.org/10.1007/978-981-96-7234-9_1

attempt, the airway was cleared with suctioning and the anatomical structures were clearly seen. Following intubation, the carbon dioxide monitor confirmed that the endotracheal tube was correctly placed, and Rowena's heart rate and oxygen saturations improved. Rowena was transferred to the neonatal intensive care unit (NICU).

3 Discussion

Providing effective ventilation is an essential skill for medical staff working in neonatal units or attending births. With increasing use of non-invasive respiratory support measures, opportunities to acquire and maintain intubation skills are limited. In 2022, 24.8% of preterm infants <32 weeks gestational age registered with the Australian and New Zealand Neonatal Network (ANZNN) were intubated in the immediate birthing environment and 3.8% of all ANZNN registrants had a 5-min Apgar score less than 4 [1]. Predictors for requiring resuscitation at birth include:

(a) Maternal factors—hypertension, maternal infection, bleeding in the second or third trimesters.
(b) Foetal factors—multiple gestation, prematurity, post-term gestation.
(c) Intrapartum factors—abnormal presentation, prolonged labour, instrumental birth [2].

Positive pressure ventilation is the mainstay of neonatal resuscitation and is the first line of intervention following stimulation [3]. Effective mask ventilation requires good technique and appropriate equipment (for example, the correct-sized mask). Some infants may not respond to or will deteriorate with mask ventilation or may require a more secure airway. Laryngeal masks are being increasingly used in neonatal resuscitations as they are relatively easy to insert with minimal training and can provide a safe and effective airway [4]. However, their use is usually limited to babies who are 34 weeks gestation or more and who weigh more than 2 kg.

Intubation success is dependent on correctly identifying anatomical landmarks. In many NICUs, intubations are frequently performed using a videolaryngoscope that allows an observer to assist with identifying anatomical structures and confirming correct endotracheal tube placement. A good rule of thumb is that if only one opening is seen, it is much more likely to be the oesophagus than the vocal cords, as the oesophagus sits posterior to the vocal cords and will be visible, particularly if the laryngoscope blade has been advanced too far and is not positioned correctly to see the more anterior laryngeal structures.

If intubation is required and you are not confident of the procedure, consider other staff who may be available to assist (such as anaesthetic or intensive care staff). If the baby is not bradycardic (that is, the heart rate is above 100 bpm), there is potentially more time to gather resources or personnel.

Intubation and advanced resuscitation require teamwork in what can be a stressful environment where attendees may become distracted by tasks rather than appreciating the overall clinical situation. Simulation has a role in training staff in resuscitation scenarios and encouraging clear and respectful communication when team members are under pressure, as well as exploring other strategies to support ventilation.

4 Other Gems

- Mask ventilation is the mainstay of initial effective resuscitation but relies on appropriate equipment and technique.
- Laryngeal masks are effective at providing airway support in infants above 34 weeks or weighing 2000 g.
- Simulation training can help with fostering teamwork and procedural skills for scenarios that are uncommon.

References

1. Chow, S. S. W., Creighton, P., Holberton, J. R., Chambers, G. M., & Lui, K. (2024). *Report of the Australian and New Zealand neonatal network 2022* (p. 16). ANZNN.
2. Australian Resuscitation Council. *ANZCOR Guideline 13.1 – Introduction to resuscitation of the newborn*. Accessed 24 Sept 2024. Available from: https://www.anzcor.org/home/neonatal-resuscitation/guideline-13-2-planning-for-newborn-resuscitation-and-identification-of-the-newborn-at-risk/
3. Wyckoff, M. H., Singletary, E. M., Soar, J., et al. (2021). 2021 international consensus on cardiopulmonary resuscitation and emergency cardiovascular care science with treatment recommendations: Summary from the basic life support; advanced life support; neonatal life support; education, implementation, and teams; first aid task forces; and the COVID-19 working group. *Resuscitation, 169*, 229–311. https://doi.org/10.1016/j.resuscitation.2021.10.040
4. Schmölzer, G. M. (2022). Face mask or laryngeal mask during positive pressure ventilation for term newborns: Is one preferable than the other? *Resuscitation, 171*, 96–97. https://doi.org/10.1016/j.resuscitation.2022.01.002

Keep an Open Mind

Jeanie Cheong

1 Clinical Pearl

Always keep an open mind … you don't have to know the diagnosis straightaway.

2 Clinical Case

A male infant was born by forceps-assisted delivery, complicated by shoulder dystocia. He was "flat" at birth, and received mask ventilation, chest compressions and 2 doses of adrenaline. His Apgar scores were 0 at 1 min, 3 at 5 min, and 3 at 10 min. His admission diagnosis was mild Stage 1 neonatal encephalopathy and thus, he did not receive hypothermia treatment. An initial cranial ultrasound was normal.

Over the next 2 days, his main symptoms consisted of severe irritability, "jitteriness" and feeding difficulties. His body and limb tone were generally increased, despite normal deep tendon reflexes. By Day 4, the clinical team revised the working diagnosis to consider the possibility of maternal drug withdrawal. His mother had been on quetiapine and lamotrigine for bipolar disorder. Phenobarbitone was administered (10 mg/kg loading dose, followed by 5 mg/kg daily) with near resolution of symptoms within 24 h. Using the modified Finnegan scoring tool to guide treatment, phenobarbitone was ceased after 5 days.

J. Cheong (✉)
Department of Neonatal Services, The Royal Women's Hospital, Parkville, VIC, Australia

Clinical Sciences, Murdoch Children's Research Institute, Parkville, VIC, Australia

Department of Obstetrics, Gynaecology and Newborn Health, & Department of Paediatrics, University of Melbourne, Parkville, VIC, Australia

C. F. Lynch et al. (eds.), *The Art of Paediatric Medicine Beyond the Evidence Base*,
https://doi.org/10.1007/978-981-96-7234-9_2

3 Discussion

Approximately 3.5% of mothers in high-income nations are treated with psychotropic medications, and thus, it is important to recognise poor neonatal adaptation (PNA) or "withdrawal." PNA manifests as sleeping and feeding difficulties, agitation, and respiratory distress [1]. Polypharmacy is becoming increasingly common in the management of mental health disorders and has been associated with an increased risk of PNA [2]. Although the evidence base was scant at the time of the above illustrative case, there has been increasing recognition of quetiapine as a possible cause of PNA [3, 4].

This case illustrates some important aspects of diagnostic reasoning:

(a) It was important to keep questioning "why" when the infant did not present with a clinical course entirely consistent with the initial diagnosis of mild hypoxic-ischaemic encephalopathy. If the team had not questioned this, the infant would have remained symptomatic for much longer, causing more neonatal morbidity and escalating parental stress.
(b) The clinical treating team were prepared to say "I don't know" and kept considering alternative diagnoses for the baby's presentation. Exploring the possibility of drug withdrawal was difficult to confirm, as there was limited literature at the time linking quetiapine to PNA.
(c) Finally, keeping an open mind was what prompted the treating team to commence the infant on phenobarbitone for possible PNA. There was a rapid response, and an excellent outcome for the infant and family.

4 Other Gems

- Neonatal encephalopathy can be due to many causes, not just hypoxia/ischaemia.
- Always get a full clinical history from the family.

References

1. Kieviet, N., Dolman, K. M., & Honig, A. (2013). The use of psychotropic medication during pregnancy: How about the newborn? *Neuropsychiatric Disease and Treatment, 9*, 1257–1266.
2. Sadowski, A., Todorow, M., Yazdani Brojeni, P., et al. (2013). Pregnancy outcomes following maternal exposure to second-generation antipsychotics given with other psychotropic drugs: A cohort study. *BMJ Open, 3*, e003062.
3. Brajcich, M. R., Palau, M. A., Messer, R. D., Murphy, M. E., & Marks, J. (2021). Why the maternal medication list matters: Neonatal toxicity from combined serotonergic exposures. *Pediatrics, 147*(2), e20192250.
4. Lau, C., Watson, H., & Cheong, J. (2015). Poor neonatal adaptation following in-utero exposure to quetiapine and lamotrigine. *Journal of Obstetrics and Gynaecology, 35*(6), 646.

I Thought It Was a Soft Murmur!

Lindsay Carrigan and Srinidhi J. V. Rao

1 Clinical Pearl

Cardiac murmurs change with shifts in neonatal physiology.

2 Clinical Case

A male infant, Leroy, was born at 42 weeks gestation weighing 4 kg. Antenatal scans and serology were unremarkable. Postnatal examination was suspicious for a pathological murmur, and he was transferred to a tertiary centre for further assessment. His heart rate, 4-limb blood pressure and pre/post ductal pulse-oximetry were within normal limits.

Examination on day 2 of life revealed normal first and second heart sounds, a soft ejection click and a grade 2–3/6 ejection systolic murmur loudest at the left upper sternal edge and radiating to the back. There were no dysmorphic features, his respiratory and abdominal examinations were unremarkable, and his femoral pulses were normal.

Echocardiography demonstrated a dysplastic, doming pulmonary valve with moderate pulmonary stenosis, a small patent ductus arteriosus and normal right ventricular function. The mean pressure gradient across the pulmonary valve (PV MG; the difference in pressure between the right ventricle and pulmonary artery)

L. Carrigan
The Royal Children's Hospital, Parkville, VIC, Australia

S. J. V. Rao (✉)
Monash Children's Hospital, Clayton, VIC, Australia

C. F. Lynch et al. (eds.), *The Art of Paediatric Medicine Beyond the Evidence Base*,
https://doi.org/10.1007/978-981-96-7234-9_3

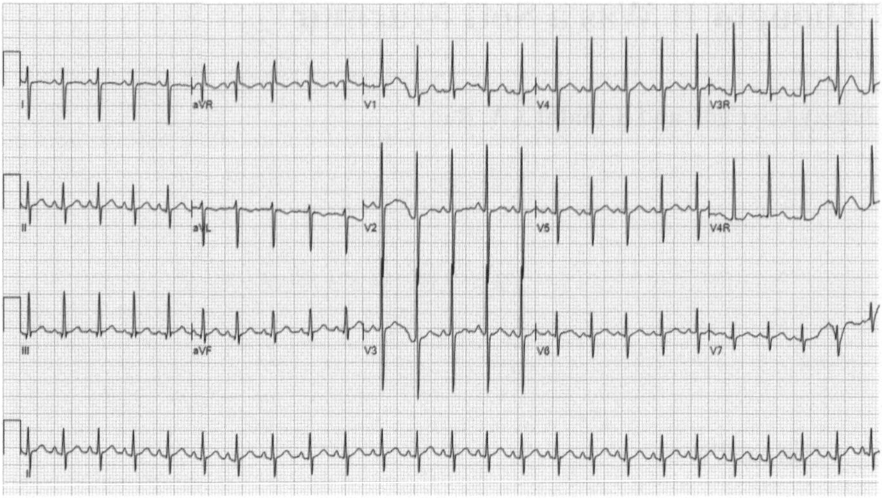

Fig. 1 Electrocardiogram (ECG) of the infant demonstrating sinus rhythm with right ventricular hypertrophy

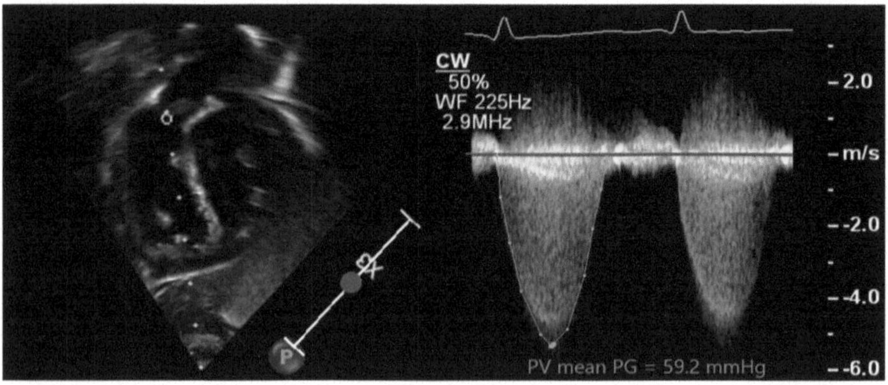

Fig. 2 Transthoracic echocardiogram demonstrating high pressures across the pulmonary valve, confirming haemodynamically significant stenosis

was 38 mmHg, falling below the threshold for intervention. After a period of observation, he was discharged home.

On review in the clinic at 24 days of age, Leroy remained asymptomatic, was feeding well and thriving. Whilst the rest of his examination was unremarkable, his murmur changed to grade 4/6 with an associated thrill on palpation. His electrocardiogram (ECG) findings revealed persistence of upright T-waves in leads V1 and V2 beyond the first week of life and prominent rightward chest lead forces indicating right ventricular hypertrophy (Fig. 1). Echocardiography demonstrated progression of his PV MG to 59 mmHg, meeting the threshold for intervention (Fig. 2). The ductus arteriosus was closed and heart function preserved despite severe obstruction.

At 7 weeks of life, Leroy's PV MG was 70 mmHg and he underwent a successful percutaneous balloon pulmonary valvuloplasty. His supra-systemic right ventricular pressure normalised with intervention (85 mmHg to 28 mmHg). There was only minimal residual pulmonary valve gradient (11 mmHg) with trivial pulmonary regurgitation. These improvements persisted over 5 years of follow-up to date with a persistent grade 1/6 pulmonary murmur and resolution of markers of right ventricular hypertrophy on ECG.

3 Discussion

In 1961, Lucas et al. [1] mused "in few structures in the infant does a little growth alter performance so profoundly as in the pulmonary vessels." The drastic change in physiology of pulmonary blood flow in the first months of life remains a central concept in paediatric cardiology. It is demonstrated in the above case by the progression of clinical, ECG and echocardiographic findings over the first 2 months of life. The escalation in intensity of murmur and PV MG reflects an unmasked pressure difference, not a change in the severity of the underlying lesion.

In the foetus, the pulmonary vascular bed remains constricted in the unexpanded, liquid-filled lungs. It only receives 10–20% of the foetal cardiac output [2] with the ductus arteriosus providing a convenient shortcut to the lower body. The minimal venous return to the left atrium ensures a low pressure compared to the right atrium. This, combined with angulation from the Eustachian valve and ridge, streams highly oxygenated blood from the ductus venosus through the foramen ovale and ultimately to the head and neck vessels and brain.

With the first breaths there is a dramatic drop in pulmonary vascular resistance. A combination of physical expansion of vessels suspended in the lung interstitium and the vasodilation effect of oxygen and other mediators allows a 20–30-fold increase in pulmonary blood flow [3]. Increased left atrial pressure from the expanding venous return closes the foramen ovale. Umbilical cord clamping causes a sharp rise in systemic pressures due to loss of the low-resistance placental circulation. The pulmonary pressures remain high as the ductus arteriosus transmits aortic pressures to the main pulmonary artery. With exposure to highly saturated blood, reversal of the direction of blood flow and the loss of placental prostaglandins, the ductal tissue gradually constricts and closes. Right ventricular output then becomes the only source of pulmonary circulation and a more gradual phase of falling pulmonary vascular resistance and pressure can begin.

The thick, muscular medial layer of the pulmonary vessels gradually thin. The pulmonary vascular surface area increases with the arborisation of new alveoli and increasing vessel diameter with somatic growth. These factors combine to cause a gradual fall in the resistance to pulmonary flow and pulmonary pressures in the first 3 months of life [2, 4]. This dramatic change in physiology drives the evolving clinical signs, ECG changes and echocardiography findings in pulmonary valve stenosis and other congenital heart disease.

Fundamentally (excluding compliance), the flow of blood across an obstruction or communication depends on the respective pressures before and after. The fall of the distal pulmonary pressures with time alters the flow dynamics in various scenarios [5]:

(a) In right sided obstruction, the elevated distal pressure (resistance) will lessen the murmur and mask the severity of the lesion.
(b) A ventricular septal defect or large patent ductus arteriosus will not shunt significantly until pulmonary pressures fall, leading to high pulmonary flow and clinical signs. Thus, even infants with large ventricular septal defects may not become symptomatic in the first few weeks of life.
(c) The initial surgery of neonatal cyanotic heart disease with poor pulmonary flow relies on an arterial source of pulmonary blood flow to overcome high pulmonary pressures.
(d) An anomalous coronary artery from the pulmonary artery can maintain short term adequate perfusion due to raised pulmonary artery diastolic pressure. Ischaemia develops with falling perfusion pressure in the first 3 months of life. Understanding this phenomenon reinforces the need for repeating the newborn examination at 6–8 weeks of life. It also clarifies the expected time course of symptoms, the appropriate timing of surgical intervention and serves to demystify much of the management of congenital heart disease.

References

1. Lucas, R. V., Geme, J. W. S., Anderson, R. C., Adams, P., & Ferguson, D. J. (1961). Maturation of the pulmonary vascular bed: A physiologic and anatomic correlation in infants and children. *American Journal of Diseases of Children, 101*(4), 467–475.
2. Rudolph, A. (2011). *Congenital diseases of the heart: Clinical-physiological considerations*. Wiley.
3. Hooper, S. B., Te Pas, A. B., Lang, J., van Vonderen, J. J., Roehr, C. C., Kluckow, M., Gill, A. W., Wallace, E. M., & Polglase, G. R. (2015). Cardiovascular transition at birth: A physiological sequence. *Pediatric Research, 77*(5), 608–614.
4. Chakkarapani, A. A., Roehr, C. C., Hooper, S. B., Te Pas, A. B., & Gupta, S. (2023). ESPR neonatal resuscitation section writing group. Transitional circulation and hemodynamic monitoring in newborn infants. *Pediatric Research, 96*, 595–603.
5. Haworth, S. G. (1988). Pulmonary vascular remodelling in neonatal pulmonary hypertension. State of the art. *Chest, 93*(3 Suppl), 133S–138S.

Collapse on Day Three of Life

Michael Clifford

1 Clinical Pearl

Always treat for sepsis, consider cardiac lesions and don't forget metabolic disease.

2 Clinical Case

A term male newborn, Hugo, has become very unwell on the postnatal ward on day three. There were no concerns antenatally, and the mother is well. The midwives comment that the baby has been slow to attach and suck but seemed otherwise normal. Hugo appears pale, grey and mottled, is gasping and has poor peripheral pulses. Initial capillary blood gas demonstrates significant metabolic acidosis with an elevated lactate and a borderline low blood sugar. Urgent transfer to the Special Care Unit occurs where intravenous access is obtained, blood cultures are taken, antibiotics and dextrose 10% infusion commenced. PGE1 (prostaglandin E1 or "alprostadil") is prepared whilst a second intravenous cannula is sited. The Neonatal Retrieval Service is contacted for advice and potential transfer to a tertiary centre.

M. Clifford (✉)
Departments of Paediatric Intensive Care, Anaesthesia and Pain Management,
The Royal Children's Hospital Melbourne, Parkville, VIC, Australia

C. F. Lynch et al. (eds.), *The Art of Paediatric Medicine Beyond the Evidence Base*,
https://doi.org/10.1007/978-981-96-7234-9_4

3 Discussion

Early and late onset neonatal sepsis is common—even in infants without maternal risk factors [1, 2]. Prior to 48 h (day 2), early onset disease is likely to be due to Group B streptococcus (GBS)—which is still susceptible to penicillin (60 mg/kg IV 12-hourly), or *Escherichia coli.* (gentamicin 5mg/kg 24 hourly) - both are covered by a third generation cephalosporin (eg cefotaxime 50 mg/kg 12 hourly). After 48 h (day 3), organisms such as *Listeria monocytogenes* and *Staphylococcus aureus* should be considered [3]. Listeria is susceptible to penicillin and ampicillin (50 mg/kg IV 6-hourly) but not covered by cephalosporins [3]. *S. aureus* is more likely if the umbilicus is infected, or if the infant has been exposed to hospital interventions (e.g. venous access) and should be covered by flucloxacillin (50 mg/kg IV12-hourly). Herpes simplex virus can also cause severe encephalopathy and metabolic acidosis [1, 2]. Any seizures should prompt the addition of acyclovir (20 mg/kg IV 8-hourly) [3].

Always check your local hospital guidelines for the most appropriate antibiotic selection for both early onset sepsis (EOS <48 hours) and late onset sepsis (LOS > 48 hours).

The first week of life finalises the transition from in-utero to ex-utero existence that commences with the first breath. Over the first few minutes, marked changes to cardiorespiratory dynamics occur. Right to left shunts close and the pulmonary vascular resistance falls. With closure of the ductus arteriosus (often delayed until day 3–5), the systemic circulation is now dependent on left ventricular outflow via the aortic valve and arch [4]. If a neonate has any of the "duct dependent" left ventricular outflow tract lesions (i.e. hypoplastic left heart syndrome, critical aortic stenosis, interrupted aortic arch and severe coarctation), closure of the ductus arteriosus will precipitate circulatory collapse [4, 5]. Differential pulses may not be appreciated and there may not be a murmur if the baby is in shock. Intravenous access and commencement of PGE1 (alprostadil) infusion (10–30 nanograms/kg/min) should occur before other cardiovascular investigations are obtained [2, 4, 5]. Increasing doses of PGE1 may be required to "open the duct" after the diagnosis has been confirmed on echocardiography and this may precipitate apnoea, necessitating intubation and ventilation [4, 5].

Similarly, transplacental nutrition and metabolic waste management are now being replaced by oral provision of carbohydrate, protein and fat in breast milk—this metabolic support is accelerated on days 3–5 when the breast milk production "comes in". Inability to metabolise any of these elements leads to accumulation of substrate and a deficiency of downstream energy production. Hypoglycaemia and metabolic acidosis (with or without raised lactate) are hallmarks of neonatal metabolic disease—either defects of carbohydrate metabolism, amino acid or fatty acid oxidation defects [1, 6]. Hyperammonaemia should be measured if encephalopathy is present (particularly if respiratory alkalosis coexists) and suggests a urea cycle abnormality. Feeds should be stopped, and intravenous dextrose commenced to provide 6 mg/kg/min (i.e. 3.6 ml/kg/h of dextrose 10%). Blood and urine should be collected and sent immediately to your laboratory for processing or storage (a metabolic diagnosis may take time, and these complex tests often require a specialised laboratory and the oversight of a metabolic paediatrician) [6]. Similarly, intravenous bicarbonate, specific amino acid free feed and sodium benzoate should only be considered once shock, sepsis and cardiac lesions have been evaluated and the metabolic team are involved [1, 2, 5, 6].

4 Other Gems

- Antibiotic dosing to cover GBS and *E. coli* should take precedence over other therapies. A single dose of cefotaxime will cover both organisms and penetrate the cerebrospinal fluid (CSF), whilst the addition of penicillin will also cover Listeria.
- A prostaglandin infusion is unlikely to harm a newborn but may cause apnoea.
- Dextrose 10% at 3.6 mls/kg/h will correct hypoglycaemia, suppress ketogenesis and protein catabolism—it will very rarely make a metabolic syndrome worse.

References

1. Fox, G., Hoque, N., & Watts, T. (2017). *Oxford handbook of neonatology* (2nd ed.). Oxford University Press.
2. Royal Children's Hospital: Clinical Practice Guidelines. (2025). *Recognition of the seriously unwell neonate and young infant.* https://www.rch.org.au/clinicalguide/guideline_index/Recognition_of_the_seriously_unwell_neonate_and_young_infant/. Accessed 17 Jun 2025.
3. Royal Children's Hospital: Clinical Practice Guidelines. (2025). *Antimicrobial guidelines.* https://www.rch.org.au/clinicalguide/guideline_index/Antimicrobial_guidelines/. Accessed 17 Jun 2025.
4. Park, M. K., & Salamat, M. (2020). *Park's paediatric cardiology for practitioners* (7th ed.). Elsevier Health Sciences.
5. Marchant, J., & McKinlay, C. (2023). Acute neonatal emergencies. In P. Cameron, G. J. Browne, B. Mitra, S. Dalziel, & S. Craig (Eds.), *Textbook of paediatric emergency medicine-e-book* (pp. 57–65). Elsevier Health Sciences.
6. Safer Care Victoria. Best practice & improvement. Metabolic disease in neonates. (2016). https://www.safercare.vic.gov.au/best-practice-improvement/clinical-guidance/neonatal/metabolic-disease-in-neonates Accessed 17 Jun 2025.

When Salt Is Vital

Sathyakala Vijayanand

1 Clinical Pearl

Salt loss secondary to congenital adrenal insufficiency must be considered in an infant with failure to thrive.

2 Clinical Case

A term neonate, Edmund, was referred to the Emergency Department by the Maternal Child Health Nurse with jaundice. Edmund had an uneventful birth however was noted to have weight loss of more than 10% of his birth weight. He was on exclusive breast feeds. He was started on phototherapy and referred to a lactation consultant. Despite being on a feeding plan with top-up feeds, Edmund had lost 13.5% of his birth weight by Day 5 of life. He appeared well clinically.

A blood test revealed his serum sodium was normal at 138 mmol/L. The blood sample was haemolysed and as a result, the patient's potassium level was unable to be interpreted. He was discharged home the following day with a plan to be reviewed in 48 hours.

Edmund was readmitted to hospital on Day 8 of life due to 15% weight loss. He was hemodynamically stable and euvolemic on examination. However, at this stage, Edmund was irritable to examine. Repeat blood tests demonstrated significant electrolyte abnormalities. He was hyponatremic with a sodium of **120** (132–147) mmol/L, hyperkalaemic with a potassium of **7.0** (3.3–6.5) mmol/L and a normal blood glucose of 4.8 (3.0–6.9) mmol/L.

S. Vijayanand (✉)
Bendigo Health, Monash Children's Hospital, Clayton, VIC, Australia

C. F. Lynch et al. (eds.), *The Art of Paediatric Medicine Beyond the Evidence Base*,
https://doi.org/10.1007/978-981-96-7234-9_5

Due to these results, Edmund was investigated for possible adrenal insufficiency. The hyperkalemia was managed immediately with intravenous (IV) actrapid insulin and a salbutamol nebuliser. He was treated with IV fluids (0.9% Normal saline +10% dextrose) at the maintenance rate and IV hydrocortisone. His sodium and potassium levels were monitored closely with blood tests repeated every 4 h.

Further investigations are listed below:

- Cortisol 89 (20–800) nmol/L
- 17-Hydroxy-progesterone (17OHP) **2842** (<21) nmol/L
- 21-Deoxy-cortisol (21DOC) **582** (<1) nmol/L

The elevated 17OHP and 21DOC confirmed the diagnosis of Congenital Adrenal Hyperplasia (CAH). The patient was treated with hydrocortisone, fludrocortisone and salt supplements, making a good clinical recovery.

3 Discussion

A neonate with poor weight gain or failure to regain birth weight must be investigated for decreased calorie intake due to feeding issues and decreased milk supply, inadequate absorption of nutrients or increased metabolism due to underlying organic pathology.

21-hydroxylase deficiency (21OHD) is the most common cause of CAH [1]. 21OHD leads to increased 17OHP levels which is shunted to produce increased androgens such as testosterone (Fig. 1). The accumulated intra-adrenal 17OHP is converted to 21-DOC, which is a specific marker for 21OHD. Salt losing CAH due

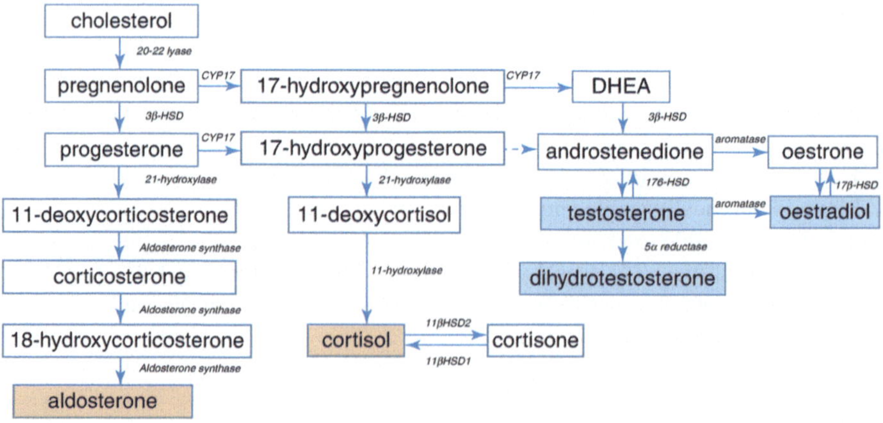

Fig. 1 Biosynthetic pathway for steroid hormones [2]*3β-HSD* 3-beta-hydroxysteroid dehydrogenase, *17β-HSD* 17-beta-hydroxysteroid dehydrogenase, *11β HSD 1&2* 11-beta-hydroxysteroid dehydrogenase

to 21OHD is an autosomal recessive disorder and leads to significant electrolyte disturbances due to aldosterone and cortisol deficiency (Fig. 1).

The incidence of 21OHD is estimated at approximately 1 in 12,500 live births. In classical CAH, a neonate may present with failure to gain weight. If unrecognised, the neonate usually presents during the second week of life in adrenal crisis with hypovolemic shock, hypoglycaemia, hyponatremia and hyperkalemia. Males can present with pigmentation of the scrotum and females with ambiguous genitalia.

An elevated 17 hydroxy-progesterone confirms the diagnosis of CAH.

In Australia, CAH is part of the newborn bloodspot screening test to prevent babies presenting with severe illness. Timely diagnosis allows early institution of appropriate treatment. However in any neonate presenting with failure to gain weight, hypovolemic shock, hypoglycaemia, hyponatremia and hyperkalemia, the diagnosis of CAH should be entertained and consideration of empirical treatment with steroids and intravenous fluids.

In non-classical CAH, the clinical presentation may differ. Children may present with early onset adrenarche and advanced bone age. Adolescents may develop signs of virilisation. In these non-classical variants, cortisol and aldosterone deficiency may not be present and hence treatment with steroids may not be required.

4 Other Gems

- Adrenal insufficiency due to CAH should be considered in a newborn presenting with electrolyte abnormalities.
- Newborn screening helps in early detection of classical CAH and prevents neonates presenting with severe illness.
- Late onset CAH can present with early onset adrenarche in older children.

References

1. Speiser, P. W., Arlt, W., Auchus, R. J., et al. (2018). Congenital adrenal hyperplasia due to steroid 21-hydroxylase deficiency: An endocrine society clinical practice guideline. *The Journal of Clinical Endocrinology & Metabolism, 103*(11), 4043–4088. https://doi.org/10.1210/jc.2018-01865
2. Woodward, G. M., & Rumsby, G. (2019). Overview of adrenal physiology and steroid biochemistry. In G. Rumsby & G. Woodward (Eds.), *Disorders of steroidogenesis*. Springer. https://doi.org/10.1007/978-3-319-96364-8_1

Think Outside the Box

Laura Rishanghan and Rupert Hinds

1 Clinical Pearl

Not all jaundiced babies who are breastfed have breast milk jaundice.

2 Clinical Case

A 9-week-old male infant, Sam, was referred to the gastroenterology team by the emergency department for investigation of prolonged jaundice. Sam was one of twins born at 37 weeks after an uncomplicated pregnancy. His growth had been along the 25th centile and he was otherwise well. Sam had been seen at 4 weeks and 6 weeks by a paediatrician in the community who had not performed any blood tests and had documented normal stool colour (according to the mother). Sam's stool colour in emergency was pale (acholic). Sam's mother, for whom the twins were her first children, articulated that she thought this was normal for a baby. Sam's blood test revealed a conjugated hyperbilirubinemia with an obstructive pattern of liver enzymes. Ultrasound and liver biopsy confirmed a diagnosis of biliary atresia and he was referred for surgical management.

L. Rishanghan · R. Hinds (✉)
Department of Gastroenterology, Monash Children Hospital, Clayton, VIC, Australia

C. F. Lynch et al. (eds.), *The Art of Paediatric Medicine Beyond the Evidence Base*,
https://doi.org/10.1007/978-981-96-7234-9_6

3 Discussion

Biliary atresia (BA) is one of the most common causes of neonatal cholestasis and yet remains difficult to diagnose [1]. The incidence in Australia is approximately 1 in 20,000 [2].

The proposed pathophysiology of BA is a combination of injury and a response to injury within the bile ducts. Due to absent or damaged bile ducts, bile is unable to drain effectively and accumulates in the liver and if not treated, eventually progresses to fibrosis and cirrhosis [3].

BA remains the leading indication for liver transplant in children worldwide. Early detection is crucial and prompt investigations should be triggered by clinical features such as conjugated jaundice, acholic stools and dark urine. As assessment of stool colour may be subjective, online resources may help to provide more objective measurements [1].

First line investigations should include bilirubin (conjugated and total), liver enzymes (ALT, AST, GGT, ALP), INR, and an abdominal ultrasound [1]. Abdominal ultrasound will often show an absent, small or contracted gallbladder however it is very important to note that the presence of a gallbladder itself does not exclude BA [4]. Further investigation will depend on the level of clinical suspicion. Referral to a paediatric gastroenterologist is recommended [1].

Due to the importance of age on the success of surgical intervention, the Kasai porto-enterostomy (KPE), early diagnosis is critical [5]. Studies show neonates having KPE at <30 days old have clearance of jaundice (CoJ) rates of >70%, while those >100 days old have CoJ rates of <40%. Even with a successful Kasai procedure (normal bilirubin at 6 months post KPE), many patients will require liver transplantation [2].

This case highlights the importance of performing basic investigations such as blood tests when seeing a neonate with altered stool colour. Early discussion with a tertiary referral centre should occur in cases where BA is considered as a potential diagnosis. This will allow earlier diagnosis and management, leading to better outcomes for the neonate.

This case illustrates some important aspects of diagnostic reasoning:

1. Don't rely on someone else's description of an important clinical finding.
2. Common things do occur commonly but not always.

4 Other Gems

- Don't forget to perform an INR on a baby with conjugated jaundice. Late-onset vitamin K deficiency may occur with liver disease in infancy and have catastrophic outcomes including intracranial haemorrhage.

References

1. Starship Child Health. *Biliary Atresia (BA): Guidelines and management [internet]*. Starship; [cited 2024 Aug 11]. Available from: https://starship.org.nz/guidelines/biliary-atresia-ba-guidelines-and-management-of/
2. Elliot, E., Dorney, S., Davidson, G., Redmond, D., Shepherd, R., Smith, A. *Extrahepatic Biliary Atresia [internet]*. Australian Paediatric Surveillance Unit; [cited 2024 Aug 11]. Available from: https://apsu.org.au/assets/past-studies/ehba.pdf
3. Tam, P. K. H., Wells, R. G., Tang, C. S. M., et al. (2024). Biliary atresia. *Nature Reviews Disease Primers, 10*(1), 47. https://doi.org/10.1038/s41572-024-00533-x
4. Singh, G., Sharma, R., Kogan, J., et al. (2024). *Biliary atresia*. Radiopaedia.org. [cited 2024 Sept 1]. Available from: https://doi.org/10.53347/rID-5176
5. Siddiqui, A. I., & Ahmad, T. (2024, January). Biliary atresia. StatPearls [Internet]. StatPearls Publishing; [Updated 2023 June 26; cited 2024 Aug 12]. Available from: https://www.ncbi.nlm.nih.gov/books/NBK537262/

Ubiquitous and Quietly Consuming

Steve Graham

1 Clinical Pearl

When the chest X-ray looks worse than the child, think of tuberculosis (TB).

2 Clinical Case

Beatrice, a two-month-old girl, was referred for assessment following exposure to her grandmother, recently diagnosed with sputum smear-positive tuberculosis, who was living in the same household as the infant at the time she became symptomatic. Beatrice had not received newborn BCG vaccination as she was born in a low tuberculosis incidence country; her grandmother was a resident in a high tuberculosis incidence country and was visiting from overseas to spend time with her new grandchild and family. Beatrice had a tuberculin skin test at home, as part of contact investigation, which was positive—induration of 18 mm. As she was asymptomatic with normal weight gain since birth at initial assessment, she was referred to the local child TB clinic for assessment the following week.

On presentation to the clinic, Beatrice's mother reported that she had developed a mild cough in the previous 2 days and was a little fussier with feeds, but was otherwise well. Examination was unremarkable. Her weight was 6kgs and she looked to be thriving since birth. Beatrice was afebrile with normal respiratory rate for age of 40 breaths per minute and no subcostal or intercostal indrawing. There were no

S. Graham (✉)
Centre for International Child Health, University of Melbourne, Parkville, VIC, Australia

University of Melbourne Department of Pediatrics, Royal Children's Hospital, Parkville, VIC, Australia

C. F. Lynch et al. (eds.), *The Art of Paediatric Medicine Beyond the Evidence Base*,
https://doi.org/10.1007/978-981-96-7234-9_7

signs of respiratory distress. Auscultation of her chest was normal with symmetrical and normal breath sounds. There was no hepatosplenomegaly or lymphadenopathy.

As clinical examination was normal, Beatrice was considered for tuberculosis preventive treatment (TPT). It was considered that her recent acute symptoms were unlikely to be tuberculosis-related but rather due to a viral upper respiratory tract infection. However, a chest X-ray was done to ensure that there was no evidence of active tuberculosis before commencing TPT.

The chest X-ray was abnormal with marked parenchymal changes in the right lung (Fig. 1). Therefore, gastric aspirates were performed which were positive for *Mycobacterium tuberculosis*. Abdominal ultrasound showed multiple nodules in the spleen and given this evidence of dissemination, a lumbar puncture was performed which found 30 lymphocytes and raised protein.

Beatrice was treated for bacteriologically confirmed drug-susceptible pulmonary tuberculosis and had an uneventful treatment course and excellent outcome. Despite strong evidence of disseminated disease including abnormal imaging of the lungs and spleen as well as findings from cerebrospinal fluid consistent with miliary tuberculosis and early tuberculous meningitis, it is likely that the excellent outcome was associated with early detection and treatment of disease.

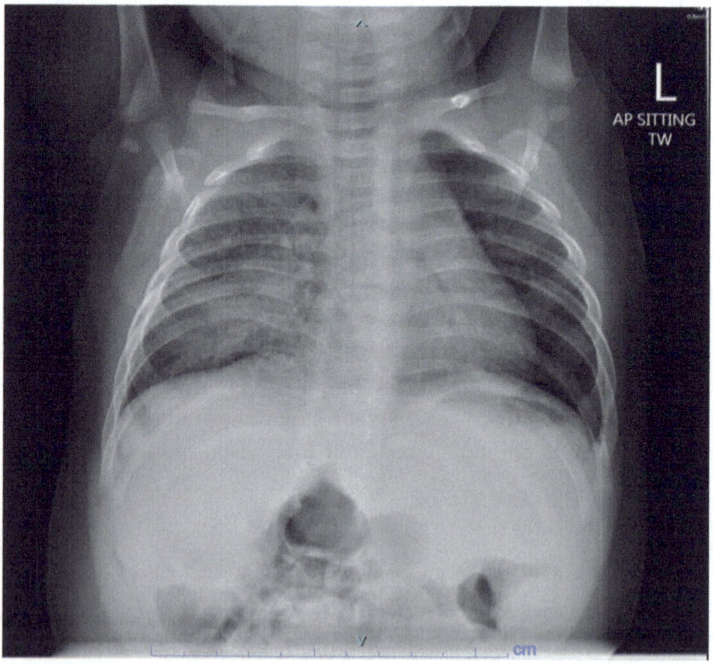

Fig. 1 Chest X-ray demonstrating right lung consolidation

3 Discussion

Mycobacterium tuberculosis is a major cause of illness and death globally that can present in all age groups [1]. In low and middle-income countries where tuberculosis is endemic, the clinical presentation of tuberculosis in young children often overlaps with other common causes of severe illness such as pneumonia, malnutrition or invasive sepsis [2]. Therefore, clinical diagnosis can be challenging especially as bacteriological confirmation is often difficult in children [3]. Even with increasing availability of molecular rapid diagnostics such as the Xpert Ultra assay, the paucibacillary nature of pulmonary tuberculosis in children as well as the challenge of obtaining sputum for testing means that most young children (<5 years) with tuberculosis require a clinical diagnosis [4, 5]. Furthermore, tuberculosis may be a comorbidity with pneumonia, malnutrition or HIV [6, 7].

Chest X-ray is the main diagnostic tool used to support clinical diagnosis of intrathoracic disease due to *M. tuberculosis* [5]. Tuberculosis-related abnormalities may be quite specific (perihilar lymph node enlargement with airway compression in children or a miliary pattern) but are also often quite non-specific [8]. The typical radiological abnormality that characterises pulmonary tuberculosis in older adolescents and adults of upper lobe cavitation, which can also be bacteriologically confirmed on sputum sample, is very unusual in children of less than 10 years.

Following infection with *M. tuberculosis*, the transition to disease can take months to years, if it occurs at all. Most infected people do not develop disease though young children, adolescents or those living with HIV are at higher risk [9]. Mycobacterial infection provokes a predominantly cell-mediated immune response [10] with lymphocytes and macrophages causing inflammatory tissue damage that is usually insidious; not only for tuberculosis but also other mycobacterial disease such as leprosy or Buruli ulcer. This is different to the acute inflammatory humoral response with neutrophil migration and cytokines caused by bacterial pathogens such as *Streptococcus, Staphylococcus* or Gram-negatives that are the major invasive bacterial pathogens causing disease in children. For example, an important characteristic that distinguishes cervical lymph node enlargement due to tuberculosis from suppurative lymphadenitis is that tuberculous lymphadenitis is not usually tender, erythematous or particularly painful even when visible and large.

Tuberculosis is an important cause of intrathoracic disease in children. Young age is a major risk factor for development of disease following infection, including disseminated disease, and for relatively rapid onset of disease [11]—as illustrated in this case. Tuberculosis commonly causes parenchymal abnormalities on Chest X-ray such as infiltration or consolidation as well as pleural effusions, but these are non-specific and are also commonly caused by bacterial pathogens. However, children with pneumonia or effusions due to non-tuberculous bacteria will usually look quite sick with tachypnoea, high fevers and evidence of respiratory distress such as subcostal indrawing. This is often not the case for tuberculosis so “when the chest X-ray looks worse than the child, think of TB”.

4 Other Gems

- The immunopathology associated with tuberculosis is often characterised by an extensive cell-mediated lymphocytic inflammatory response without causing the acute inflammatory manifestations of invasive bacterial disease such as high fever, marked lassitude or pain.
- Severe disease due to tuberculosis can also cause immunosuppression and result in a false negative tuberculin skin test. Treatment of tuberculosis can cause an immune-mediated inflammatory response whereby the child deteriorates clinically following initiation of treatment and their imaging findings worsen, requiring temporary treatment with corticosteroids [3]. This can occur in HIV-uninfected children especially in those with severe malnutrition, a comorbidity common with tuberculosis which itself causes marked immunosuppression especially of cell-mediated rather than humoral immunity.
- Childhood malnutrition is very common in low-income settings and affects the epidemiology of childhood diseases. For example, wheeze whether due to asthma or bronchiolitis is common in children from high-income settings but is rarely seen/heard in undernourished children or infants. Therefore, if you detect wheeze in a malnourished child, think beyond asthma in your differential diagnosis. A chest X-ray may be indicated especially if there is poor response to treatment with an inhaled bronchodilator. Tuberculosis can cause wheeze (or stridor) due to airway compression from enlarged lymph nodes compressing the main bronchi (or trachea).

References

1. WHO Global TB Report. (2023). World Health Organization, Geneva.
2. Graham, S. M., Sismanidis, C., Menzies, H. J., Detjen, A. K., Marais, B. J., & Black, R. E. (2014). Importance of tuberculosis control to address child survival. *Lancet, 383*, 1605–1607.
3. Chiang, S. S., Graham, S. M., Schaaf, H. S., et al. (2023). Clinical standards for drug-susceptible tuberculosis in children and adolescents. *The International Journal of Tuberculosis and Lung Disease, 27*, 584–598.
4. Gunasekera, K. S., Vonasek, B., Oliwa, J., et al. (2022). Diagnostic challenges in childhood pulmonary tuberculosis—Optimizing the clinical approach. *Pathogens, 11*, 382.
5. The Union. (2023). Diagnosis and management of tuberculosis in children and adolescents. In *A desk guide for primary health care workers* (4th ed.). The Union.
6. Oliwa, J. N., Karumbi, J. M., Marais, B. J., Madhi, S. A., & Graham, S. M. (2015). Tuberculosis as a cause or comorbidity of childhood pneumonia in tuberculosis endemic settings: A systematic review. *The Lancet Respiratory Medicine, 3*, 235–243.
7. Chabala, C., Roucher, C., Ton Nu Nguyet, M. H., et al. (2024). Development of tuberculosis treatment decision algorithms in children below 5 years hospitalised with severe acute malnutrition in Zambia and Uganda: A prospective diagnostic cohort study. *EClinicalMedicine, 73*, 102688.

8. The Union. (2022). Diagnostic CXR atlas for tuberculosis in children. In *A guide to chest X-ray interpretation*. The Union.
9. Marais, B. J., et al. (2004). The natural history of childhood intra-thoracic tuberculosis: A critical review of literature from the pre-chemotherapy era. *The International Journal of Tuberculosis and Lung Disease, 8*, 392–402.
10. Tebruegge, M., Ritz, N., Donath, S., et al. (2019). Mycobacteria-specific mono- and poly-functional CD4+ T cell profiles in children with latent and active tuberculosis: A prospective proof-of-concept study. *Frontiers in Immunology, 10*, 431.
11. Martinez, L., Cords, O., Horsburgh, C. R., et al. (2020). The risk of tuberculosis in children after close exposure: A systematic review and individual-participant meta-analysis. *Lancet, 395*, 973–984.

Keep Your Eyes, Ears and Mind Open

Alyce Horstman and Joanna Tully

1 Clinical Pearl

Young infants with minor skin or soft tissue injuries are at high risk of subsequent more serious physical abuse, but the significance of these injuries is often missed, particularly when the family appears to be "just like us."

2 Clinical Case

James was the second child. His mother was a nurse and his father a teacher, and the family were well known to their general practitioner (GP) and maternal and child health nurse (MCHN) because of James' brother's autism. The family were viewed as exceptionally caring parents. James was 4 weeks old when his mother took him to the emergency department (ED) because she had noticed a "sore" next to his mouth. He was diagnosed with a staphylococcal infection and given antibiotic cream.

At 6 weeks of age, James had his immunisations with the MCHN and was observed to have a small bruise on his left cheek. Although unsure of the cause, his mother attributed the bruise to holding James' face while burping him.

A. Horstman
The Royal Children's Hospital, Melbourne, VIC, Australia

Department of Forensic Medicine, Monash University, Melbourne, VIC, Australia

J. Tully (✉)
Department of Forensic Medicine, Monash University, Melbourne, VIC, Australia

Victorian Forensic Paediatric Medical Service, The Royal Children's and Monash Children's Hospital, Melbourne, VIC, Australia

C. F. Lynch et al. (eds.), *The Art of Paediatric Medicine Beyond the Evidence Base*,
https://doi.org/10.1007/978-981-96-7234-9_8

At 7 weeks of age James was observed to have a subconjunctival haemorrhage in his left eye for which the GP prescribed chloramphenicol.

At 9 weeks of age James attended a virtual ED appointment because his saliva was blood-stained, and his mother had observed a "hole" under his tongue. The doctor missed the frenulum injury and reassured James' mother, advising her that she should discuss this with James' private paediatrician at an appointment scheduled in a week's time. James never attended that appointment.

Several days before the scheduled appointment James collapsed at home, received cardiopulmonary resuscitation, and was transferred to a tertiary children's hospital where a computed tomography scan demonstrated bilateral subdural haemorrhages and a catastrophic brain injury. Further investigation revealed that James also had extensive bilateral retinal haemorrhages, ligamentous injury to his neck, and three posterior rib fractures. A medical diagnosis of inflicted head injury was made. Child Protection and police were alerted. James' father admitted to forcefully shaking James out of frustration and exhaustion during a night-time feed.

3 Discussion

Sentinel injuries are visible, minor, but poorly explained injuries in pre-mobile infants that can signal clinically occult but more serious injuries, or precede more significant inflicted trauma, including inflicted head injury. When a sentinel injury is identified, the response should include forensic evaluation searching for occult injury, usually with brain and spine imaging, a skeletal survey, and an ophthalmological examination, as well as involving protective services in line with mandatory reporting requirements.

When the medical records of infants diagnosed with inflicted trauma were retrospectively reviewed and compared with the medical records of non-abused infants, over a quarter had previously presented with a sentinel injury that had not been recognised to be significant by medical providers [1]. None of the non-abused infants had a history of a sentinel injury [1]. The most common sentinel injury is bruising, with intra-oral injury and subconjunctival haemorrhage also identified as being important [1]. Injuries identified during early infancy carry the strongest association with subsequent risk of abuse [2].

While the significance of sentinel injuries in heralding abuse was recognised as early as the 1970s, there has been no clear improvement in the rate at which medical providers recognise and respond to sentinel injuries since this time [3]. It has been estimated that, if the significance of sentinel injuries were better appreciated, many infants would be protected from further abusive injury and up to 4 in 5 fatalities resulting from inflicted head injury could be prevented [3].

Cognitive bias affects us all and there are particularly powerful cognitive biases at play when professionals encounter the possibility of non-accidental injury. Abuse is diagnosed more frequently in families of low socioeconomic status or of non-white ethnicity, and this reflects stereotyping that child abuse only occurs in certain families. It seems that little has changed since 1966 when two Australian doctors published a cardinal paper highlighting the extent to which children were being physically abused in Australia, the reluctance of medical professionals to acknowledge the problem, and their attitude of disbelief, particularly "*when faced by a neatly dressed and plausible husband or wife*" [4]. Child abuse still remains "*unseen and ignored*" in the community; a national survey finding that the public rated it less concerning than petrol prices, transport, and roads. This is reflected in the reluctance of doctors to accept that a parent could have harmed their child [5]. Certainly, as forensic paediatricians, the case scenario presented above is all too familiar. Statements from doctors minimising the significance of a bruise in an infant are all too commonly heard, often made, it seems, on the basis of the social background or presentation of the parents. Failure to look for, or consider trauma as a differential, will result in missed opportunities to recognise abuse and to change the trajectory of children and families' lives.

In addition to cognitive biases, there are systemic barriers to the identification of sentinel injuries. Children present to a variety of healthcare settings and may be assessed by providers without sufficient paediatric training. This means that providers may encounter forensically significant injuries in young children but be unaware of their significance due to gaps in their knowledge about child development, paediatric medical conditions and injury epidemiology. They may also be unfamiliar with the response recommended following identification of injuries in infants, leading to delays in or absence of protective intervention. Furthermore, increased demand for acute health services has led to an emergence of 'waiting room medicine' where infants are seen briefly, often without a complete assessment or examination, and discharged home if they are deemed low risk of serious illness. Additionally, the emergence of telehealth and virtual consultations presents a new challenge for ensuring careful examination of infants and detection of injuries.

There are tools available that aim to improve the rate of recognition of sentinel injuries. The use of such tools may overcome the tendency of doctors to employ intuitive reasoning, encourage objectivity, and help to overcome cognitive bias. The simple phrase "*those who don't cruise, don't bruise*" acts as an easy aide memoir when encountering an infant with bruises [2]. For those working in emergency departments, simple quality improvement initiatives such as "*one and down, in a gown*" could help encourage a top to toe examination for every infant less than 12 months [6, 7].

The TEN4FACESp mnemonic (available at https://www.luriechildrens.org/globalassets/media/pages/research/tricam/ten-4/lch-2386-ten-4-facesp-8.5x11_final_r1.pdf) is helpful in keeping nonaccidental trauma at the forefront of our minds when evaluating and treating children for any and all complaints, and is a screening tool to help practitioners identify when bruising in children under 4 years of age is more likely to be caused by abuse than accidental injury [8, 9]. The tool reminds clinicians that bruising on the Torso, Ear or Neck, Frenulum injuries, bruising to the Angle of the jaw and soft part of the Cheek, Eyelid bruising, Subconjunctival haemorrhages and Patterned bruises in children less than 4 years of age should always prompt consideration of inflicted trauma [8, 9]. Any bruise in an infant less than 4 months of age, no matter how small and no matter the location, should be further investigated [8].

For James, the medical system failed him. So too, the medical system failed his father, who faces years in prison. So too, the medical system failed his mother, who now cares for a severely disabled child and his sibling alone. We can do better, and we can do better by keeping our eyes and our minds open.

4 Other Gems

- **Never** ignore bruising in pre-mobile infants.
- Examine infants top-to-toe, every consult, every time.
- Keep child abuse in the forefront of your mind, it is far more common than you might think.

References

1. Sheets, L. K., Leach, M. E., Koszewski, I. J., Lessmeier, A. M., Nugent, M., & Simpson, P. (2013). Sentinel injuries in infants evaluated for child physical abuse. *Pediatrics, 131*(4), 701–707.
2. Oral, R., Yagmur, F., Nashelsky, M., Turkmen, M., & Kirby, P. (2008). Fatal abusive head trauma cases: Consequence of medical staff missing milder forms of physical abuse. *Pediatric Emergency Care, 24*(12), 816–821.
3. Jenny, C., Hymel, K. P., Ritzen, A., Reinert, S. E., & Hay, T. C. (1999). Analysis of missed cases of abusive head trauma. *Journal of the American Medical Association, 281*(7), 621–626.
4. Birrell, R. G., & Birrell, J. H. (1968). The maltreatment syndrome in children: A hospital survey. *The Medical Journal of Australia, 2*(23), 1023–1029.
5. Tucci, J., & Mitchell, J. (2022). Still unseen and ignored: Tracking community knowledge and attitudes about child abuse and child protection in Australia. *Frontiers in Psychology, 2*(13), 860212.
6. Crichton, K. G., Spencer, S., Shapiro, R., McPherson, P., Izsak, E., McDavid, L. M., Baker, C., & Thackeray, J. D. (2023). Timely recognition of abusive injuries (TRAIN): Results from a statewide quality improvement collaborative. *Pediatric Quality & Safety, 8*(2), e637.
7. Greene, H. M., Letson, M. M., Spencer, S. P., Dolan, K., Foster, J., & Crichton, K. G. (2023). Recognizing nonaccidental trauma in a pediatric tertiary hospital: A quality improvement imperative. *Pediatric Quality & Safety, 8*(2), e644.
8. Pierce, M. C., Kaczor, K., Acker, D., Webb, T., Brenzel, A., Lorenz, D. J., Young, A., & Thompson, R. (2017). History, injury, and psychosocial risk factor commonalities among cases of fatal and near-fatal physical child abuse. *Child Abuse & Neglect, 69*, 263–277. https://doi.org/10.1016/j.chiabu.2017.04.033. Epub 2017 May 10.
9. Pierce, M. C., Kaczor, K., Lorenz, D. J., Bertocci, G., Fingarson, A. K., Makoroff, K., Berger, R. P., Bennett, B., Magana, J., Staley, S., Ramaiah, V., Fortin, K., Currie, M., Herman, B. E., Herr, S., Hymel, K. P., Jenny, C., Sheehan, K., Zuckerbraun, N., Hickey, S., Meyers, G., & Leventhal, J. M. (2021). Validation of a clinical decision rule to predict abuse in young children based on bruising characteristics [published correction appears in *JAMA Network Open*. 2021;4(9):e2130136]. *JAMA Network Open, 4*(4), e215832.

Unsettled/Irritable Babies—Is It Angina?

Ngai Lam Woo and Srinidhi Rao

1 Clinical Pearl

Consider anomalous origin of the left coronary artery from pulmonary artery (ALCAPA) in infants presenting with intermittent irritability, sweatiness, and respiratory distress.

2 Clinical Case

A 3-month-old infant, Ayesha, presents to emergency after multiple visits to different general practitioners with a constellation of non-specific symptoms. The parents report that Ayesha has been more unsettled for the past 5 days, with interrupted sleeping patterns and only settling when held upright. They also noticed some increasing breathlessness and respiratory distress when Ayesha is unsettled, in addition to some wheezy noises. A detailed feeding history reveals that oral intake has additionally been an issue, with breastfeeds lasting short periods before their baby becomes fussy and breathes faster. The frequency of wet nappies is unchanged, albeit lighter in volume.

On examination, Ayesha is tachypnoeic without increased work of breathing. The peripheral pulses are normal, including the femoral pulses. A soft 2/6 systolic murmur is heard apically, with the liver edge palpable 2 cm below the right costal margin. The respiratory examination is otherwise unremarkable.

N. L. Woo
The Children's Hospital at Westmead, Westmead, NSW, Australia

S. Rao (✉)
Monash Children's Hospital, Clayton, VIC, Australia

C. F. Lynch et al. (eds.), *The Art of Paediatric Medicine Beyond the Evidence Base*,
https://doi.org/10.1007/978-981-96-7234-9_9

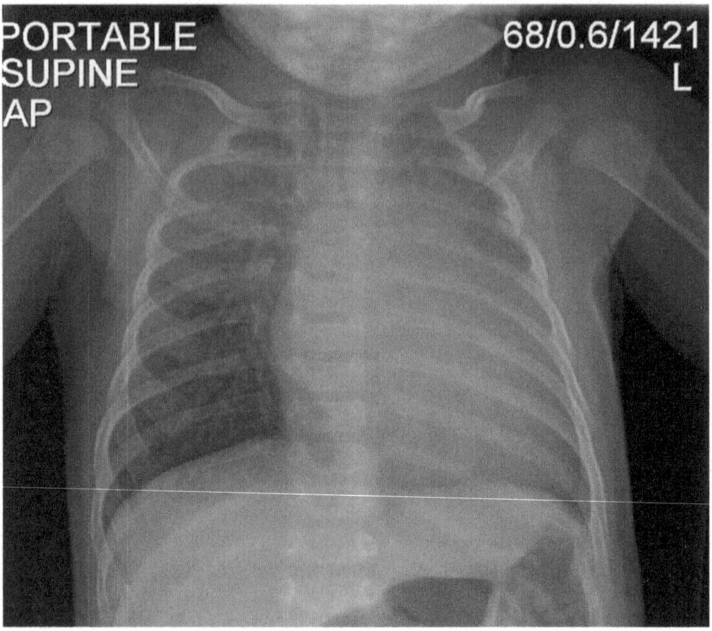

Fig. 1 Chest X-ray of the infant at ED presentation showing significant cardiomegaly

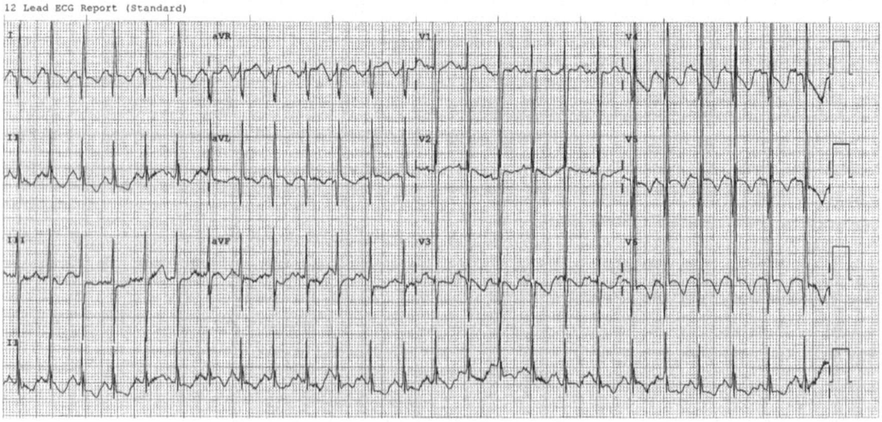

Fig. 2 Electrocardiogram (ECG) of the infant

The chest X-ray (Fig. 1) shows cardiomegaly with otherwise clear lung fields.

The electrocardiogram (ECG) (Fig. 2) reveals sinus rhythm (upright P-waves in leads I and AVF), left axis deviation (QRS axis more leftward than normal for age), biventricular hypertrophy (high amplitude diphasic QRS waves in the precordial leads) and left ventricular strain (ST depression and T-wave inversion in the lateral leads).

While Ayesha is feeding, you note that she also appears to be sweaty and breathing faster than before.

3 Discussion

Anomalous left coronary artery from the pulmonary artery (ALCAPA) is a rare congenital heart disease (0.25–0.5%), with an incidence of approximately 1 per 300,000 births [1]. In this lesion, the perfusion of the left coronary artery is dependent upon desaturated blood at low pressures, coming from the pulmonary artery. This results in progressive coronary artery steal as pulmonary vascular resistance drops and blood preferentially flows into the lower pressure pulmonary arteries from the myocardium, causing myocardial ischaemia [2].

Clinically, patients typically present at 2–3 months of age with intermittent pallor, irritability, as well as cold sweating due to ischaemic angina during the exertion of feeding. Over time, the infants go on to develop symptoms of heart failure (tachycardia, tachypnoea, poor feeding, and diaphoresis) [3].

The symptomatology has significant overlap with features of respiratory illnesses and other childhood conditions such as gastro-oesophageal reflux or even colic.

A high index of suspicion should therefore be held in recurrent presentations in which a clear diagnosis or pathogen is not identified. Careful examination and timely investigation in this instance established the diagnosis.

4 Other Gems

- Prompt surgical intervention is crucial in minimising long-term myocardial damage. Long term outcomes of surgery are good with up to 98% reported survival at 20 years [4].
- A subset of ALCAPA present later in life due to the presence of collateral supply to the myocardium, and can present as dilated cardiomyopathy, sudden cardiac death or significant arrhythmias in adolescence and adulthood.

References

1. Lardhi, A. (2010). Anomalous origin of left coronary artery from pulmonary artery: A rare cause of myocardial infarction in children. *Journal of Family and Community Medicine., 17*(3), 113–116.
2. Blickenstaff, E. A., Smith, S. D., Cetta, F., Connolly, H. M., & Majdalany, D. S. (2023). Anomalous left coronary artery from the pulmonary artery: How to diagnose and treat. *Journal of Personalized Medicine [Internet]., 13*(11), 1561. [cited 2024 July 8]. Available from: https://www.ncbi.nlm.nih.gov/pmc/articles/PMC10672344/

3. Hauser, M. (2005). Congenital anomalies of the coronary arteries. *Heart, 91*(9), 1240–1245.
4. Naimo, P. S., Fricke, T. A., d'Udekem, Y., Cochrane, A. D., Bullock, A., Robertson, T., et al. (2016). Surgical intervention for anomalous origin of left coronary artery from the pulmonary artery in children: A long-term follow-up. *The Annals of Thoracic Surgery [Internet]., 101*(5), 1842–1848.

Strawberry Birthmarks: When Early Treatment Counts

Sangho Lee and Ann Boyapati

1 Clinical Pearl

Infantile haemangiomas located on critical anatomical sites (such as the eyelid, nose and lip) should be treated early to prevent deformity.

2 Clinical Case

A 2-month-old girl, Florence, was referred to the dermatology clinic with a solitary, 7 mm infantile haemangioma affecting the vermillion border of the lip. She is the first child of a Caucasian couple and was born at 34 weeks. Her parents noticed an erythematous macule appearing 1 week after birth, which rapidly increased in size and became raised. There was no associated ulceration or feeding difficulties. Her parents had used topical timolol gel for 1 month with minimal response.

After screening for cardiovascular risk factors, Florence was commenced on oral atenolol 0.5 mg/kg daily. Within 2 weeks, her parents reported an arrest in growth and regression of the haemangioma. The medication was well tolerated. The dose was increased to 1 mg/kg daily and continued until the patient reached 12 months of age.

S. Lee
Monash Health, Clayton, VIC, Australia

A. Boyapati (✉)
Department of Dermatology, Monash Health, Clayton, VIC, Australia

C. F. Lynch et al. (eds.), *The Art of Paediatric Medicine Beyond the Evidence Base*,
https://doi.org/10.1007/978-981-96-7234-9_10

3 Discussion

Infantile haemangiomas are the most common vascular tumour of infancy, occurring in up to 10% of infants [1]. They present as flat erythematous macules soon after birth. The lesions increase in size and become raised during the proliferative phase, which takes place over the first 3–5 months of life. This is followed by a plateau phase, with most haemangiomas reaching maximal growth by 12 months. Resolution of infantile haemangiomas gradually occurs over the course of infancy and childhood [2].

In the majority of resolved infantile haemangiomas, there is minimal scarring and dyspigmentation [3]. As such, infantile haemangiomas can often be safely managed with surveillance alone or topical timolol.

Infantile haemangiomas can become problematic in high-risk areas, with the following possible complications:

- Periorbital: amblyopia, visual axis obstruction, astigmatism, ptosis, proptosis, strabismus.
- Perinasal: ulcerative destruction of nasal septum, nasal obstruction.
- Perioral: feeding difficulties, ulceration.
- Periauricular: external auditory canal obstruction.
- Cervicofacial (chin, anterior neck, lower lip): airway obstruction, stridor, hoarseness, aspiration.

Additionally, haemangiomas located on cosmetically significant sites can lead to deformity, with resultant psychological distress [1, 4].

Although in the case presented the haemangioma was small, it was located on the lip, at the cosmetically significant vermillion border. Due to the potential for feeding difficulties, ulceration and deformity, oral treatment was indicated.

Patients with high risk or cosmetically significant haemangiomas should be considered for treatment with oral beta blockers such as atenolol and propranolol. Beta blockers are most beneficial during the rapid proliferative phase, as most haemangiomas reach 80% of their final size by 5 months [3]. Hence, early identification and referral is important for the treatment to have meaningful results.

4 Other Gems

- When treating infantile haemangiomas conservatively, reassuring and educating parents regarding the natural course and prognosis is important. Up to 50% of infantile haemangiomas completely resolve by 5 years of age, 70% by seven and 90% by nine [2].
- Ulceration is the most common complication of infantile haemagioma, with greater risk in intertriginous areas such as the lip, neck, axillae and anogenital region [1]. Prompt management is required to prevent complications such as

pain, infection and scarring. Analgesia, regular emollients, barrier products (e.g. containing zinc oxide) and non-adhesive dressings are the first line of treatment [1].

- Visceral involvement and syndromic presentations such as PHACES (**p**osterior fossa anomalies, **h**aemangioma, **a**rterial anomalies, **c**ardiac anomalies, and **e**ye anomalies) **s**yndrome should be considered in cases of multiple or large (>5 cm) haemangiomas, particularly those located over the face [2]. If PHACES is suspected, patients must not be started on a beta blocker until imaging is performed due to the risk of stroke secondary to reduced cardiac output [5].

References

1. Rodríguez Bandera, A. I., Sebaratnam, D. F., Wargon, O., & Wong, L. C. F. (2021). Infantile hemangioma. Part 1: Epidemiology, pathogenesis, clinical presentation and assessment. *Journal of the American Academy of Dermatology, 85*(6), 1379–1392.
2. Leung, A. K. C., Lam, J. M., Leong, K. F., & Hon, K. L. (2021). Infantile hemangioma: An updated review. *Current Pediatric Reviews, 17*(1), 55–69.
3. Harter, N., & Mancini, A. J. (2019). Diagnosis and management of infantile hemangiomas in the neonate. *Pediatric Clinics of North America, 66*(2), 437–459.
4. Darrow, D. H., Greene, A. K., Mancini, A. J., & Nopper, A. J. (2015). Section on dermatology, section on otolaryngology-head and neck surgery, and section on plastic surgery. Diagnosis and management of infantile hemangioma. *Pediatrics, 136*(4), e1060–e1104.
5. Sebaratnam, D. F., Rodríguez Bandera, A. L., Wong, L. C. F., & Wargon, O. (2021). Infantile hemangioma. Part 2: Management. *Journal of the American Academy of Dermatology, 85*(6), 1395–1404.

Birthmarks: Should We See the Surgeon?

Will Alexander

1 Clinical Pearl

Most 'birthmarks' aren't here to stay.

2 Clinical Case

Arthur, a 6-month-old boy, has a bright red lesion on his trunk. His parents deny that it was present at birth but upon closer inspection of the newborn photos there does, in fact, seem to be a small telangiectatic 'bruise' in that area, albeit quite a lot paler. It has subsequently grown significantly, as well as becoming a bright 'cherry' pink, with a raised non-compressible plaque-like consistency. It is non-tender, and not itchy nor bleeding.

Arthur's parents are keen to have it removed and are asking for a referral to a surgeon. They fear that the longer it is left, the larger it will grow, and the resultant scar will be longer.

3 Discussion

'Birthmark' is an umbrella term used by lay and medical professionals alike, that encompasses a very wide range of conditions. The preferred term is vascular anomaly.

W. Alexander (✉)
Royal Children's Hospital, St Vincent's Private and Public Hospital, Monash Health, Epworth Freemasons, Victorian Hand Surgery Associates, Fitzroy, VIC, Australia

C. F. Lynch et al. (eds.), *The Art of Paediatric Medicine Beyond the Evidence Base*,
https://doi.org/10.1007/978-981-96-7234-9_11

Vascular anomalies can be divided into:

(a) Vascular tumours including the classic haemangioma/'strawberry birthmark', as well as some other, rarer and more aggressive lesions. Vascular tumours involve endothelial cell proliferation and can therefore be benign or, rarely, malignant.
(b) Vascular malformations which can involve deeper tissue layers, and may be arterial, venous, lymphatic, or a mix of these vessel types. Vascular malformations are congenital malformations of vessels, and are generally thought to be present at birth, although not necessarily clinically evident.

The classification and nomenclature of vascular anomalies has been the subject of great debate, and this debate is ongoing [1].

The described lesion in this case is most likely to be an 'infantile haemangioma', which is the most common of the vascular anomalies, affecting ~5% of infants, particularly girls [2, 3]. Most of these are isolated, and most appear in the first month of life as a subtle lesion (as opposed to congenital haemangiomas, which are present at birth). These lesions will go through a proliferative phase for 3–9 months, where the lesion is plump and red, a plateau and then an involuting phase for 1–7 years where the lesions gradually fade and will then be 'involuted'. Involuted does not mean 'completely gone', and some of these lesions (~20–50%) will have residual bulk, skin redundancy, or colour disparity.

Most infantile haemangiomas can be monitored, and the parents reassured. If there is a residual lesion after involution, it can be managed as an elective aesthetic issue, typically with surgical excision or laser. In rare circumstances the location, behaviour, or size of the lesion demands more urgent treatment. Concerning features include visual field obstruction or pressure on the globe, airway involvement, obstruction of the auditory canal, or risk of permanent cosmetic damage. Similarly, bleeding or ulceration may trigger earlier interventions. In these situations, systemic beta-blockers (propranolol or atenolol), topical timolol [4], or more rarely ACE-inhibitors, are the usual first line treatment. Surgical excision is sometimes useful for small, ulcerated lesions but otherwise generally not indicated in the growth phase.

Particularly large or deep vascular anomalies may need further investigation to exclude complex associated conditions (thrombocytopaenia, or PHACE syndrome), or vascular malformations (deeper lesions that are present at birth and will not involute). This group of patients should be referred to a multidisciplinary vascular anomaly service with dermatology, plastic surgery, interventional radiology, and paediatric input.

4 Other Gems

- A useful generalisation for infantile haemangiomas is that 50% of lesions will have involuted by the age of 5, and 90% by the age of 9 [2].

- Surgical excision is typically reserved as an elective option, for residual aesthetic concerns. Laser, similarly, can be used to improve any colour discrepancy.
- Haemangiomas behave very differently to vascular malformations which are present at birth, do not involute, and may undergo acute changes with intralesional haemorrhage, infection, or thrombus. These are typically managed in a multidisciplinary team setting.
- Severe thrombocytopaenia due to platelet trapping (Kasabach-Merritt phenomenon) is seen in infants with the lesion Kaposiform Haemangioendothelioma (KHE), sometimes confused with haemangioma, but which requires urgent diagnosis and treatment.

References

1. Andrews, L., Shope, C., Lee, L. W., & Hochman, M. (2022). Vascular anomalies: Nomenclature and diagnosis. *Dermatologic Clinics, 40*(4), 339–343. https://doi.org/10.1016/j.det.2022.06.007
2. Janis, J. (2014). *Essentials of plastic surgery* (2nd ed.). Thieme Medical Publishers Inc.
3. Drolet, B. A., Esterly, N. B., & Frieden, I. J. (1999). Hemangiomas in children. *The New England Journal of Medicine, 341*(3), 173–181. https://doi.org/10.1056/NEJM199907153410307
4. Phillips, R. J., Penington, A. J., Bekhor, P. S., & Crock, C. M. (2012). Use of propranolol for treatment of infantile haemangiomas in an outpatient setting. *Journal of Paediatrics and Child Health, 48*(10), 902–906. https://doi.org/10.1111/j.1440-1754.2012.02521.x

Anaesthetic Safety in Children

Will Alexander

1 Clinical Pearl

How young is too young for non-urgent surgery?

2 Clinical Case

Kai, a 9-month boy, has an underdeveloped (hypoplastic) thumb, and the Plastic Surgery team have booked him for a thumb reconstruction. The procedure aims to augment the relatively deficient muscles and ligaments that support the thumb and allow the child to develop his thumb opposition fine motor skills. Kai is otherwise developing well, with no syndromic associations.

Kai's parents are concerned about the safety of the anaesthetic on his developing brain. They are wanting to delay the surgery until he is older. The surgeons are concerned that thumb-pinch and opposition development typically occurs around 12–18 months, and if his thumb surgery is significantly delayed beyond this point, he may grow up neglecting this thumb/hand. They are also concerned that compliance with dressings/splints decreases from 18 months of age, until the child is around 4–5 years old.

W. Alexander (✉)
Royal Children's Hospital, St Vincent's Private and Public Hospital, Monash Health, Epworth Freemasons, Victorian Hand Surgery Associates, Fitzroy, VIC, Australia

C. F. Lynch et al. (eds.), *The Art of Paediatric Medicine Beyond the Evidence Base*,
https://doi.org/10.1007/978-981-96-7234-9_12

3 Discussion

The safety of an anaesthetic in infants and toddlers is of utmost concern to parents and clinicians alike. Many times, there is no choice; trauma and infections often necessitate early surgery, which simply must proceed. Conversely, elective surgery can be planned, and often a compromise between surgical urgency and anaesthetic safety must be reached.

There are two issues at play here:

1. The effect of anaesthetic agents on neurodevelopment.
2. The simple logistics of operating on a smaller human.

3.1 The Effect of Anaesthetic Agents on Neurodevelopment

Anaesthetic agents reliably disrupt neurodevelopment in animal models, but the evidence in humans is less convincing [1]. Recently there have been some excellent studies which have quite convincingly suggested that a single anaesthetic exposure is not harmful to a child's intelligence. The GAS trial, published in the Lancet (2019) compared regional with general anaesthetic for infantile hernia repairs and found no difference in neurodevelopmental outcomes at 5 years of age [2]. The Mayo Anaesthesia Safety in Kids (MASK) study retrospectively reviewed patients with nil, single, or multiple anaesthetic exposures under the age of 3 years, and found no difference in intelligence, but slightly lower scores for processing speed and fine motor abilities in multiply exposed children [3]. A sibling matched-cohort study (the 'PANDA trial') compared siblings within 3 years of age, in whom one had a general anaesthetic before 3 years of age, and the other did not. The median duration of surgery was 80 minutes and there were no statistically significant differences in intelligence or behavioural outcomes [4]. Unfortunately, there is not clear evidence regarding children with repeated nor prolonged anaesthetic exposures.

Based on this evidence, one can confidently support surgery in this young cohort if deemed necessary or beneficial.

3.2 The Simple Logistics of Operating on a Smaller Human

The logistics of operating on smaller children should also be considered. Factors such as blood volume, diameter of the airway and peripheral veins for cannulation, and risk of hypothermia are important anaesthetic considerations, especially below 10 months of age.

4 Other Gems

- Whilst no surgeons nor anaesthetists will push to operate younger than necessary, parents are often hungry for some evidence-based reassurance that by consenting to an early operation, they are not committing their child to harm. The GAS, MASK, and PANDA studies are useful for these conversations [2–4].
- There are occasionally other factors to consider, such as the psychological impact of multiple operations on both the child and/or their parent(s).

References

1. Ing, C., Warner, D. O., Sun, L. S., et al. (2022). Anesthesia and developing brains: Unanswered questions and proposed paths forward. *Anesthesiology, 136*(3), 500–512. https://doi.org/10.1097/ALN.0000000000004116
2. McCann, M. E., de Graaff, J. C., Dorris, L., et al. (2019). Neurodevelopmental outcome at 5 years of age after general anaesthesia or awake-regional anaesthesia in infancy (GAS): An international, multicentre, randomised, controlled equivalence trial. *Lancet (London, England)., 393*(10172), 664–677. https://doi.org/10.1016/S0140-6736(18)32485-1
3. Warner, D. O., Zaccariello, M. J., Katusic, S. K., et al. (2018). Neuropsychological and behavioral outcomes after exposure of young children to procedures requiring general anesthesia: The Mayo Anesthesia Safety in Kids (MASK) study. *Anesthesiology, 129*(1), 89–105. https://doi.org/10.1097/ALN.0000000000002232
4. Sun, L. S., Li, G., Miller, T. L. K., et al. (2016). Association between a single general anesthesia exposure before age 36 months and neurocognitive outcomes in later childhood. *Journal of the American Medical Association, 315*(21), 2312–2320. https://doi.org/10.1001/jama.2016.6967

Food Allergy Is an Uncommon Cause of Eczema

Sangho Lee and Ann Boyapati

1 Clinical Pearl

It is common for eczema to flare when solid foods are being introduced. However, eczema is uncommonly caused by food allergy.

2 Clinical Case

A 9-month-old boy, Omar, was brought to the dermatology clinic by his parents for review post an admission to hospital with widespread, impetiginized eczema. He has a strong family history of eczema, asthma and food allergies. Omar's parents observed worsening of his eczema when gluten, dairy and eggs were introduced, and subsequently excluded these from his diet. They denied any history of urticaria or angioedema and had not sought allergist or dietician input. Omar's parents requested investigations to evaluate for food allergies, believing it was the cause of the boy's eczema.

After counselling regarding the limited value of such investigations, Omar's parents were encouraged to gradually reintroduce the excluded foods under supervision. The eczema was treated with general skin care measures (including bath oils, bleach baths and a greasy emollient) as well as a moderately potent topical corticosteroid. Upon review 2 months later, there was significant improvement in Omar's eczema.

S. Lee
Monash Health, Clayton, VIC, Australia

A. Boyapati (✉)
Department of Dermatology, Monash Health, Clayton, VIC, Australia

C. F. Lynch et al. (eds.), *The Art of Paediatric Medicine Beyond the Evidence Base*,
https://doi.org/10.1007/978-981-96-7234-9_13

3 Discussion

Eczema in infancy commonly occurs around the age of 6–12 months, which coincides with the introduction of solid foods. Patients with eczema frequently have multiple co-existing atopic conditions, with up to a third of patients with moderate to severe eczema reported to have concurrent food allergies [1]. Therefore, it can be easily interpreted by parents (and health professionals) that allergenic foods are the cause of the child's eczema.

Patients with atopic diseases have multiple concomitant immune dysregulations including increased T helper 2 cell activation and IgE sensitisation [1, 2]. This helps to explain the positive correlation between eczema and food allergies. However, eczema is caused by a complicated interaction between many other genetic and environmental factors, including epidermal barrier dysfunction and disruption in the cutaneous microbiome [2]. Therefore, the causal relationship between eczema and food allergy is tenuous.

In practice, the vast majority of patients do not see a notable clinical improvement in their eczema after dietary modifications alone. Furthermore, patients report less flares associated with foods when their eczema is well-controlled. Current evidence suggests that introducing allergenic foods in the first year of life does not increase the risk of atopic dermatitis or food allergy [3, 4]. In fact, it is recommended that infants with eczema be introduced to peanut-containing foods as early as 4–6 months to reduce the risk of peanut allergy [5].

In the clinical case, the parents excluded foods they believed were causing the infant's eczema. However, in infants and children who need robust nutrition for their rapid growth and development, the implication of dietary exclusion is significant [2, 3]. Furthermore, if allergenic foods that a child previously did not react to are excluded, there is a greater risk of developing allergy when such foods are reintroduced later in life [2, 3]. If, as in our case, the parents have already excluded allergenic foods from the patient's diet, they should be gradually and safely reintroduced with supervision. This allows for true clinical assessment of immediate and delayed cutaneous reactions post ingestion to determine whether the food is actually contributing to eczema flares (known as oral food challenge) [5].

Further allergy testing may be useful in a small group of patients who show a high enough clinical suspicion for a relationship between food allergies and eczema flares—that is, if there is a convincing demonstration of eczema flares post ingestion of certain foods despite a prolonged trial of adequate lifestyle modifications and topical therapies [5]. When referring patients for food allergy testing, it is important to be mindful that many findings can be coincidental or irrelevant. Most children with eczema have positive skin prick findings to several foods, but only about one third correlate with positive food challenges [1]. The RAST test and skin prick tests have high negative predictive values but low specificities and positive predictive values, reflecting the fact that IgE sensitisation does not always lead to clinical manifestations of food allergy [5]. Therefore, it is important to closely consider the clinical history when interpreting test results and deciding on dietary exclusions.

4 Other Gems

- Food allergy can present in either immediate or delayed phenotypes [2, 5]. The majority of food allergy cases are IgE-mediated, immediate hypersensitivity reactions where patients experience acute symptoms such as urticaria, itch and flushing 1–2 h post exposure to food [2]. This is different to delayed, non-IgE-mediated reactions where patients show gradual worsening of redness, dryness and itchiness 6–48 h post ingestion of food [2, 5]. Delayed food allergies are thought to be due to food allergens activating the Th2 pathway, which is also directly implicated in eczema pathogenesis [2]. Since these reactions are not caused by IgE antibodies, RAST and skin prick tests are not useful in their prediction.
- Food allergens in the environment can penetrate through the impaired cutaneous barrier of patients with eczema and promote IgE sensitisation [2]. This can occur well before infants are exposed to such allergens via the gastrointestinal tract. On the other hand, early oral exposure to food allergens via the intestinal mucosa has been found to inhibit Th-2-dependent allergic responses and is hence protective against food sensitisation [2]. This "dual-antigen-exposure hypothesis" highlights that good eczema treatment and early introduction of allergenic foods are important in preventing food allergies in infants with atopic dermatitis.
- Although any food can potentially trigger an allergic response, 90% of clinically relevant food allergies are caused by a small number of foods—namely cow's milk, eggs, peanut, wheat and soy [1]. Of these, most children outgrow their allergies to milk, eggs, wheat and soy by childhood [1]. Therefore, dietary exclusion of allergenic foods in patients with eczema is neither relevant nor necessary in most cases and should only be considered after critically evaluating the relationship with eczema flares.

References

1. Sicherer, S., & Sampson, H. (1999 Sep). Food hypersensitivity and atopic dermatitis: Pathophysiology, epidemiology, diagnosis, and management. *The Journal of Allergy and Clinical Immunology, 104*(3), S114–S122.
2. Papapostolou, N., Xepapadaki, P., Gregoriou, S., & Makris, M. (2022). Atopic dermatitis and food allergy: A complex interplay what we know and what we would like to learn. *Journal of Clinical Medicine, 11*(14), 4232.
3. Obbagy, J. E., English, L. K., Wong, Y. P., Butte, N. F., Dewey, K. G., Fleischer, D. M., et al. (2019). Complementary feeding and food allergy, atopic dermatitis/eczema, asthma, and allergic rhinitis: A systematic review. *The American Journal of Clinical Nutrition, 109*, 890S–934S.
4. Waidyatillake, N. T., Dharmage, S. C., Allen, K. J., Bowatte, G., Boyle, R. J., Burgess, J. A., et al. (2018). Association between the age of solid food introduction and eczema: A systematic review and a meta-analysis. *Clinical and Experimental Allergy, 48*(8), 1000–1015.
5. McAleer, M., O'Regan, G., & Irvine, A. (2018). Atopic dermatitis. In *Dermatology* (4th ed., p. 224). Elsevier.

Children May Have Hidden Congenital Issues

Sari Hayllar

1 Clinical Pearl

Infants have yet to prove themselves anatomically and metabolically normal.

2 Clinical Cases

2.1 Case 1

Hana, an 8-month-old girl, was being followed up in a general paediatric clinic for culture-negative bacterial meningitis diagnosed at 11 weeks of age. She was making pleasing developmental progress but was consistently bothered by constipation. Past treatment included a stool softener and cow's milk protein exclusion advice. An insistent grandmother was in attendance on this occasion, and she was not leaving the consultation without answers. The history of the stooling pattern was of distress with the passage of ribbony stool. Rectal examination noted a very narrow anal canal with a prominent bony ridge. Further history from the grandmother included information about her own history of surgery in childhood for spina bifida.

Hana had two X-rays including pelvis and lower spine, which revealed an unusual sickle-shaped hemi-sacrum which pointed to a rare, autosomal dominant form of sacral agenesis (Currarino syndrome).

Subsequent surgery confirmed the final element of the triad, a presacral mass (anterior meningocoele) which was ultimately resected along with an associated rectothecal fistula, the likely aetiology of her meningitis.

S. Hayllar (✉)
West Gippsland Healthcare, Warragul, VIC, Australia

C. F. Lynch et al. (eds.), *The Art of Paediatric Medicine Beyond the Evidence Base*,
https://doi.org/10.1007/978-981-96-7234-9_14

This diagnosis had implications for the broader family. Grandma's "spina bifida" was confirmed to show classic, sickle-shaped hemi sacrum, consistent with Currarino syndrome. Both of her daughters were subsequently diagnosed with Currarino syndrome and required surgery which included resection of a premalignant sacral teratoma.

2.2 *Case 2*

A 3-year-old boy, named Walter, with Trisomy 21 was transferred from a small regional hospital with pneumonia. Walter was unwell on arrival with an oxygen requirement, moderate work of breathing and bilateral crackles. There was no cardiac history (previously normal echocardiogram). The only other past history was grommet insertion.

Chest X-ray showed bilateral opacifications, an elevated left hemidiaphragm and an enormous gastric bubble with an air-fluid level. A nasogastric tube was passed in the hope that some of his respiratory compromise would be alleviated. Foul debris-containing fluid was drained with some clinical improvement. A diagnosis of duodenal stenosis was subsequently confirmed by barium swallow. Further history from Walter's mother revealed a history of non-bilious vomiting in infancy. This had been diagnosed as gastroesophageal reflux and managed with positioning and massaging of his distended abdomen with successful reduction in symptoms. Walter recovered well after abdominal surgery.

3 Discussion

As paediatricians we are acutely aware of the need to consider congenital anomalies in our differential diagnoses, particularly in the critically unwell neonate. Time critical recognition of duct-dependent cardiac defects, upper and lower airway malformations, obstructive causes of bilious vomiting and metabolic derangements from congenital adrenal conditions are frequently highlighted in our training.

Considering rare congenital causes of much less dramatic and commonplace symptoms can be challenging. Whilst these cases showcase unusual conditions, they are a reminder to consider congenital variants in differential diagnoses of even the most mundane presentations. This is a pearl to share with our junior doctors and medical students. The paediatric population is different to the adult cohort in a very particular way.

4 Other Gems

- Always listen to grandmas.
- Always take a detailed three generational family tree.

It's Not Inappropriate

Sarah McNab

1 Clinical Pearl

Unwell children frequently require less fluid than "maintenance volume" to achieve hydration.

2 Clinical Case

Harold, an 8-month-old baby, is admitted to hospital with meningitis. He has an intravenous line for antibiotics. He is irritable and refusing any feeds and you are asked to prescribe fluids.

3 Discussion

Maintenance fluid requirement is the daily volume of fluid needed to maintain hydration. This is best delivered orally when possible. When children are unable to drink, they may be prescribed this fluid to be given either by a nasogastric tube or intravenously.

S. McNab (✉)
The Royal Children's Hospital Melbourne, Parkville, VIC, Australia

Department of Paediatrics, University of Melbourne, Parkville, VIC, Australia

Murdoch Children's Research Institute, Parkville, VIC, Australia

C. F. Lynch et al. (eds.), *The Art of Paediatric Medicine Beyond the Evidence Base*,
https://doi.org/10.1007/978-981-96-7234-9_15

Table 1 The 4,2,1 Rule for calculating maintenance fluids

Body weight	Fluid requirement (mL/h)
<10 kg	4 mL/kg/h
10–20 kg	40 mL/h + (2 mL/kg/h for each kg over 10 kg)
>20 kg	60 mL/h + (1 mL/kg/h for each kg over 20 kg)

In paediatrics, maintenance fluid rate is generally calculated via a weight-based equation (known as the 4,2,1 rule)—see Table 1. This calculation is based on a paper from the 1950s and was derived from fluid requirements for well children [1].

However, when we're prescribing fluid to hospitalised children, we frequently ask for fluid restriction—typically to "2/3 of maintenance rate."

3.1 Why Do We Do This?

Hospitalised children are more likely to have excess secretion of antidiuretic hormone (or ADH). This hormone is exactly as described: as an anti-diuretic it will reduce the urine output of the child, causing them to retain fluid. Some children are at higher risk of excess ADH secretion. This includes children with neurological conditions (such as meningitis or those who have undergone craniofacial surgery) or significant respiratory conditions (such as pneumonia or bronchiolitis). However, research has shown that ADH may be high in a much wider group of situations, including in children with nausea, anxiety or pain [2].

This phenomenon is sometimes described as the Syndrome of Inappropriate ADH secretion (or SIADH). However, this is a misnomer: secreting ADH in response to significant illness is an appropriate evolutionary response to help survive dehydration.

If you imagine being unwell without ready access to food or water, you would first need to survive the illness **and** survive dehydration while too unwell to source water. In this context, ADH is released to reduce urine output and help conserve fluid.

The consequence is that the fluid rates for healthy children (the 4,2,1 rule) are excessive for many hospitalised children. When hospitalised patients with high circulating levels of ADH are administered fluids at rates recommended for healthy children, there is a risk of fluid overload. There is also a risk of hyponatraemia, particularly if the fluid is hypotonic (containing less sodium than plasma) as the fluid essentially "dilutes" the plasma. This is further exacerbated if children are receiving fluid in addition to the maintenance rates prescribed, either through their own oral intake or through the, sometimes quite substantial, volumes of fluid co-administered with intravenous medication [3].

3.2 Where Does This Leave Us?

When children are admitted to hospital and require fluid to be prescribed, they need a thorough clinical assessment and consideration of prescribing a lesser volume than the 4,2,1 rule. This is due to the **very appropriate** secretion of ADH in unwell children. Monitor the child's fluid status closely with regular weights (at least daily, and more frequently if the child is more unwell), clinical assessment, and electrolytes, and adjust the fluid prescription accordingly.

4 Other Gems

- There are some children who will need higher volumes of fluid. For example, a child with gastroenteritis who may present with dehydration and with ongoing gastrointestinal losses.
- Please refer to local clinical guidelines as this chapter is not intended to be a comprehensive summary of fluid management in children.

References

1. Holliday, M. A., & Segar, W. E. (1957). The maintenance need for water in parenteral fluid therapy. *Pediatrics, 19*(5), 823–832.
2. Moritz, M. L., & Ayus, J. C. (2015). Maintenance intravenous fluids in acutely ill patients. *New England Journal of Medicine, 373*(14), 1350–1360.
3. Brossier, D. W., Goyer, I., Verbruggen, S. C., Chaparro, C. J., Rooze, S., Marino, L. V., Schlapbach, L. J., Tume, L. N., & Valla, F. V. (2024). Intravenous maintenance fluid therapy in acutely and critically ill children: State of the evidence. *The Lancet Child & Adolescent Health, 8*, 236–244.

Persistent Fever in Babies

Linny K. Phuong and David A. Foley

1 Clinical Pearl

Kawasaki Disease (KD) should be considered in a child with prolonged fever and clinical findings suggestive of systemic inflammation especially those less than 6 months of age, regardless of ethnicity.

2 Clinical Case

A 4-month-old female, Saoirse, born in Australia to parents of European ancestry, presented with a 6-day history of fever. Despite multiple visits to her general practitioner, no clear source of infection was able to be identified. On the third visit and due to ongoing fever and clinical concerns, the child was referred to the local hospital for further assessment. Saoirse was noted to have non-exudative conjunctivitis and a diffuse erythematous exanthem (rash).

L. K. Phuong (✉)
Infection and Immunity Theme, Murdoch Children's Research Institute, Royal Children's Hospital, Parkville, VIC, Australia

Department of Paediatrics, University of Melbourne, Parkville, VIC, Australia

D. A. Foley
Department of Microbiology, PathWest Laboratory Medicine WA, Nedlands, WA, Australia

Wesfarmers Centre of Vaccines and Infectious Diseases, Telethon Kids Institute, University of Western Australia, Perth, WA, Australia

School of Medicine, University of Western Australia, Perth, WA, Australia

C. F. Lynch et al. (eds.), *The Art of Paediatric Medicine Beyond the Evidence Base*,
https://doi.org/10.1007/978-981-96-7234-9_16

3 Discussion

Kawasaki Disease (KD) is an acute vasculitis that primarily affects children and can lead to significant long-term cardiac complications if not recognised and treated promptly. Although it is more frequently diagnosed in children of Asian descent, KD can occur in children of any ethnicity. The primary goal in diagnosing and managing KD is to reduce systemic inflammation and prevent the formation of coronary artery aneurysms (CAAs). Without treatment, up to 25% of children with KD may develop CAAs. With appropriate therapy, including intravenous immunoglobulin (IVIg) and low-dose aspirin, this risk can be reduced to 3–5% [1].

Diagnosing KD can be challenging because there is no specific diagnostic test. Clinicians must maintain a high index of suspicion, especially in cases of prolonged fever without a clear source [2]. A thorough history and systematic clinical examination are crucial in recognising KD early.

The mnemonics 'CRASH' and 'BURN' may be helpful to recall the associated five principal features of acute KD (CRASH), in addition to the prolonged fevers 'BURN' (Table 1). It is important to remember that it is likely that not all features will be present concurrently. BURN is also a reminder of the potential cardiac consequences.

A diagnosis of classic KD can be made when a child has a prolonged fever with at least four of the five principal features. Incomplete KD should be considered in children, particularly those under 6 months, who have prolonged fever but fewer than four principal features. The presence of associated symptoms, such as neurological, gastrointestinal, or joint manifestations, may also raise suspicion for KD [1–3]. Laboratory tests are non-specific, however may display signs of inflammation, including an elevated C-reactive protein (CRP) and erythrocyte sedimentation rate (ESR) at baseline. There may also be evidence of sterile pyuria. Sepsis is an important differential diagnosis; empiric antibiotics are recommended whilst investigations are underway.

Treatment with IVIg (2 g/kg) is most effective if given within 10 days of the onset of fever. This is started in conjunction with aspirin (3–5 mg/kg daily). A baseline echocardiogram may be obtained, but should not delay therapy, and may be normal at baseline. Once IVIg has been given, ESR is no longer a useful marker of inflammation, as it will be elevated due to the prior IVIg administration [1].

Table 1 The five principal features of Kawasaki disease

C	Conjunctivitis	Non-exudative conjunctivitis, sparing the limbus (border between the cornea and sclera)
R	Rash	Typically extensive and can be non-specific (including maculopapular, urticarial, erythema multiforme-like)
A	Adenopathy (cervical)	Usually unilateral, >1.5 cm in diameter
S	'Strawberry tongue' (referring to oral changes)	Includes cracking and dryness and/or 'lipstick-sign' of the lips, a 'strawberry tongue'
H	Hands/feet (peripheral changes in the palms and soles)	Erythema, pain and swelling initially Desquamation is a later sign

4 Other Gems

- Parents should be encouraged to seek further medical evaluation if their child has persistent fever or evolving symptoms.
- A useful sign to help diagnose acute KD in children who have had BCG vaccination, is erythema or swelling at the injection site (BCG-itis).

References

1. McCrindle, B. W., Rowley, A. H., Newburger, J. W., et al. (2017). Diagnosis, treatment, and long-term management of Kawasaki disease: A scientific statement for health professionals from the American Heart Association. *Circulation, 135*, e927–e999.
2. Phuong, L. K., Chen, K. Y., Burgner, D. P., & Curtis, N. (2020). What paediatricians need to know about the updated 2017 American Heart Association Kawasaki disease guideline. *Archives of Disease in Childhood, 105*(1), 10–12.
3. Yoon, Y. M., Yun, H. W., & Kim, S. H. (2016). Clinical characteristics of Kawasaki disease in infants younger than six months: A single-center study. *Korean Circulation Journal, 46*(4), 550–555.

Not All Thermometers Are Created Equal

Linny K. Phuong and David A. Foley

1 Clinical Pearl

Understanding the differences in thermometer types and their accuracy is essential to determine if fever is present.

2 Clinical Case

Jordan, a 9-month-old boy, appeared grizzly and felt warm to the touch. He had been attending childcare for the past 3 days, and his mother, Mary, had not received any notifications about other unwell children in his room. Concerned, Mary checked her medicine cabinet and found two thermometers: an infrared forehead thermometer and a tympanic thermometer. Since Jordan was grizzly, Mary opted to take his temperature using the infrared forehead thermometer, which showed a reading of 37.5 °C. Unsure if this indicated a fever, she used the tympanic thermometer, which gave a reading of 38.2 °C.

L. K. Phuong (✉)
Infection and Immunity Theme, Murdoch Children's Research Institute, Royal Children's Hospital, Parkville, VIC, Australia

Department of Paediatrics, University of Melbourne, Parkville, VIC, Australia

D. A. Foley
Department of Microbiology, PathWest Laboratory Medicine WA, Nedlands, WA, Australia

Wesfarmers Centre of Vaccines and Infectious Diseases, Telethon Kids Institute, University of Western Australia, Perth, WA, Australia

School of Medicine, University of Western Australia, Perth, WA, Australia

C. F. Lynch et al. (eds.), *The Art of Paediatric Medicine Beyond the Evidence Base*,
https://doi.org/10.1007/978-981-96-7234-9_17

3 Discussion

Fever, defined as a core body temperature of 38 °C or higher, can arise from various causes, including infections, malignancies, and inflammatory conditions [1]. Fever is a common source of anxiety for parents and caregivers [2, 3], who often seek reliable methods to measure their child's temperature. While parental subjective assessments of their child's temperature can sometimes be accurate, objective measurements using thermometers are preferred in clinical decision-making [1, 4].

Temperature can be measured using contact and non-contact thermometers, each with distinct advantages and limitations regarding their accuracy, ease of use, and the discomfort they may cause [5, 6]. Accurate temperature measurement is particularly crucial in specific populations, such as children under 3 months of age or those with immunodeficiencies, as the presence of fever in these groups typically warrants urgent medical evaluation [1].

Infrared forehead thermometers are non-contact devices that are popular due to their ease of use, particularly in young children. However, their accuracy can be affected by external factors such as room temperature, perspiration, or improper positioning. Notably, non-contact forehead thermometers have a higher false-positive rate for detecting fever in children than other methods [7].

Tympanic thermometers measure the infrared heat emitted from the ear canal, providing a more reliable estimate of core temperature compared to non-contact devices. Accurate measurement requires proper placement, which can be challenging with young, irritable children like Jordan, as these devices may also cause discomfort.

Axillary (underarm) thermometers are non-invasive and easy to use, but they can underestimate core body temperature by up to 1 °C [1], potentially leading to underdiagnosis of fever.

Rectal thermometers are considered the gold standard for measuring core temperature due to their accuracy, but their use is limited by concerns over discomfort and the risk of injury, especially in neonates and infants.

In addition to variations in accuracy based on the site and method of measurement, thermometers are subject to both fixed and random errors. Random errors are unpredictable and can be influenced by environmental factors or human handling, while fixed errors are consistent biases inherent to the device itself. These errors can cumulatively lead to clinically significant discrepancies in temperature readings [1, 7–10].

With respect to Jordan in the case above, the exact type and accuracy of the thermometer used are less critical than his overall clinical appearance. Fever is a physiological response to infection; healthcare professionals no longer routinely recommend interventions to reduce fever, such as cold baths or regular antipyretic use. Instead, decisions around using an antipyretic will be more about managing his discomfort.

The choice of the thermometer, if needed, should be guided by the purpose of temperature measurement, balancing accuracy, cost, and practicality. For children under 3 months of age, axillary thermometers are generally a reasonable option as they are affordable, relatively easy to use, and are relatively accurate in this group. Tympanic thermometers are preferred in older children living with comorbidities where a fever would warrant medical evaluation. For other children, a wider range of options are acceptable, including tympanic and forehead thermometers. Most importantly, parents should be encouraged to seek medical attention if they are concerned about their child's health, regardless of the temperature reading on the thermometer.

4 Other Gems

- The height of the fever does not necessarily correlate with the severity of the illness.
- Temperature can be in normal range or low (hypothermia) in critical illness.

References

1. Pecoraro, V., Petri, D., Costantino, G., et al. (2021). The diagnostic accuracy of digital, infrared and mercury-in-glass thermometers in measuring body temperature: A systematic review and network meta-analysis. *Internal and Emergency Medicine, 16*(4), 1071–1083.
2. Morris, E., Glogowska, M., Ismail, F. A., et al. (2021). Parents' concerns and beliefs about temperature measurement in children: A qualitative study. *BMC Family Practice, 22*(1), 9.
3. El-Radhi, A. S. (2012). Fever management: Evidence vs current practice. *World Journal of Clinical Pediatrics, 1*(4), 29–33.
4. Edwards, G., Fleming, S., Verbakel, J. Y., van den Bruel, A., & Hayward, G. (2022). Accuracy of parents' subjective assessment of paediatric fever with thermometer measured fever in a primary care setting. *BMC Prim Care., 23*(1), 30.
5. Thermometers: Understand the options. Available from: https://www.mayoclinic.org/diseases-conditions/fever/in-depth/thermometers/art-20046737
6. Hayward, G., Verbakel, J. Y., Ismail, F. A., et al. (2020). Non-contact infrared versus axillary and tympanic thermometers in children attending primary care: A mixed-methods study of accuracy and acceptability. *The British Journal of General Practice, 70*(693), e236–ee44.
7. Kim, Y. M., Jang, M. R., Moon, J. R., et al. (2022). Clinical accuracy of non-contact forehead infrared thermometer measurement in children: An observational study. *Children (Basel)., 9*(9), 1389.
8. Non-contact thermometers for detecting fever: A review of clinical effectiveness-CADTH Rapid Response Reports. Ottawa (ON): Canadian Agency for Drugs and Technologies in Health; 20 Nov 2014.
9. Alayed, Y., Kilani, M. A., Hommadi, A., et al. (2022). Accuracy of the axillary temperature screening compared to Core rectal temperature in infants. *Global Pediatric Health, 9*, 2333794x221107481.
10. Dunne, E. A., Cunningham, K., O'Donnell, C. P. F., & McCarthy, L. K. (2021). Bench-top comparison of thermometers used in newborn infants. *Archives of Disease in Childhood. Fetal and Neonatal Edition, 106*(4), 435–437.

They Aren't Going to Melt

Anastasia Mutic, Rouzanna Aganesova, and Simon Craig

1 Clinical Pearl

Fever is a normal, adaptive response to infection, and does NOT necessarily need treatment.

2 Clinical Case

Xavier is a 2-year-old boy with a history of febrile convulsions 6 months earlier. He is otherwise well, on no regular medications, and is immunised. He presents to the Emergency Department (ED) with his concerned parents as he has developed a temperature this evening. He is alert and interactive, with normal vital signs, apart from a temperature of 38.2 °C. You are asked by one of the nurses to chart paracetamol and ibuprofen.

A. Mutic
Department of Paediatrics, School of Clinical Sciences at Monash Health, Monash University, Clayton, VIC, Australia

R. Aganesova
Paediatric Emergency Department, Monash Medical Centre, Monash Health, Clayton, VIC, Australia

S. Craig (✉)
Department of Paediatrics, School of Clinical Sciences at Monash Health, Monash University, Clayton, VIC, Australia

Paediatric Emergency Department, Monash Medical Centre, Monash Health, Clayton, VIC, Australia

C. F. Lynch et al. (eds.), *The Art of Paediatric Medicine Beyond the Evidence Base*,
https://doi.org/10.1007/978-981-96-7234-9_18

3 Discussion

Fever, defined as a temperature >38 °C [1], is a common symptom of childhood illness. It is part of an acute phase response, most frequently as a result of infection, and is characterised by *controlled* elevation of the hypothalamic set point for body temperature [2].

The controlled elevation in body temperature creates an unfavourable environment for pathogen growth and proliferation [3]. The development of fever as a useful and adaptive response to infection has been thought to be present in both warm-blooded and cold-blooded vertebrates for more than 600 million years of evolution [4], much longer than paracetamol and ibuprofen have been available! Specific elements of the innate and adaptive immune responses facilitated by fever include increased mobilisation of immune cells, augmented antibody production and activation of heat shock proteins [5].

Fever phobia, exaggerated concerns about the consequences of childhood fever, was first described 45 years ago [6] however, is still common in both parents and healthcare professionals [7–11].

Specific areas where there is a disconnect between available evidence, clinical guidelines and day-to-day practice include:

- **The administration of antipyretics to a febrile child in the absence of pain or distress.** As outlined above, fever is an adaptive response. It does not require treatment.
- **The administration of antipyretics to a child with fever and tachycardia.** This doesn't necessarily help make a diagnosis. A study of 740 children in a single UK Emergency Department demonstrated that persistent tachycardia after the administration of antipyretics was not an independent predictor of serious bacterial infection [12].
- **The administration of antipyretics to prevent a febrile convulsion.** If a child has had a febrile convulsion in a previous illness, there is no evidence that antipyretic administration will reduce the risk of convulsions with a future febrile illness [13].

A single study from Japan compared regular rectal paracetamol to administration of no antipyretics to children following a febrile seizure and found a reduced rate of recurrent febrile convulsions within the same illness in those who received regular paracetamol [14]. However, this finding has not been replicated, and completely withholding antipyretics from the other treatment arm (which would be quite different to usual practice) may have exaggerated any possible benefit.

- **The use of alternating or combined antipyretics.** A 2013 Cochrane review suggests that there is some evidence that alternating paracetamol/ibuprofen or administering both medications may be more effective at reducing temperatures than monotherapy alone [15]. However, treatment of fever alone does not appear to be a useful therapeutic endpoint. There is inconclusive evidence regarding whether or not this approach makes the child feel better, and insufficient evidence to recommend one approach over another [15].

Patient information handouts routinely provide advice on appropriate treatment for fever in children. Typical advice recommends treatment with antipyretics only if the child is unwell, miserable, or in pain. However, these messages are often undermined by well-meaning clinicians who attempt to "get the fever under control" with aggressive and unnecessary use of antipyretics. This non-evidence-based practice can reinforce fever phobia, leading to increased parental anxiety, more healthcare seeking behaviour (pharmacy visits, GP visits, emergency department visits), and greater healthcare expenditure. It is incumbent on all paediatric clinicians to understand the existing literature, provide evidence-based information, rational prescribing, and education to colleagues and parents/caregivers.

References

1. The Royal Children's Hospital, Melbourne, Australia. *Clinical practice guideline on febrile child* [Internet, last updated September 2022; cited 8 Sept 2024]. Available from: https://wwww.rch.org.au/clinicalguide/
2. Niehues, T. (2013). The febrile child: Diagnosis and treatment. *Deutsches Ärzteblatt International, 110*(45), 764–73; quiz 774. https://doi.org/10.3238/arztebl.2013.0764. (In eng).
3. Richardson, M., & Purssell, E. (2015). Who's afraid of fever? *Archives of Disease in Childhood, 100*(9), 818–820. https://doi.org/10.1136/archdischild-2014-307483. (In eng).
4. Evans, S. S., Repasky, E. A., & Fisher, D. T. (2015). Fever and the thermal regulation of immunity: The immune system feels the heat. *Nature Reviews. Immunology, 15*(6), 335–349. https://doi.org/10.1038/nri3843. (In eng).
5. Zampronio, A. R., Soares, D. M., & Souza, G. E. (2015). Central mediators involved in the febrile response: Effects of antipyretic drugs. *Temperature (Austin), 2*(4), 506–521. https://doi.org/10.1080/23328940.2015.1102802. (In eng).
6. Schmitt, B. D. (1980). Fever phobia: Misconceptions of parents about fevers. *American Journal of Diseases of Children, 134*(2), 176–181. (In eng).
7. Martins, M., & Abecasis, F. (2016). Healthcare professionals approach paediatric fever in significantly different ways and fever phobia is not just limited to parents. *Acta Paediatrica, 105*(7), 829–833. https://doi.org/10.1111/apa.13406. (In eng).
8. Raffaeli, G., Orenti, A., Gambino, M., et al. (2016). Fever and pain management in childhood: healthcare providers' and parents' adherence to current recommendations. *International Journal of Environmental Research and Public Health, 13*(5). https://doi.org/10.3390/ijerph13050499. (In eng).
9. Clericetti, C. M., Milani, G. P., Bianchetti, M. G., et al. (2019). Systematic review finds that fever phobia is a worldwide issue among caregivers and healthcare providers. *Acta Paediatrica, 108*(8), 1393–1397. https://doi.org/10.1111/apa.14739. (In eng).
10. MacMahon, D., Brabyn, C., Dalziel, S. R., McKinlay, C. J., & Tan, E. (2021). Fever phobia in caregivers presenting to New Zealand emergency departments. *Emergency Medicine Australasia, 33*(6), 1074–1081. https://doi.org/10.1111/1742-6723.13804. (In eng).
11. Tan, E., Beck, S., Haskell, L., et al. (2022). Paediatric fever management practices and antipyretic use among doctors and nurses in New Zealand emergency departments. *Emergency Medicine Australasia, 34*(6), 943–953. https://doi.org/10.1111/1742-6723.14022. (In eng).

12. Wittmann, S., Jorgensen, R., Oostenbrink, R., et al. (2023). Heart rate and respiratory rate in predicting risk of serious bacterial infection in febrile children given antipyretics: Prospective observational study. *European Journal of Pediatrics, 182*(5), 2205–2214. https://doi.org/10.1007/s00431-023-04884-7. (In eng).
13. Hashimoto, R., Suto, M., Tsuji, M., et al. (2021). Use of antipyretics for preventing febrile seizure recurrence in children: A systematic review and meta-analysis. *European Journal of Pediatrics, 180*(4), 987–997. https://doi.org/10.1007/s00431-020-03845-8. (In eng).
14. Murata, S., Okasora, K., Tanabe, T., et al. (2018). Acetaminophen and febrile seizure recurrences during the same fever episode. *Pediatrics, 142*(5). https://doi.org/10.1542/peds.2018-1009. (In eng).
15. Wong, T., Stang, A. S., Ganshorn, H., et al. (2013). Combined and alternating paracetamol and ibuprofen therapy for febrile children. *Cochrane Database System Review, 2013*(10), Cd009572. https://doi.org/10.1002/14651858.CD009572.pub2. (In eng).

Urine Trouble

Simon Craig

1 Clinical Pearl

Is this a "nice to have" or a "need to have" urine sample?

2 Clinical Case

Jasmine is a previously well 18-month-old girl who has presented to the Emergency Department (ED) with a two-day history of runny nose, cough, fever, and vomiting. She is immunised, and on no regular medications.

She is reviewed by a junior registrar who notes clear coryza, pharyngeal erythema and a dry cough. Jasmine has normal vital signs apart from a temperature of 38.5 °C. Her chest is clear, and she has a non-tender abdomen. It is decided that a urine sample be collected.

An hour later, Jasmine remains in an ED cubicle. She has had her nappy off for the past 40 min, and her father is encouraging her to drink, while simultaneously attempting to catch a urine sample. Jasmine is well enough to run around the cubicle, and her father's patience is wearing thin. You enter the cubicle to review her, only to see her squat down and urinate on the floor.

S. Craig (✉)
Paediatric Emergency Department, Monash Medical Centre, Monash Health, Clayton, VIC, Australia

Department of Paediatrics, School of Clinical Sciences at Monash Health, Monash University, Clayton, VIC, Australia

C. F. Lynch et al. (eds.), *The Art of Paediatric Medicine Beyond the Evidence Base*,
https://doi.org/10.1007/978-981-96-7234-9_19

3 Discussion

Although a urinary tract infection (UTI) is a potentially important diagnosis in a young child, its likelihood varies according to the child's age and the clinical picture [1]. A child with a clear alternative focus for infection (short history of fever, associated cough, runny nose, red throat) is much more likely to have a viral illness. However, a child with a history of recurrent UTI, prolonged high fever, vomiting, and no alternative focus, requires a definitive urine sample.

Collection of a "clean" urine sample in a young child can be a challenging and frustrating task. In a study of over 100 pre-continent children requiring a urine sample in a single ED, the average time to pass urine was over 1 h, with 80% of children passing urine within 2 h [2]. A study comparing methods of bladder stimulation in over 300 infants (aged 1–12 months) resulted in around 80% of children not having a successful clean catch sample taken [3]. Interpretation is also not straightforward. Observational studies and randomised trials demonstrate between 27% and 40% of "clean catch" urine samples are contaminated [3, 4].

An online and freely accessible UTI risk calculator has been developed in Pittsburgh, USA, which provides pre-test probability for UTI based on duration and height of the fever, age and sex of the child, history of UTI, and presence of an alternative focus of the fever [5]. The risk calculator (accessible at www.uticalc.pitt.edu) was derived from a nested case-control study of over 2000 children aged 2 to 23 months of age with a documented temperature of 38 °C or higher [5]. A subsequent validation study in a single Chicago emergency department demonstrated acceptable sensitivity (90.2%) and specificity (42.9%) [6].

If you do decide to collect a urine sample in a non-toilet-trained child, then set a time limit (e.g., 30 min). At that time, ask yourself—*"Does this child need a definitive sample? Should we do a catheter specimen?"* If the answer is "yes", then you have a "need to have" urine sample. If the answer is "no", then the urine sample is not urgent, or may not be indicated at all.

If, after the time has elapsed, you have a child with a "need to have" urine sample, then strong consideration should be given to a definitive sample under appropriate sedation (e.g. in-out catheter specimen with nitrous oxide or intranasal/oral midazolam sedation).

If you have decided that the urine sample falls into the "nice to have" category, then do not persist with attempts at a clean catch in the emergency department. If the child is well and there is no clear indication for the test, reconsider the need for a urine sample at all. If you decide that it still might be useful, provide the parent with a few urine pots and sterile wipes to attempt at home, with a view to visiting their GP for reassessment and urine testing if indicated. If a sample is taken at home, the pot should be placed in a plastic bag and refrigerated until it can be taken for testing [7].

4 Other Gems

- Current Australian guidelines recommend against collecting urine to exclude a UTI if there is another clear focus of fever and the child is not unwell [8].
- A randomised trial of the Quick-Wee method (gauze soaked in cold fluid placed on the suprapubic area) in over 350 infants aged <12 months demonstrated that it led to a significantly higher rate of voiding within 5 min (33%) compared with standard clean catch urine (12%) [3]. However, even under study conditions, a large proportion of infants did not have a urine sample successfully obtained.

References

1. Barola, S., & Grossman, O. K., & Abdelhalim, A. (2024). *Urinary tract infections in children.* [Updated 2024 Jan 11]. *StatPearls* [Internet]. Treasure Island (FL): StatPearls Publishing; 2024 Jan-. Available from: https://www.ncbi.nlm.nih.gov/books/NBK599548/
2. Davies, P., Greenwood, R., & Benger, J. (2008). Randomised trial of a vibrating bladder stimulator--the time to pee study. *Archives of Disease in Childhood, 93*(5), 423–424. https://doi.org/10.1136/adc.2007.116160. (In eng).
3. Kaufman, J., Fitzpatrick, P., Tosif, S., et al. (2017). Faster clean catch urine collection (quick-wee method) from infants: Randomised controlled trial. *BMJ, 357*, j1341. https://doi.org/10.1136/bmj.j1341. (In eng).
4. Tosif, S., Baker, A., Oakley, E., Donath, S., & Babl, F. E. (2012). Contamination rates of different urine collection methods for the diagnosis of urinary tract infections in young children: An observational cohort study. *Journal of Paediatrics and Child Health, 48*(8), 659–664. https://doi.org/10.1111/j.1440-1754.2012.02449.x. (In eng).
5. Shaikh, N., Hoberman, A., Hum, S. W., et al. (2018). Development and validation of a calculator for estimating the probability of urinary tract infection in young febrile children. *JAMA Pediatrics, 172*(6), 550–556. https://doi.org/10.1001/jamapediatrics.2018.0217. (In eng).
6. Smith, A. G., Kshetrapal, A., Boles, L., et al. (2023). External validation of the UTICalc with and without race for pediatric urinary tract infection. *The Journal of Pediatrics, 263*, 113681. https://doi.org/10.1016/j.jpeds.2023.113681. (In eng).
7. Clinpath Pathology [online]. *Urine sample collection.* Available at https://www.clinpath.com.au/patients/patient-resources/testing-information/urine-sample-collection/. Accessed 5 Sept 2024.
8. The Royal Children's Hospital, Melbourne, Australia. Clinical practice guideline on urinary tract infection [Internet, last updated July 2019; cited 5 Sept 2024]. Available from: https://wwww.rch.org.au/clinicalguide/

When Little Girls Will Not Pee

Tom Solan and Franz E Babl

1 Clinical Pearl

Urinary retention is usually due to vaginal irritation.

2 Clinical Case

Hannah is a 3-year-old girl who presents to the emergency department with her parents at 3 a.m., inconsolable. Her parents report that she has been refusing to pass urine for most of the day and holding at her vagina. She is afebrile but clearly in pain and distressed. It is difficult to assess her, but you think you can palpate a full bladder. Her abdomen is otherwise soft; when distracted, there is no guarding or peritonism. Hannah has seen her GP during the day, who felt that her vagina was irritated and she likely has vulvovaginitis. You also note that she has some vaginal erythema and inflammation but no obvious visible foreign body. Her family has attempted at-home treatments including paracetamol, ibuprofen, and topical lignocaine, without success. A warm bath administered in the emergency department helps her to urinate successfully. However, you are concerned that the same thing will happen again and want to provide her family with the best practice guidance.

T. Solan
Emergency Department, The Royal Chidren's Hospital Melbourne, Parkville, VIC, Australia

F. E. Babl (✉)
Emergency Department, The Royal Chidren's Hospital Melbourne, Parkville, VIC, Australia

Departments of Paediatrics and Critical Care, The University of Melbourne, Parkville, VIC, Australia

Clinical Sciences, Murdoch Children's Research Institute, Parkville, VIC, Australia

C. F. Lynch et al. (eds.), *The Art of Paediatric Medicine Beyond the Evidence Base*,
https://doi.org/10.1007/978-981-96-7234-9_20

3 Discussion

Paediatric urinary retention is an uncommon condition defined by the inability to void despite a full bladder. It can be caused by various factors, including anatomical, neurological, and psychological conditions, or infections. Among pre-pubescent girls, vaginal irritation—often due to infection and inflammation—is the most frequent cause, with vulvovaginitis being the leading contributor. Balanitis is the leading cause of acute urinary retention in boys [1].

Urinary retention in children can present acutely or chronically. Acute retention manifests as the sudden inability to urinate, often accompanied by abdominal pain and distension. Chronic retention involves incomplete bladder emptying over time, which may go unnoticed until complications such as infections or incontinence arise [2, 3].

In Hannah's case, urinary retention was secondary to irritation from vulvovaginitis, where the sting of urine on the irritated vulval area caused enough discomfort to inhibit her normal voiding reflex. This condition can be caused by poor hygiene, the use of irritants (e.g., soaps, bubble baths), or wearing tight or synthetic clothing [2].

When assessing paediatric urinary retention, it is important to consider the following conditions as possible causes:

- **Urinary Tract Infection (UTI):** UTIs may lead to urinary retention in girls who are more susceptible to infections due to their shorter urethra. UTIs typically present with symptoms such as fever, vomiting, dysuria, urgency, and sometimes abdominal pain [3, 5].
- **Constipation:** Constipation is a frequent cause of urinary retention in children, as a full rectum can exert pressure on the bladder, causing functional obstruction. Constipation can directly cause bladder dysfunction, leading to incomplete voiding or retention [3].
- **Trauma or Foreign Body:** Trauma or the presence of a foreign body in the vaginal area can cause significant irritation, resulting in retention. Vaginal foreign bodies, such as toilet paper or small objects, can lead to symptoms like vaginal discharge, bleeding, and difficulty urinating [6].
- **Neurogenic Bladder:** Neurological conditions, such as tethered spinal cord syndrome or spina bifida, may cause urinary retention by disrupting the normal neural pathways controlling the bladder. Although less common, these conditions should be considered if no other cause is apparent [3].
- **Psychological Causes:** Urinary retention can also be psychogenic in nature, with anxiety or fear contributing to the inability to void. Children may refuse to urinate if they associate it with pain, as in cases of vulvovaginitis [2].

Warm baths are highly effective in reducing the sting from urine on the irritated vulvar and vaginal mucosa as well as relaxing the pelvic muscles and relieving discomfort, allowing the child to void [2]. In Hannah's case, the warm bath was sufficient to resolve the retention. A similar effect can often be achieved by voiding into a warm shower.

Clinical practice guidelines recommend avoiding irritants such as soaps, bubble baths, and synthetic fabrics that can exacerbate vulvovaginitis. Encouraging the use of loose cotton underwear, practicing good hygiene, and ensuring the child changes out of wet clothing quickly are important measures for preventing further irritation.

Another suggested method for managing irritation is the use of vinegar baths, where half a cup of white vinegar is added to a shallow bath. This has been shown to provide symptomatic relief in children with vulvovaginitis. Additionally, educating caregivers on the importance of front-to-back wiping is important for long-term prevention [4].

While non-pharmacological measures are often sufficient, more severe cases of vaginal irritation may require pharmacological interventions. Mild vulvovaginitis can be treated with topical emollients to soothe irritated skin, but in cases of significant inflammation, the application of low-dose steroid creams (e.g., hydrocortisone 1%) may be necessary [5].

In Hannah's case, paracetamol and ibuprofen were administered at home to manage her pain and inflammation, but they were ineffective. The use of lignocaine, a topical anaesthetic, was also attempted but failed to alleviate the discomfort. Given the role of psychological distress in exacerbating the symptoms, the lack of success with these medications could have been influenced by her anxiety and fear.

Although rare, infections are sometimes associated with vulvovaginitis, and antibiotics should be prescribed based on the causative organism. Common pathogens include *Staphylococcus aureus*, *Escherichia coli*, and group A streptococci [1].

For cases where pinworms are suspected (due to nocturnal itching or discomfort), mebendazole is the treatment of choice. Pinworms can exacerbate vulvovaginitis by causing the child to scratch the irritated area, leading to further inflammation and discomfort. Treatment is often recommended for the entire household to prevent reinfection [6].

4 Other Gems

- Voiding into warm baths is highly effective for relieving urinary retention caused by vulvovaginitis and should be considered first-line therapy.
- Psychological factors can play a significant role in paediatric urinary retention, particularly in children who associate urination with pain. Treating the psychological aspect through reassurance and stress-relief techniques may be helpful.
- Vulval skincare is important to prevent recurrent irritation. Caregivers should be instructed on the proper care of the sensitive skin around the vulva, including avoiding harsh cleansers and maintaining dryness with loose cotton clothing.
- Clinicians should avoid performing internal vaginal examinations in prepubescent children and should refrain from taking internal swabs unless absolutely necessary.

References

1. Loveless, M., & Myint, O. (2018). Vulvovaginitis: Presentation of more common problems in pediatric and adolescent gynecology. *Best Practice & Research Clinical Obstetrics and Gynaecology, 48*, 14–27. https://doi.org/10.1016/j.bpobgyn.2017.08.014
2. Romano, M. E. (2020). Prepubertal vulvovaginitis. *Clinical Obstetrics and Gynecology, 63*(3), 479–485. https://doi.org/10.1097/GRF.0000000000000542
3. Schäfer, F.-M., et al. (2020). Acute urinary retention in children. *Journal of Pediatric Urology, 16*, 842.e1–842.e6. https://doi.org/10.1016/j.jpurol.2020.08.014
4. Starks, J. (2020). Vaginal irritation in prepubertal girls: Age-specific considerations in primary care. *The Journal for Nurse Practitioners, 16*, e35–e39.
5. GOSH NHS Foundation Trust. (2017). *Urinary retention: Causes, symptoms, and treatment*. Great Ormond Street Hospital for Children NHS Foundation Trust.
6. The Royal Children's Hospital Melbourne. (2022). *Vulval and vaginal conditions: Clinical practice guidelines*. https://www.rch.org.au/clinicalguide/guideline_index/Vulval_and_Vaginal_Conditions/

Not as Clear as It May Seem

Johanna Ramírez-Romero and Santiago Mintegi

1 Clinical Pearl

Be careful with a child brought to the Emergency Department after the ingestion of an unknown substance. Identify the substance before sending this child home.

2 Clinical Case

A 2-year-old child, Sofia, was brought to the paediatric emergency department (ED) after accidental ingestion of an undetermined amount of liquid her parents kept in a previously used water bottle.

The mother reported that Sofia had ingested the liquid and vomited immediately. She brought the bottle to the ED. The bottle did not have any identification of the liquid. Sofia appeared well and was asymptomatic upon the arrival to the ED.

The paediatricians on duty examined the liquid. It was semitransparent with a strong odour. Sofia's father worked as a window and blind installer, thus he used to store different liquid products pertaining to work at home. The treating doctor talked to her father, who claimed it was paraffin oil, which is non-toxic in small amounts. Of note 1 year prior, the parents brought Sofia to ED after a detergent ingestion without any toxic effect.

A strong smell from the liquid led to suspicion that the substance might be a hydrocarbon, so it was decided to keep Sofia in the observation area due to the risk of complications (mainly respiratory). It was initially difficult to convince her father

J. Ramírez-Romero · S. Mintegi (✉)
Pediatric Emergency Department, Cruces University Hospital, University of Basque Country, Bilbao, Spain

C. F. Lynch et al. (eds.), *The Art of Paediatric Medicine Beyond the Evidence Base*,
https://doi.org/10.1007/978-981-96-7234-9_21

but, finally, Sofia was admitted to the Observation Area of the ED for monitoring as identification of the toxicant was not possible.

Activated charcoal was not given as in some children, it can induce vomiting, and if the toxicant was a hydrocarbon, aspiration can result, causing chemical pneumonitis from direct injury to the lung parenchyma. Other consequences of aspiration are pulmonary oedema, bronchospasm, and resultant hypoxia.

Sofia's father was asked to check for substances that were stored at home while the mother stayed with her daughter.

One hour later, Sofia began vomiting and showed a progressive decrease in the level of consciousness, bilateral miosis, bradycardia and generalised hyporeflexia. This was compatible with a cholinergic substance poisoning, very commonly found in insecticides containing organophosphates. Her father was alerted and he exclaimed: "The ants!", and recalled that he bought diazinon, an insecticide that belongs to the group of organophosphates.

Intravenous (IV) atropine was administered and Sofia was admitted to the paediatric intensive care unit (PICU). Plasma cholinesterase value was **63** mU/ml (normal values 4600–14,400 mU/ml) with normal full blood examination and other routine blood tests. In the PICU, Sofia required another dose of IV atropine and five doses of IV pralidoxime. The cholinesterase value 2 days after admission was 4231 mU/ml and she was discharged from the PICU. Sofia was discharged home 2 days later with paediatric neurology follow-up due to the potential risk of long-term sequelae, such as peripheral neuropathies. Fortunately, Sofia had no long term clinical consequences.

3 Discussion

Poisoning exposures (mainly ingestions) are a frequent reason for consultation in the ED. One out of every 200–300 ED child presentations are related to poisoning exposures, most of them non-intentional ingestion of a toxicant [1].

Although most patients do well, some of them require prompt treatment and admission to hospital, even to PICU.

In young patients, most intoxications occur unintentionally, since, due to the child's eagerness to explore, they may accidentally ingest drugs or household products [1]. Storage of the toxicant in containers other than the original may facilitate accidental ingestion as children might find them familiar.

Unintentional pesticide poisoning is common in rural areas. The term "pesticide" encompasses a broad group of chemical substances intended to kill unwanted insects, plants, or rodents. Organophosphate and carbamate poisoning are the most widely known types of poisoning [2].

Organophosphate pesticide poisoning can occur related to skin contact, inhalation, or ingestion of pesticides. Organophosphate pesticides act as irreversible cholinesterase inhibitors since organophosphate-cholinesterase binding is not spontaneously reversible without pharmacological intervention. This inhibition leads to the accumulation of acetylcholine, and thus to the activation of muscarinic and nicotinic receptors. This results in cholinergic syndrome and decreased blood acetyl cholinesterase levels [3].

Clinical signs of organophosphate poisoning begin 30 minutes to 2 hours after contact, depending on the route of entry, dose, type of organophosphate, and individual susceptibility. 24–48 h after poisoning, the "intermediate syndrome" may appear as weakness/paralysis of the respiratory muscles, limbs, face, and neck, in the absence of cholinergic symptoms. It may persist for several days, leading to severe respiratory failure that requires mechanical ventilation. Binding of the organophosphate to acetylcholinesterase is irreversible; therefore, symptoms may persist for up to 3 months, which is the time it takes for the enzyme to regenerate. In addition, neurotoxic organophosphates inhibit neurotoxic esterase activity (>80%), which is found in the brain, medulla, peripheral nervous system, heart, spleen, and lymphocytes and is responsible for delayed polyneuropathy [4].

The management of children with organophosphate pesticide poisoning should always begin with initial stabilisation using the ABC approach (maintaining a patent airway and adequate breathing and circulation with control of brady-arrhythmias). Respiratory failure is the most frequent cause of death. Patients with moderate-to-severe intoxication may show a decreased level of consciousness, increased secretions, and respiratory failure (due to respiratory muscle paralysis) and may require mechanical ventilation. For intubation, non-depolarising muscle blockers should be used, and the use of succinylcholine (metabolized by butyrylcholinesterase, which is inhibited by the organophosphate and may cause prolonged relaxation) is not recommended [5].

When the entry route is digestive, gastrointestinal decontamination and administration of activated charcoal at a dose of 1 g/kg should be performed.

Administration of antidotes should begin during the initial approach. Atropine (a muscarinic antagonist) is administered at doses of 0.05 mg/kg and the dose can be doubled every 5–10 minutes until symptoms disappear. The use of oximes (such as pralidoxime), an antidote to nicotinic effects, can be considered with a loading dose of 25–50 mg/kg in slow infusion followed by a continuous infusion diluted in saline at 10–20 mg/kg/hr. [6, 7].

Most patients recover without any subsequent sequelae. However, it is necessary to observe these children in hospital for 36–48 hours. It is essential to monitor the appearance of the symptoms of intermediate syndrome and delayed polyneuropathy. Organophosphates are included in the group of hazardous chemical emergencies and poisonings [4].

Accidental poisoning is preventable, and the reduction in consultations due to poisoning exposures can be achieved with the implementation of adequate prevention measures. Although most patients do well, many children require interventions in the ED, such as gastrointestinal decontamination procedures, antidotes or support. Strategies such as placing safety caps on medications should be designed and implemented. Health education is essential, highlighting the importance of correct storage of drugs and household products to keep them out of the reach of children and in their original containers. In addition, patients presenting for a poisoning exposure with an unknown substance should always be cautiously managed, even if the patient appears well.

4 Other Gems

- Toddlers love to place everything they find in their mouths, no matter what the object is. This increases the risk for unintentional poisoning.
- Storage of the toxicant in containers other than the original may facilitate accidental ingestion as children might find them familiar.
- Organophosphate pesticide poisoning is common in rural areas.
- Accidental poisoning is potentially preventable with the implementation of correct prevention measures:
  - Adequate storage of medications and household products and keeping them out of the reach of children is essential.
  - Physicians should always inquire about the nature of the potentially toxic substances of unknown origin, even if the patient appears well and is asymptomatic when evaluated.

References

1. Mintegi, S., Azkunaga, B., Prego, J., Qureshi, N., Dalziel, S. R., Arana-Arri, E., Acedo, Y., Martinez-Indart, L., Urkaregi, A., Salmon, N., Benito, J., & Kuppermann, N. (2019). Pediatric emergency research networks (PERN) poisoning working group. International epidemiological differences in acute poisonings in pediatric emergency departments. *Pediatric Emergency Care, 35*(1), 50–57.
2. Roberts, J. R., Karr, C. J., Paulson, J. A., Brock-Utne, A. C., Brumberg, H. L., Campbell, C. C., et al. (2012). Pesticide exposure in children. *Pediatrics, 130*(6), e1765–e1788.
3. Seltzer, J. A., Friedland, S., Friedman, N. A., Winkler, G. A., Foreman, E., Al Mubarak, Y., et al. (2022). Accidental organophosphate poisoning: A case series of 2 pediatric coumaphos exposures. *Journal of the American College of Emergency Physicians Open, 3*(6), e12859.
4. Henretig, F., Kirk, M. A., & McKay, A. (2019). Hazardous chemical emergencies and poisonings. *The New England Journal of Medicine, 380*, 1638–1655.
5. Hulse, E. J., Haslam, J. D., Emmett, S. R., & Woolley, T. (2019). Organophosphorus nerve agent poisoning: Managing the poisoned patient. *British Journal of Anaesthesia, 123*(4), 457–463.
6. Bocanegra, M. A., Campanario, I., Moreno Perulero, M. L., Araujo, F., & Encinas, B. C. (2009). Pralidoxima en intoxicación por organofosforados: a propósito de dos casos en pediatría. *Farmacia Hospitalaria., 33*(6), 336–337.
7. Marruecos-Sant, L., & Martín-Rubí, J. C. (2007). Uso de oximas en la intoxicación por organofosforados. *Medicina Intensiva, 31*(5), 258–260.

Collateral Damage Caused by Thumb Sucking

Roderic Phillips

1 Clinical Pearl

Scarring, not thumb sucking causes concern.

2 Clinical Case

As a consultant paediatric dermatologist, I was asked to review a 3-year-old girl, Eleanor, with a history of thumb sucking, and secondary facial scratching to the point of scarring. Eleanor sucked either thumb and with her spare index finger would pick at her skin on either cheek. Eleanor's parents were very distressed by the scarring that were appearing on each cheek. She had been reviewed by multiple practitioners with little change.

The family were trying to stop Eleanor from sucking her thumb. They were placing a thumb guard (a plastic guard with some movement that encloses the thumb down to the thenar eminence) on both hands during the day, and a protective sleeve at night time. Intensive moisturising, steroid cream and wound care had healed the wounds, but she sometimes would sneak her thumb out of the thumb guard, suck it, and scratch her face to bleeding within minutes. Eleanor had no other sensory behaviours, and she was developmentally appropriate and normal.

R. Phillips (✉)
Department of Paediatrics, Monash University, Clayton, VIC, Australia

Royal Childrens Hospital, Parkville, VIC, Australia

C. F. Lynch et al. (eds.), *The Art of Paediatric Medicine Beyond the Evidence Base*,
https://doi.org/10.1007/978-981-96-7234-9_22

3 Discussion

I have seen many young children with a similar story. When assessing this problem, it has three distinct parts.

1. She is sucking her thumbs.
2. She is rubbing her skin
3. Her fingernails are damaging her skin.

In a three-year-old, thumb sucking is quite common and normal. It is rarely related to stress, or underlying family issues. Non-nutritive sucking in infants is nearly universal and is considered normal. It is a natural way for babies to soothe themselves and may start before birth. In preterm infants, non-nutritive sucking may have benefits of its own [1]. Most children spontaneously discontinue thumb sucking sometime between 2 and 4 years of age [2]. Some toddlers use a dummy for the same purpose. It may be easier to remove these than address thumb sucking. Cultural practices influence the degree of parental concern about the practice [3].

When secondary skin problems are present, as with Eleanor, the family may be much more concerned. To address this, explain to the parents that it is Eleanor's fingernails that will be the cause of any permanent scarring. This needs to be the central and immediate focus of management. Measures to reduce 1 and/or 2 are fine if you want to try them, and if these work, great. However, the actual problem is 3. Focusing on 3 is useful.

Nails damage skin because the sharp cut edge of the nail can dig up the epidermis. Eleanor's parents had already been trying to keep her nails short, but not effectively. Cutting them shorter doesn't fully solve the problem as the nail still has the sharp cut edge to damage skin.

Ask the parents to buy a good quality diamond encrusted or similar manicure nail file. Or one of the many electric nail files sold for toddlers. Cut the nails short (once). Then use the nail files to make the nail really short and to chamfer off the edge, so the nail tip ends up with a rounded smooth profile. You can show parents how to do this, but as long as they know what they are aiming to do (i.e. remove any edge on the nail profile), it's pretty simple. It is easy. It takes approximately 30–40 s in total (3–4 s per nail) every night, because all that needs to be filed off is the tiny amount of nail that grew in 1 day. The parents will take 30 s to do all the nails on their child, provided they do it every night. They can check the effect by using the child's nail to try and scratch the parent's forearm—they will recognize the difference once the edge is rounded off.

This method immediately and dramatically reduces/stops the skin damage—which is the primary problem.

References

1. Pinelli, J., & Symington, A. J. (2005). Non-nutritive sucking for promoting physiologic stability and nutrition in preterm infants. *Cochrane Database of Systematic Reviews*, Issue 4. Art. No.: CD001071. https://doi.org/10.1002/14651858.CD001071.pub2. Accessed 31 Jan 2025.
2. Viggiano, D., Fasano, D., Monaco, G., & Strohmenger, L. (2004). Breast feeding, bottle feeding, and non-nutritive sucking; effects on occlusion in deciduous dentition. *Archives of Disease in Childhood, 89*(12), 1121–1123. https://doi.org/10.1136/adc.2003.029728. PMID: 15557045; PMCID: PMC1719762.
3. Feştilă, D., Ghergie, M., Muntean, A., Matiz, D., & Şerb, N. A. (2014). Suckling and non-nutritive sucking habit: What should we know? *Clujul Medical Journal, 87*(1), 11–14. https://doi.org/10.15386/cjm.2014.8872.871.df1mg2. Epub 2014 Jan 30. PMID: 26527989; PMCID: PMC4462418.

Optimising Scar Outcome

Will Alexander

1 Clinical Pearl

The best scar management for children after trauma is multifactorial.

2 Clinical Case

Mei, a two-year-old girl, ran into a coffee table and had a nasty forehead laceration. She did not have any concussion symptoms. The family opted for Mei to be taken to theatre for debridement and layered repair by a plastic surgeon.

Post-operatively her parents are anxious to know what the best way is to prevent hypertrophic and keloid scarring, as the mother has suffered from keloid scars after both her ear piercing and caesarean surgery.

3 Discussion

Note: This discussion will focus on how to achieve the best outcome from surgical scars and full thickness lacerations; the management of burns and grazes is a different topic.

There are many factors that influence the quality of scarring after surgery. Unfortunately, some of these cannot be modified (genetic predisposition, conditions

W. Alexander (✉)
Royal Children's Hospital, St Vincent's Private and Public Hospital, Monash Health, Epworth Freemasons, Victorian Hand Surgery Associates, Fitzroy, VIC, Australia

C. F. Lynch et al. (eds.), *The Art of Paediatric Medicine Beyond the Evidence Base*,
https://doi.org/10.1007/978-981-96-7234-9_23

such as Ehlers-Danlos, and the location of the scar—deltoid, ear, pre-sternal are high risk zones); but an awareness can influence how vigilant the clinician and parents should be in post-operative scar care.

An example of post-operative evidence-based instructions for families can be summarised as follows:

1. Immediately after the operation until the first follow-up check:
   - Follow the instructions given on the day of surgery (if in doubt, leave the dressings on).
2. From the first post-operative visit until 6 weeks post operatively:
   - Keep the scar covered with a hypoallergenic medical paper tape as much as possible [1, 2]. This can be wet in the shower and changed as often as needed (usually every 1–3 days).
   - If it is not feasible to cover the scar with tape, then twice-a-day application of soft paraffin is another option.
3. From 6 weeks onwards (until 18 months post-operatively):
   - Protect carefully from the sun **(the most important step)**.
   - Use sunscreen, clothing, or tape to physically protect the area from sun damage.
   - Moisturise and massage twice a day (can use sunscreen as the moisturiser in the mornings).

- Optional:
  - Silicone ointment/tape if the scar is raised or if there is a high risk of hypertrophic scars/keloid scars. If there is a high concern, these can be instituted even earlier, from as soon as the wound has epithelialized [1–3]. Silicone tape is more effective than ointment, but compliance with sheets/tape can be lower than with ointment. The sheet needs to be applied to the scar for 12–24 h/day and used for at least one month [4]. The mechanism of action of silicone is not well understood, but likely relates to increased temperature and collagenase activity, polarisation of the scar tissue, and improved hydration [2].
  - Compression/pressure: Pressure clip earrings and compression sleeves (often with silicone sheet lining them) have been shown to improve scar quality.
  - Laser: mainly used for improvement in colour than contour.
  - Intralesional steroid.

It should be noted that, particularly in children, the natural history of scarring is that they will typically peak in thickness/erythema at about 1–3 months after an operation and then start to settle from there onwards. The final scar outcome is seen at ~18 months post-surgery.

Problematic scars can include hypertrophic scars (raised, pink, itchy; but within the limits of the original scar) or keloid scars (as for hypertrophic but also extending outside the borders of the original scar). These are difficult to manage and therefore prevention is important. Intralesional steroid injections, silicone sheeting,

5-fluorouracil, and occasionally excision +/− low dose radiation are used in treatment of these [4].

4 Other Gems

- Good genetics, surgical technique, and early careful wound care aimed at preventing infection/dehiscence are important factors in obtaining good scar outcomes; but can often not be altered by the patient or their family.
- For the prevention of problematic scarring, tape and silicone have strong evidence early in scar maturation.
- There are treatments available for hypertrophic and keloid scarring, but prevention is ideal.

References

1. Mustoe, T. A., Cooter, R. D., Gold, M. H., et al. (2002). International clinical recommendations on scar management. *Plastic and Reconstructive Surgery, 110*(2), 560–571. https://doi.org/10.1097/00006534-200208000-00031
2. Janis, J. (2014). *Essentials of plastic surgery* (2nd ed.). Thieme Medical Publishers Inc.
3. Gold, M. H., McGuire, M., Mustoe, T. A., et al. (2014). Updated international clinical recommendations on scar management: part 2--Algorithms for scar prevention and treatment. *Dermatologic Surgery: Official Publication for American Society for Dermatologic Surgery [et al]., 40*(8), 825–831. https://doi.org/10.1111/dsu.0000000000000050
4. Del Toro, D., Dedhia, R., & Tollefson, T. T. (2016). Advances in scar management: Prevention and management of hypertrophic scars and keloids. *Current Opinion in Otolaryngology & Head and Neck Surgery, 24*(4), 322–329. https://doi.org/10.1097/MOO.0000000000000268

15 Seconds of Silence Is Golden

Roderic Phillips

1 Clinical Pearl

Stop talking and listen to your toddler.

2 Clinical Case

Most of us encounter families with toddlers who have learnt to talk and who have become pretty verbal, talking a lot. Or we have some of our own, as children or as grandchildren. Day after day, you will hear conversations like the following:

Saanvi, a toddler, comes home after going to the zoo with a grandparent.
Parent asks: "what did you do today?"
Saanvi pauses for one or two seconds, then the parent says: "Did you go to the zoo?"
Saanvi says "Yes."

What has happened here is that the parent has dumbed the question down for Saanvi and then gets an immediate answer "Yes."

Try this experiment.

Parent asks: "What did you do today?"
And waits. And waits. And waits. Just listening, staying focussed on the toddler but saying nothing.
Eventually, after a delay that can be as long or longer than 15 to 20 seconds, the toddler will start responding in a much more interesting and complex way, and

---

R. Phillips (✉)
Royal Childrens Hospital, Parkville, VIC, Australia

Department of Paediatrics, Monash University, Clayton, VIC, Australia

C. F. Lynch et al. (eds.), *The Art of Paediatric Medicine Beyond the Evidence Base*,
https://doi.org/10.1007/978-981-96-7234-9_24

will genuinely tell you something. "We were on a tram and the tram driver started the tram and a lady nearly fell over. A man helped her sit down."

Waiting 15 seconds in silence seems like a lifetime. But consider this above exchange from the toddler's viewpoint.

"What did you do today?"

The toddler starts by reviewing/remembering some aspects of the day and choosing what was interesting. Then the toddler has to work out how to describe that to the parent. What words to use? It was on a tram. What word describes the person sitting at the front of a tram? What happened? How to describe that?

This is the same process we use when trying to speak a foreign language that we are just learning. The eventual sentence will contain words and word constructions that the toddler has never used before and probably has never heard in that context.

3 Discussion

Waiting 15 seconds in silence seems like a lifetime. Most of us never get close to silence in a conversation. In a medical consultation, you will have to train the other adults around you. Parents are often eager to "tell the story" or interpret for their child. You need to explain to them what you are doing. Otherwise, they will interrupt the silence to "dumb the question down." Silence can be disconcerting for some people. There is an expected conversational "flow" between the speakers, with culture also playing a large role in how fast or slow a conversation proceeds.

Adults will often talk continuously to a child or ask rapid-fire questions without pausing for time and space to respond. Young infants and toddlers are surrounded by speech and yet rarely given adequate time to process what they are hearing. Their brains are just starting to understand the sounds used to form words and the pattern of stresses and intonation indicating a question as opposed to a statement. Before they can process what was just said, they are faced with more adult talk. During an interaction with a toddler, you also need the toddler to recognise that you are maintaining focus on them through the whole silence. Just waiting. Letting them think; giving their hardworking brains time to process all the information they are receiving from you before they can formulate a verbal response.

In paediatric practice, learning to communicate with children at different ages and stages is a core skill. Considering the child's point of view, the child's developmental stage and allowing time and space to "meet them in the middle." Communication in health care is an essential skill and the most common "procedure" in medicine [1]. In paediatric practice there are three participants; the physician, the parent and the child. This requires triadic consultation skills [1] which may be taught in medical school and honed with practice. However, it is common that the child patient is often involved for a very small proportion of the medical interview. Very young children may not even be invited to participate. Enabling effective child participation will allow a developmental continuum for children to actively participate in their own health care. It is also a lot of fun!

4 Other Gems

- Even young infants need "space" to communicate. "Watch Wait and Wonder" is therapeutic intervention to improve relationships between parent and infant [2]. Its principles are important for parents to understand this unique time of a young child's life.

References

1. Spender, Q. (2007). Talking to children. *British Journal of General Practice, 57*, 861–863.
2. Cohen, N. J. (2002). Watch, wait, and wonder: An infant-led approach to infant-parent psychotherapy. *Newsletter of the Infant Mental Health Promotion Project, 35*(Winter), 1–4.

If You Always Look, You Sometimes Find Zebras

Catherine F Lynch

1 Clinical Pearl

Always check the Blood Pressure (BP) during routine consultations for young children.

2 Clinical Cases

2.1 Case 1

Ravi, aged 3 years, attended private outpatients with his exasperated mother. Toilet training was not going well. Ravi was excellent at weeing in the potty but poo was a different matter. He refused to sit on the potty or toilet. He "held on", squirming despite tummy pain. Ravi hid behind the couch to open his bowels. He soiled his underpants on a daily basis and pretended it had nothing to do with him.

Everyone was unhappy.

Examination findings revealed a charming well grown boy. Weight was 15.1 kg (50th centile), height 97 cm (50th centile) and BMI 16 (50th centile). Ravi's abdomen was loaded with faeces but there was no organomegaly. He had normal male genitalia and anus. There was a smear of poo on his underpants. His BP was 120/75 mmHg (> **95th centile**). Dual heart sounds were noted with palpable femoral pulses and no radio-femoral delay. No skin lesions were present.

Advice about managing toileting was given and the high blood pressure noted. It was confirmed on subsequent readings in different settings. Investigations were

C. F. Lynch (✉)
Alfred Health, Melbourne, VIC, Australia

C. F. Lynch et al. (eds.), *The Art of Paediatric Medicine Beyond the Evidence Base*,
https://doi.org/10.1007/978-981-96-7234-9_25

performed and included electrolytes, urea, creatinine and a renal ultrasound. The ultrasound revealed the cause of the hypertension as congenital renal dysplasia. Ravi was commenced on antihypertensive medication. He also learned to poo on the toilet. Long term he grew well, maintained normotension throughout childhood and was discharged from paediatric care at the age of 18 years.

2.2 *Case 2*

Jessica, aged 2 ½ years, attended a clinic with her concerned parents. She had been unwell for 2 months with several episodes of intermittent vomiting without diarrhoea. Each episode lasted for a few days then resolved. Jessica had good energy levels, a comfortable daily bowel motion and a reasonable appetite. She had excellent language skills and was developmentally advanced. It was noted that she had lost 1 kg in weight over the past month.

Examination findings revealed a chatty little girl with weight 13.2 kg (50th centile), height 90 cm (50th centile), BMI 16.2 (50th centile) and BP 115/72 mmHg (> **95th centile**). Dual heart sounds were noted with palpable femoral pulses and no radio-femoral delay. Abdominal examination was normal. No skin lesions were present. Initial investigations included a FBC, EUC, LFT, and coeliac screen which were all normal. An urgent MRI brain was performed revealing a large cerebellar mass consistent with a medulloblastoma. She received surgical and oncological treatment. Long term she survived into adulthood cancer-free.

3 Discussion

Blood pressure in children, unlike adults, is dependent on age, height and gender. There are normed scales which help identify children with elevated blood pressure [1].

Measuring blood pressure in children may seem more difficult than in adults. For example, readings are likely to be falsely high in crying toddlers, normal ranges for blood pressure are often not displayed on the clinic wall, and an appropriately sized cuff may not be available in the clinic room.

BP should be measured in the right arm of a relaxed, seated child. The appropriately sized cuff should be used [2]. Very young children may be more comfortable on a parents' lap. BP measurement by auscultation is the gold standard. BP measured by an automated device correlates reasonably well with auscultation, with practical advantages of rapid measurement remote from the child and elimination of reader error. However, it is worth practising with a manual BP cuff and auscultation.

My practice is to pump up the cuff whilst feeling the pulse at the wrist. This means the cuff is not pumped up too tightly and allows for a "quick" systolic as you release the pressure. Auscultation then follows. Even young children are usually able to manage this, and it becomes a routine part of "going to the doctor". Checking the BP manually gives the clinician a chance to interact directly with the child and build the relationship.

Hypertension is defined as BP > 95th centile for age, gender and height on three or more occasions.(4)

It is recommended that all children over the age of 3 years have their BP measured routinely. The cases above illustrate that routine BP measurement for toddlers is helpful as a "red flag" in pursuing and identifying a secondary cause for hypertension. Secondary hypertension is more common in children than adults. Very young children with hypertension should be evaluated more completely than older children. There are children < 3 years who are more at risk of hypertension (Table 1) and surveillance should begin early.

Overall, hypertension in children and adolescents has become much more prevalent due to the strong link between obesity and high BP. There has been a marked increase in the prevalence of overweight and obese children [4]. Primary hypertension, defined as systolic BP or diastolic BP at or above the 95th centile on repeated measurement, is identifiable in children and adolescents.

There may be a positive family history, a BMI >95th centile and evidence of metabolic syndrome (i.e. insulin resistance with high triglycerides, low high density lipoprotein, truncal obesity and hyperinsulinemia). In these cases, other cardiovascular risk factors should be identified. Checking for sleep disorders is particularly important. Evaluating the presence of other comorbidities is important for planning and implementing therapies to reduce the cardiovascular risk and help control BP. The physical examination in children with hypertension is often otherwise normal.

In medical training we are taught, "If you hear hooves, think of horses, not zebras." If measuring BP becomes a routine part of clinical assessment for young children, when high blood pressure is noted the level of suspicion of a "zebra" will be heightened, allowing timely investigation of an underlying cause.

Table 1 Risk Factors for hypertension in children

Neonatal period	History of prematurity, very low birthweight, or other neonatal complication requiring intensive care
Cardiac	Congenital heart disease (repaired or not)
Renal	Recurrent urinary tract infections, haematuria, or proteinuria Family history of congenital renal disease Known renal disease or urologic malformations
Transplant	Bone marrow or solid organ
Other systemic illnesses known to be associated with hypertension	Tuberous sclerosis, Neurofibromatosis

4 Other Gems

- Over the period of childhood, the trend is for average heart rate and respiratory rate to decrease and blood pressure to increase. It is important to be aware of the normal ranges for vital signs [3] and how they change across childhood.
- Unlike weight or height growth charts where the trajectory is always upwards, BMI changes over time include a reduction during the toddler years before a steady rise across childhood and adolescence.

References

1. Team DFTB. (2021). *Blood pressure centiles, don't forget the bubbles*. Available at: https://doi.org/10.31440/DFTB.1149
2. National High Blood Pressure Education Program Working Group on High Blood Pressure in Children and Adolescents. (2004). The fourth report on the diagnosis, evaluation and treatment of high blood pressure in children and adolescents. *Pediatrics, 114*, 555–576. May 2005.
3. Fleming, S., et al. (2011). Normal ranges of heart rate and respiratory rate in children from birth to 18 years of age: A systematic review of observational studies. *The Lancet, 377*(9770), 1011–1018.
4. Jeong, S. I., & Kim, S. H. (2024). Obesity and hypertension in children and adolescents. *Clinical Hypertension, 30*, 23. https://doi.org/10.1186/s40885-024-00278-5

Have You Thought About Quitting?

Rob Roseby

1 Clinical Pearl

Parent and carer smoking is harmful to a child, even when they smoke outside. You can reduce harm to children by helping parents or carers who smoke move towards a quit attempt.

2 Clinical Case

An 18-month-old child, Jun, is admitted to hospital with a viral lower respiratory tract infection. On history, you find their older sibling recently had an adenotonsillectomy and grommets, and that Jun's father smokes "but only outside".

As Jun starts to improve and you can think about when discharge may be possible, the family asks if there is anything that can reduce the risk of Jun getting sick again. You bring up the issue of parental smoking, but the father emphasises that he only smokes outside.

Do you have anywhere to go in this conversation?

R. Roseby (✉)
Respiratory Paediatrician and Service Director, Medical Specialties, Monash Childrens Hospital, Clayton, Vic, Australia

Department of Paediatrics, Monash University, Clayton, Vic, Australia

C. F. Lynch et al. (eds.), *The Art of Paediatric Medicine Beyond the Evidence Base*,
https://doi.org/10.1007/978-981-96-7234-9_26

3 Discussion

Parent and carer smoking, even if outside, is associated with harms to children [1], seemingly with a dose-response relationship [2]. The risk of most respiratory illnesses, and odds for a child undergoing adenotonsillectomy and tympanic membrane ventilation tube insertion, are roughly doubled if they live with a parent or carer who smokes [2]. The odds of sepsis and serious bacterial infection are even higher [3].

Parent and carer smoking cessation helps everyone in the household, but our job is not to *make* them quit! It's tempting to push hard, given that at any moment in time, 80% of smokers want to quit. However, quitting is a process not an action. Remember the famous Prochaska and di Clemente stages of change model of behaviour change? Their "Transtheoretical Model" postulates that behaviour change involves movement through five stages of precontemplation, contemplation, preparation, action, and maintenance. Using this model, our job is to help nudge a smoker closer to a quit attempt.

Brief smoking cessation advice works [4, 5]. Just one sentence from a GP such as "We both know smoking is not good for your health, maybe you should think about quitting" can result in a 12-month quit rate of a few percent higher than if nothing was said. Depending on the setting and intensity of intervention, clientele can be even more receptive to such messages [5].

So, what do we do as child health professionals, where the smoker is not our patient?

For delivery of smoking cessation messages, the child health context is different from that of adult health, where the smoker is generally the patient themselves [6]. In child health, we know that if done poorly, parent smokers can become more entrenched and less likely to quit than if no cessation message had been delivered [7].

The skill is in choosing the right time and using a non-confrontational approach.

Particularly for admitted patients, but also for many ambulatory patients, parents as carers are receptive to prevention messages and may even ask if there's anything to stop this sort of illness from happening again. This is your moment, but what brief message do you deliver?

Being directive might make you feel as though you've been staunch about it, but that doesn't work. A motivational interviewing approach eg. "Have you thought about quitting? [pause for answer] What gets in the way?", "How committed to smoking are you?" is likely to be more successful. I like the line "I know you know smoking is not good for you and you probably know it's not good for [XX/ XY] either. Is there anything I can do to help you move closer to a quit attempt?"

I'm generally positive about their response, almost regardless of what they say. If I meet a dead end I go no further, but this often leads to a brief conversation about the average number of quit attempts before success (it's 6!) and that nicotine replacement or Bupropion can be helpful. I send them back to their General Practitioner for follow up, including a letter that outlines the conversation, and sometimes provides the Quitline phone number [8].

References

1. Brown, N., et al. (2015). Interventions to reduce harm from smoking with families in infancy and early childhood: A systematic review. *International Journal of Environmental Research and Public Health, 12*(3), 3091–3119.
2. Jones, L. L., et al. (2011). Parental and household smoking and the increased risk of bronchitis, bronchiolitis and other lower respiratory infections in infancy: Systematic review and meta-analysis. *Respiratory Research, 12*(1), 5.
3. Iles, K., Poplawski, N., & Couper, R. (2001). Passive exposure to tobacco smoke and bacterial meningitis in children. *Journal of Paediatrics and Child Health, 37*(4), 388–391.
4. Lancaster, T., et al. (2000). Effectiveness of interventions to help people stop smoking: Findings from the Cochrane library. *BMJ, 321*(7257), 355–358.
5. Cornuz, J. (2007). Smoking cessation interventions in clinical practice. *European Journal of Vascular and Endovascular Surgery, 34*(4), 397–404.
6. Behbod, B., et al. (2018). Family and carer smoking control programmes for reducing children's exposure to environmental tobacco smoke. *Cochrane Database of Systematic Reviews, 1*, CD001746.
7. Irvine, L., et al. (1999). Advising parents of asthmatic children on passive smoking: Randomised controlled trial. *British Medical Journal, 318*(7196), 1456–1459.
8. Quitline. *Quit smoking*. Quitline Australia. Available at: https://www.quit.org.au. Accessed 24 Jan 2025.

Enhancing Attachment Between Young Children with Autism and Their Parents

Jennifer Harrison

1 Clinical Pearl

Relationship development should be considered alongside other allied health development-enhancing strategies for autistic children and their parents.

2 Clinical Case

A three-year-old female child, Imogen, was referred to the local child psychiatry service for assessment. She was conceived by IVF to a solo parent who was undergoing regular psychiatric care for depression and generalised anxiety. Imogen was born healthy but was described as being a difficult baby.

From birth, Imogen was irritable, difficult to soothe, difficult to settle, demanding and difficult to breastfeed (requiring help from a lactation consultant). Imogen was also prone to developing health complications, such as viral infections and reflux.

Concerns were present from birth, but features of autism were increasingly noted by age two years including a delay in speech acquisition, increasing 'meltdowns', a preoccupation with numbers and counting, severe separation anxiety, a strong preference for her own agenda in play, and food fussiness when she'd transitioned to solids.

The care team included a paediatrician, private psychiatrist and attachment specialist, but they were unclear about the diagnosis of autism in the face of evident mother-child relationship issues. There had been a stressed relationship between the

J. Harrison (✉)
Neurodevelopmental Team, Developmental Assessment and Management Program, Neuropsychiatry Clinic, Alfred ICYAMHWS, Melbourne, VIC, Australia

C. F. Lynch et al. (eds.), *The Art of Paediatric Medicine Beyond the Evidence Base*,
https://doi.org/10.1007/978-981-96-7234-9_27

mother and her own mother (who was described as possibly having undiagnosed autism) since early childhood with periods of estrangement.

Referral concerns centred around the diagnostic dilemma, but also the worry that gains in relationship development in the community therapy were not generalising to the home.

Our multidisciplinary developmental assessment indicated that Imogen was indeed autistic, but that symptoms were elevated due to the relationship difficulties between the mother and her child, including severe separation anxiety.

With her mother's permission and following a period of psychoeducation about autism and care team support, eight sessions of Wait Watch Wonder therapy [1] were provided. This included four sessions of child-led Wait Watch Wonder play, interspersed with four parent sessions with the two therapists encouraging reflections on the previous week's session, including open discussion about microevents that had happened in the playroom.

The intervention was non-threatening and playful. It demonstrated the loneliness of parenting and the excellence of the physical aspects of mothering but highlighted the significant problems in the emotional engagement between mother and child.

Imogen presented with many anxious, angry behaviours in the first play session but as the sessions progressed, progress was made. Meltdowns became less frequent, and Imogen was increasingly able to separate from her mother's safe base with increasing curiosity in the play and enjoyable interactions. Her mother was encouraged to set gentle but firm limits on unacceptable behaviour. Following the intervention, Imogen and her mother were referred back to their private relationship therapist.

3 Discussion

Often autism and the relationship with a caregiver are seen as dichotomous, either/or entities, rather than in need of being understood together. The literature on attachment in autism indicates that most autistic children are securely attached to their preferred care giver but at a rate that is slightly less than that seen in non-autistic populations [2]. Children with autism often show their attachment behaviours in different ways to neurotypical securely attached children [3].

The children appear to be less adept at reading and giving social cues, such as eye contact, and they "refuel" emotionally in unusual ways (such as backing up to the parent, rather than reaching for the parent). One of the strongest memories of my career has been watching parents reaching out to their autistic children with exaggerated loving gestures despite the minimal feedback they might be receiving from their child.

More recently, a systematic review of maternal sensitivity in populations of autistic children and their mothers suggests that maternal sensitivity does indeed affect the security of attachment. The authors also indicate that more research is needed to better understand the way mothers/parents adapt to a child's autism [4].

The Wait Watch Wonder approach is only one of several possible attachment-enhancing interventions we could have chosen (none of which have been well studied in autism). In our experience, the chosen approach enhanced the mother and child's trust in us and in each other and improved the fun and enjoyment within their relationship. The child was still autistic but happier and more explorative. The mother felt better able to 'read' her child. A final meeting with the mother's extended family to discuss the diagnosis and the best ways to support the family was also helpful.

In our team, we receive mainly complex referrals where attachment disruption, mental health conditions and trauma often occur in conjunction with neurodevelopmental presentations. We are developing an interview to help shape the discussion about relationship development, always with parent permission. We are very aware of the 1960s history of blaming parenting (when terms such as 'the refrigerator mother' were applied), but we find that this gentle approach is acceptable and helpful to families.

4 Other Gems

- Relationship development is important for all families including those with an autistic child.
- Some parent-child relationships need extra help, often when there is a history of intergenerational attachment difficulties, and the parent is eager to understand this better.
- There needs to be more research into relationship development throughout the lifespan but particularly early in the family's journey with autism (e.g. what are the most effective interventions).

References

1. Cohen, N., Muir, E., Lojkasek, M., et al. (1999). Wait watch and wonder: Testing the effectiveness of a new approach to mother-infant psychotherapy. *Infant Mental Health Journal, 20*, 429–451.
2. Teague, S., Gray, K., Tonge, B., & Newman, L. (2017). Attachment in children with autism spectrum disorder: A systematic review. *Research in Autism Spectrum Disorders, 35*, 35–50.
3. Dissanayake, C., & Crossley, S. (1997). Autistic children's responses to separation and reunion with their mothers. *Journal of Autism and Developmental Disorders, 27*(3), 295–312.
4. Cossette-Côté, F., Bussières, E., & Dubois-Comtois, K. (2022). The association between maternal sensitivity/availability and attachment in children with autism spectrum disorder. *Current Psychology, 41*, 8236–8248.

Define Normal

Paul Monagle

1 Clinical Pearl

Until one understands normal, it is impossible to diagnose disease accurately.

2 Clinical Case

Felix is a 4-year-old developmentally normal boy with no past history, a normal western diet, who presented to his General Practitioner (GP) with lethargy just over 12 months ago. Initial blood tests showed a haemoglobin (Hb) of 130 g/l (Reference Range 110–140 g/L), mean cell volume (MCV) 89 fl (Reference range 75–90 fL), Ferritin **10** mcg/L (Lab reported ferritin reference range 20–150 mcg/L).

Felix was diagnosed as iron deficient and commenced on oral iron replacement (3 mg/kg/day elemental iron).

Repeat blood tests after 3 months demonstrated a Hb 130 g/l, MCV 89 and a Ferritin of **15**. Felix was given a further 3 months of oral iron at 6 mg/kg/day. Repeat blood tests reported a Hb 130 g/l, MCV 89 and a Ferritin of **15**. He was then given IV ferric carboxymaltose 15 mg/kg iron at the GP procedure centre, unfortunately complicated by anaphylaxis requiring adrenaline and a 24-h admission to hospital.

One month post infusion his ferritin was 140 and FBE unchanged, but 6 months later his blood tests again reported a Hb 129, MCV 88 and a Ferritin of **11**. Felix was referred for paediatric management of refractory iron deficiency.

P. Monagle (✉)
Department of Paediatrics, University of Melbourne, Parkville, VIC, Australia

Clinical Haematology, Royal Children's Hospital, Parkville, VIC, Australia

Haematology Research, Murdoch Children's Research Institute, Parkville, VIC, Australia

C. F. Lynch et al. (eds.), *The Art of Paediatric Medicine Beyond the Evidence Base*,
https://doi.org/10.1007/978-981-96-7234-9_28

3 Discussion

Iron deficiency is frequently misdiagnosed in children for a number of reasons [1].

While many laboratories report the lower limit of normal for ferritin as 20 or even 30, multiple studies in Australia and other countries have shown that the 2.5th centile for ferritin is approximately 10 throughout most of childhood [2, 3]. Many laboratory parameters have age specific (and sometime analyser specific) reference ranges.

By definition, 95% of children will have a ferritin within the age-appropriate reference range, however each person has their own physiological set point and therefore some children may have a ferritin within the reference range yet not be normal or physiological for them. Conversely, 2.5% of children will have a ferritin below the reference range and yet be physiologically normal.

Iron studies are often misleading and misdiagnosis of iron deficiency because of inappropriate interpretation is frequent. Serum iron is not useful in the diagnosis of iron deficiency, in part due to diurnal variation and fluctuations related to iron intake over the previous 24 h. In community-based children, ferritin alone is the best guide to iron status, notwithstanding it is an acute phase reactant and so may be normal in iron deficient children with intercurrent infection or inflammation. Repeat testing once clinically well may be required.

Children who are iron replete (a physiologically normal ferritin for them) will excrete almost all additional oral iron and hence will appear to have minimal if any ferritin response, even when compliant with prolonged oral iron therapy.

If the Hb and MCV are normal, there is time to address any issues (Table 1).

Recent studies do not support that iron deficiency (in the absence of anaemia) has any long-term neurodevelopmental impacts [4, 5]. Stable Hb and MCV across a range of ferritins suggest that the ferritin results do not reflect iron deficiency for that particular child. As in the case above, the fact that Jeremy's Hb and MCV were unchanged even when his ferritin increased to 140 suggests that they were normal when his ferritin was 10.

Intravenous (IV) iron is expensive and may have significant side effects. The majority of children with iron deficiency (even in the presence of anaemia) will respond to oral iron, and IV iron should be predominantly reserved for proven

Table 1 Stages of iron deficiency

Stage of iron deficiency	Early /Mild	Moderate	Severe
Ferritin	Low	Low	Low
MCV	Normal	Low	Low
Haemoglobin	Normal	Normal	Normal
Overall haematological status	Reduced iron stores Normal haemopoiesis	Impaired haemopoiesis	Inadequate haemopoiesis

MCV mean cell volume

inflammatory bowel disease, true failure of oral iron therapy and chronic blood loss that cannot be managed with oral iron. IV iron should be given in an environment able to manage anaphylaxis in a child.

Iron deficiency in children is common in:

(a) Premature neonates (failure to gain iron stores during the third trimester).
(b) Infants fed cow's milk prior to 12 months of age (cow's milk enteritis).
(c) Infants who fail to transition to solid foods and continue high milk/formula intake beyond 12 months of age.
(d) Severe selective eating disorders.
(e) Strict vegetarians.
(f) Menstruating teenage girls.

Most of these children can be diagnosed on history alone. In the absence of such a history, iron deficiency is rare, and one should suspect malabsorption (coeliac disease) or blood loss (most often gastrointestinal). Felix had no features on history to explain iron deficiency. As a 4-year-old boy with no significant past medical history, if he had truly been iron deficient he should have been referred immediately for further investigations.

Much harm comes from over diagnosis and inappropriate treatment when normal parameters for age are not understood.

4 Other Gems

- There are multiple reasons for lethargy in children, and if related to iron deficiency, there is usually symptomatic improvement within days of commencing oral iron. If the ferritin is normal for age, then the lethargy is likely due to another cause.

References

1. Sezgin, G., Li, L., Westbrook, J., Wearne, E., Azar, D., McLeod, A., Pearce, C., Ignjatovic, V., Monagle, P., & Georgiou, A. (2021). Influence of serum iron test results on the diagnosis of iron deficiency in children: A retrospective observational study. *BMJ Open, 11*(7), e046865. https://doi.org/10.1136/bmjopen-2020-046865. PMID: 34226221; PMCID: PMC8258555.
2. Hoq, M., Matthews, S., Karlaftis, V., Burgess, J., Cowley, J., Donath, S., Carlin, J., Yen, T., Ignjatovic, V., Monagle, P., Kids, H. A. P. P. I., & study team. (2019). Reference values for 30 common biochemistry analytes across 5 different analyzers in neonates and children 30 days to 18 years of age. *Clinical Chemistry, 65*(10), 1317–1326. https://doi.org/10.1373/clinchem.2019.306431. Epub 2019 Sep 3.
3. Sezgin, G., Monagle, P., Loh, T. P., Ignjatovic, V., Hoq, M., Pearce, C., McLeod, A., Westbrook, J., Li, L., & Georgiou, A. (2020). Clinical thresholds for diagnosing iron deficiency: Comparison of functional assessment of serum ferritin to population based centiles. *Scientific Reports, 10*(1), 18233. https://doi.org/10.1038/s41598-020-75435-5. PMID: 33106588; PMCID: PMC7589482.

4. Pasricha, S. R., Hasan, M. I., Braat, S., Larson, L. M., Tipu, S. M. M., Hossain, S. J., Shiraji, S., Baldi, A., Bhuiyan, M. S. A., Tofail, F., Fisher, J., Grantham-McGregor, S., Simpson, J. A., Hamadani, J. D., & Biggs, B. A. (2021). Benefits and risks of iron interventions in infants in rural Bangladesh. *The New England Journal of Medicine, 385*(11), 982–995. https://doi.org/10.1056/NEJMoa2034187
5. Larson, L. M., Feuerriegel, D., Hasan, M. I., Braat, S., Jin, J., Tipu, S. M. U., Shiraji, S., Tofail, F., Biggs, B. A., Hamadani, J. D., Johnson, K. A., Bode, S., & Pasricha, S. R. (2023). Effects of iron supplementation on neural indices of habituation in Bangladeshi children. *The American Journal of Clinical Nutrition, 117*(1), 73–82. https://doi.org/10.1016/j.ajcnut.2022.11.023. Epub 2022 Dec 23.

Salbutamol and Elevated Lactate

Michael Clifford

1 Clinical Pearl

Consider salbutamol toxicity in the younger child with asthma, refractory to standard therapies.

2 Clinical Case

A 4-year-old boy, Alfred, is being treated for an acute episode of wheeze. He has previously been salbutamol responsive and has a "puffer" at home. Alfred has received several "bursts" of bronchodilator via metered dose inhaler (MDI) with a spacer and is now receiving a second nebulised dose of salbutamol in oxygen. His heart rate is 140 beats per minute, respiratory rate 30 breaths per min, non-invasive blood pressure 110/60 mmHg, pulse oximetry is 88% on air but 99% with the nebuliser running with 10 litres/min of oxygen. Alfred's pulse oximetry trace is noted to demonstrate significant "*pulsus paradoxus*"—respiratory variation of peak and baseline of the pulse oximetry waveform (Fig. 1).

Alfred has intercostal and subcostal retractions, hyperinflation with hepatic ptosis and widespread bilateral wheeze. A chest x-ray has been ordered. He has an IV in situ and a dose of magnesium sulphate is about to be administered following 20 mg of methylprednisolone. The nurses are also preparing High Flow Nasal Cannula and a Paediatric Intensive Care review (PICU) has been requested. A venous blood gas taken at the time of his IV insertion is as follows (Table 1).

M. Clifford (✉)
Departments of Paediatric Intensive Care, Anaesthesia and Pain Management, The Royal Children's Hospital Melbourne, Parkville, VIC, Australia

C. F. Lynch et al. (eds.), *The Art of Paediatric Medicine Beyond the Evidence Base*,
https://doi.org/10.1007/978-981-96-7234-9_29

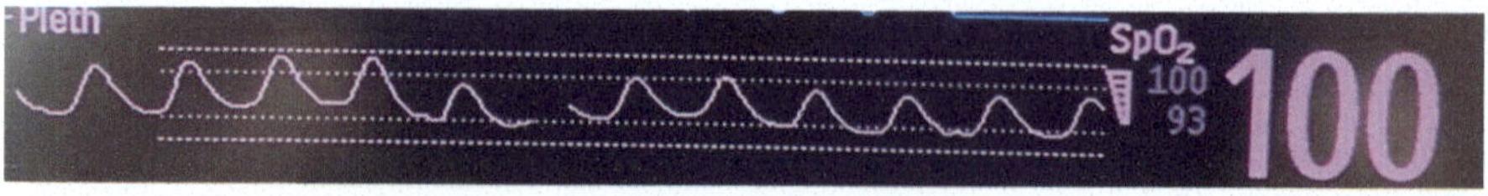

Or

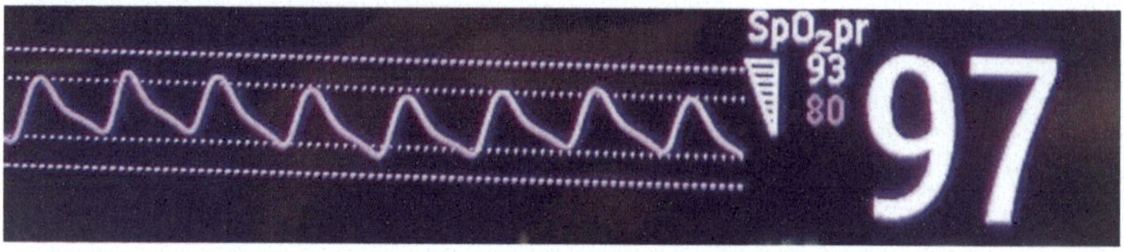

Fig. 1 Examples of pulsus paradoxus

Table 1 Summary of venous blood gas results

Investigation	Result	Reference range and units (Royal Children's Hospital, Melbourne)
pH	7.35	7.35–7.45
pO2	50	30–55 mmHg
pCO2	36	35–50 mmHg
Bicarbonate	**18***	22–28 mmol/l
Sodium	145 mmol/l	135–145 mmol/l
Potassium	**2.8*** mmol/l	3.3–5.1 mmol/l
Chloride	**110*** mmol/l	99–107 mmol/l
Glucose	**12*** mmol/l	3.6–5.4 mmol/l
Lactate	**6*** mmol/l	0.5–2.2 mmol/l

The blood gas result shows many features (marked with an *) consistent with salbutamol toxicity. A patient with worsening asthma or fatigue is unlikely to have a normal CO2—indeed the venous CO2 would be expected to be very high (> 60 mmHg).

3 Discussion

Management of the acutely unwell child with breathing difficulty is common, often stressful and the fear of failing to provide adequate therapy is ever present. The response to therapy in asthma is often non-linear, the bedside assessment tests limited, and deterioration can be difficult to identify. Initial treatment for *severe* asthma is multiple puffs (4, 6 or 10) of 100 mcg salbutamol via a spacer, with or without ipratropium bromide (4 puffs) every 20 min for 3 doses [1–3]. Corticosteroids are given as soon as possible, i.e. oral prednisolone 1 mg/kg before or intravenous methylprednisolone 1 mg/kg after intravenous access is obtained. Frequent review is recommended with escalation to second line intravenous agents such as magnesium sulphate (0.2 mmol/kg over 20 mins) or aminophylline (10 mg/kg over 30–60 mins) with continuous electrocardiographic monitoring [1–3].

Wheeze will often respond rapidly to bronchodilator therapy and even disappear in mild exacerbations of asthma, but may take considerable time if more severe, especially with a large inflammatory contribution. Time is required for steroids to enhance salbutamol response and reduce the inflammatory (secretory) component. The presence of *wheeze* (and the associated effort of breathing) or even *desaturation* (from salbutamol worsening "shunting" via an effect on mismatch) will often lead to further doses of salbutamol, even if the smooth muscle component of the acute episode has been optimally treated.

An augmentation of beta 2 responsivity will occur immediately as steroids increase stored beta 2 receptor expression on smooth muscle, augment further production of these receptors and enhance the subcellular response over the next few hours to days [3].

Salbutamol will also enhance the metabolic production of lactate within skeletal muscle (especially in the presence of corticosteroids) and this metabolite requires transfer to the liver for conversion back to glucose [4].

Lactate (or rather its associated H+ ion) generates a metabolic acidosis that stimulates respiration, both depth and rate. This will often make the child with asthma work harder for any given level of airway obstruction. The major problem is that this "worsening" often encourages more salbutamol to be given as "the child looks worse", is "working harder" or even "getting tired." Smaller children receiving salbutamol via nebuliser are often at risk, as they have a smaller minute ventilation to nebuliser flow rate [5, 6]. This means they will receive even more salbutamol with each breath as they improve. This is *even worse* if they now receive intravenous salbutamol [6].

It is not easy to identify, from the end of the bed, the child who is worsening from refractory asthma and fatigue versus the child with salbutamol toxicity. Salbutamol toxicity is often associated with tremulousness, agitation, tachycardia, tachypnoea, hyperpnoea and an increased effort of breathing—these are also the features of asthma, hypoxia and hypercapnia. The pulse oximeter may have a variation in the width of the waveform and its baseline—this is equivalent to "pulsus paradoxus" and indicates significant changes in intrathoracic pressure—from the increased effort of breathing (Fig. 1) [7].

A venous blood gas (VBG) can be very useful in this setting. A metabolic acidosis (rather than respiratory), as evidenced by a normal or low pCO2 on a VBG, essentially rules out 'worsening asthma.' An arterial pCO2 taken concurrently would invariably be lower than the venous PCO2. Elevations of lactate are expected with salbutamol toxicity, and hyperglycaemia and hypokalaemia often coexist. Beta 2 stimulation augments glycogenolysis, leading to increased blood glucose [4, 5]. The subsequent insulin release and direct beta 2 stimulation of Na/K ATPase induces the intracellular shift of K+ from the extracellular space [5].

Often the use of magnesium and/or aminophylline, high flow or even inhaled oxygen alone enables a reduction in salbutamol dosing and a clinical improvement [1–3]. This is often easiest to do in an intensive care environment where more nursing and medical staff are available to provide continuous observation and reassessment, especially during reduced salbutamol treatment [8, 9].

4 Other Gems

- Salbutamol toxicity is now the most common cause of admission to PICU with asthma.
- Salbutamol toxicity and worsening asthma are almost (but not completely) indistinguishable.
- A venous (or arterial) blood gas can often help to identify lactic acidosis and hypokalaemia—both indicative of significant salbutamol exposure.
- The presence of a low pCO2 on a venous gas is diagnostic of hyperventilation—which can only be due to salbutamol excess (or anxiety).

References

1. Victor, C., & Powell, E. (2023). Acute asthma. In P. Cameron, G. J. Browne, B. Mitra, S. Dalziel, & S. Craig (Eds.), *Textbook of paediatric emergency medicine-e-book* (pp. 165–170). Elsevier Health Sciences.
2. Royal Children's Hospital. (2023). *Clinical practice guidelines*. Acute asthma. https://www.rch.org.au/clinicalguide/guideline_index/Acute_asthma/. Accessed 17 Jun 2025.
3. National Asthma Council. (2022). *Australian asthma handbook*. Version 2.2. Edition 13. https://www.asthmahandbook.org.au/acute-asthma/clinical. Accessed 17 Jun 2025.
4. Meert, K., & L; McCaulley, LaTasha; Sarnaik, Ashok P. (2012). Mechanism of lactic acidosis in children with acute severe asthma. *Pediatric Critical Care Medicine, 13*, 28–31.
5. Andrzejowski, P., & Carroll, W. (2016). Salbutamol in paediatrics: pharmacology, prescribing and controversies. *Archives of Disease in Childhood – Education and Practice, 101*, 194–197.
6. Starkey, E. S., Mulla, H., Sammons, H. M., & Pandya, H. C. (2014). Intravenous salbutamol for childhood asthma: Evidence-based medicine? *Archives of Disease in Childhood, 99*, 873–877.
7. Krishnan, S. G., Wong, H. C., Ganapathy, S., & Ong, G. Y. (2020). Oximetry-detected pulsus paradoxus predicts for severity in paediatric asthma. *Archives of Disease in Childhood, 105*, 533–538.
8. Pilar, J., Modesto I Alapont, V., Lopez-Fernandez, Y. M., Lopez-Macias, O., Garcia-Urabayen, D., & Amores-Hernandez, I. (2017). High-flow nasal cannula therapy versus non-invasive ventilation in children with severe acute asthma exacerbation: An observational cohort study. *Medicina Intensiva, 41*, 418–424.
9. Ozer, M., Buyuktiryaki, B., Sahiner, U. M., Teksam, O., Karaatmaca, B., Soyer, O., & Sekerel, B. E. (2018). Repeated doses of salbutamol and aeroallergen sensitisation both increased salbutamol-induced hypoxia in children and adolescents with acute asthma. *Acta Paediatrica, 107*, 647–652.

Children Don't Read Textbooks

Mark Norden

1 Clinical Pearl

Gastroenteritis is a diagnosis of exclusion.

2 Clinical Case

A previously healthy 4-year-old girl, Yumi, presented with a 4-day history of vomiting, diarrhoea, and decreased appetite. Vomiting occurred intermittently, mainly after meals. She had 4–5 loose, watery bowel movements daily, without blood or mucus. Yumi's abdominal pain was sporadic and moved between the left lower abdomen, suprapubic area, and right lower abdomen/flank. She had no current respiratory or urinary symptoms but had recently recovered from a viral respiratory illness 2 weeks ago.

On presentation, Yumi was mildly febrile (37.5 °C). Her other vital signs were within normal range. She appeared well hydrated and comfortable, even cheerful. Examination revealed a soft abdomen with mild suprapubic tenderness and mild right sided abdominal/flank tenderness. Urinalysis demonstrated a trace of both nitrites and blood and significant ketones. Her BSL was 6.2.

A provisional diagnosis of gastroenteritis was made, and Yumi was commenced on nasogastric rehydration. Due to mild right-sided abdominal signs, a surgical opinion was sought before admission to the paediatric ward. On surgical review Yumi was afebrile, appeared pain-free and was asking for food. She had mild right sided abdominal tenderness without evidence of peritonitis. Yumi could walk,

M. Norden (✉)
Faculty Medicine and Health, University of New South Wales, Sydney, NSW, Australia

C. F. Lynch et al. (eds.), *The Art of Paediatric Medicine Beyond the Evidence Base*,
https://doi.org/10.1007/978-981-96-7234-9_30

perform sit ups and jump. Intravenous Augmentin was commenced for possible urosepsis.

Blood tests were taken, and an abdominal ultrasound was booked for the next morning. The following day her pain had resolved, and she had remained afebrile with normal vital signs. Urine culture was pending.

Investigations were as follows (Table 1).

Yumi continued to improve, and 24 h post presentation was afebrile, able to mobilise without discomfort and complained of being hungry.

However, her abdominal ultrasound at this time demonstrated acute appendicitis with a 40 × 20 × 25 mm peri-appendicular collection. She underwent surgery, during which she was found to have a "gangrenous appendix with an abscess walled off by omentum".

Over the next 4 days Yumi required IV fluids, antibiotics, antipyretics and targeted opiate analgesia. She was discharged home and was expected to make a full recovery.

3 Discussion

Overall, 1–8% of children presenting with abdominal pain have acute appendicitis. Less than 10% of these are pre-school children [1]. Acute appendicitis is very rare in infants <12 months. It may be rare, have an atypical presentation with very high rates of perforation, but it does occur [2].

Toddlers less than 3 years of age present with vomiting (85–90%), pain (35–81%), fever (40–60%) and diarrhoea (18–46%). The mean time interval between onset and diagnosis is 3–4 days, by which time perforation (82–92%) has likely occurred [3, 4].

In preschoolers (3–5 years) abdominal pain is the most frequent symptom (89–100%), followed by vomiting (66–100%) [1]. Perforation occurs in 43–72% of children in this age group. The younger the child, the more challenging it may be to diagnose.

The appendicular tip may be in a retrocaecal or pelvic position. *If retrocaecal,* flank or back pain is more common than anterior abdominal pain and tenderness. *If pelvic,* abdominal signs may be absent and urinary symptoms can predominate. Luminal obstruction is usually present and, the younger the child, is more likely due to lymphoid hyperplasia than a faecolith. Lymphoid hyperplasia is associated with gastroenteritis, respiratory infections and infectious mononucleosis [5].

Misdiagnosis rates are high in younger children, so the clinician must maintain a high index of suspicion [6]. Pre-school children often present late with complications including perforation, abscess formation, peritonitis, and sepsis. Peritonitis is more common than abscess formation due to the underdeveloped omentum in the younger child.

Table 1 Serial blood tests at presentation, 24 and 72 h

	White cell count (normal range 11.0–14.0)	Neutrophils (normal range 1.5–7.5)	CRP (normal range 0–10)	Lactate (normal range < 2.2)	Sodium (normal range 133–144)	Chloride (normal range 97–110)	Bicarbonate (normal range 18–30)
At presentation	13.2	**10.8**	**249**	1.1	**129**	**95**	**16**
24 h later	12.0	**9.8**	**147**	–	139	106	22
72 h later	**10.1**	6.9	**206**	–	140	103	25

High rates of **misdiagnosis** and **perforation** in younger children occur because their symptoms are **non-specific**. They often have difficulty communicating their discomfort, making abdominal examinations challenging. Symptoms overlap with those of common childhood illnesses such as:

- gastroenteritis
- intussusception
- urinary tract infections
- respiratory infections
- blunt abdominal trauma
- diabetic ketoacidosis
- obstructed hernia
- testicular torsion
- septic arthritis of the right hip
- toxic shock syndrome
- sepsis
- meningitis

In the presence of equivocal signs and history, it is prudent to admit children under 5 years of age for close observation and serial physical examination. Maintain a high level of suspicion for acute appendicitis.

On initial assessment this girl was suspected to have gastroenteritis or possible early urosepsis. The presence of mild right-sided tenderness led to the decision to perform an abdominal ultrasound. The markedly elevated CRP suggested significant inflammation.

So why did she clinically improve with a perforated appendix?

After the appendix ruptures, pain may temporarily subside, and signs of peritonitis will depend on the location of the appendix and the body's ability to contain the infection. Unusually, despite her age, she had contained any peritoneal infection within her omentum.

Gastroenteritis is usually a clinical diagnosis. It should, therefore, always be considered a diagnosis of exclusion. When faced with a child presenting with typical features of gastroenteritis, ask yourself "what else could it be?" ....and remember ***children don't read textbooks.***

References

1. Rothrock, S. G., & Pagane, J. (2000). Acute appendicitis in children: Emergency department diagnosis and management. *Annals of Emergency Medicine, 36*, 39–51.
2. Turco, R., Mauro, A., Quitadamo, P., Gaglione, G., Esposito, F., Di Nardo, G., & Tipo, V. (2023). Acute appendicitis in infants. *Journal of Pediatric Surgery Case Reports, 88*, 102508.
3. Bagłaj, M., Rysiakiewicz, J., & Rysiakiewicz, K. (2011). Acute appendicitis in children under3 years of age. Diagnostic and therapeutic problems. *Medycyna Wieku Rozwojowego, 16*, 154–161.

4. Alloo, J., Gerstle, T., Shilyansky, J., & Ein, S. H. (2004). Appendicitis in children less than 3 years of age: A 28-year review. *Pediatric Surgery International, 19*, 777–779.
5. Almaramhy, H. (2017). Acute appendicitis in young children less than 5 years of age: Review article. *Italian Journal of Paediatrics., 43*, 15.
6. Chang, Y. J., Chao, H. C., Kong, M. S., Hsia, S. H., & Yan, D. C. (2010). Misdiagnosed acute appendicitis in children in the emergency department. *Chang Gung Medical Journal, 33*, 551–557.

Part II
Children (5–12 Years)

A Masquerader of an Acute Surgical Abdomen

Sathyakala Vijayanand

1 Clinical Pearl

Diabetic ketoacidosis (DKA) is an acute medical emergency which can mimic a surgical abdomen with severe abdominal pain.

2 Clinical Case

A 5-year-old boy, Michael, presents to emergency with a 2-day history of abdominal pain and non-bilious vomiting. Initially, he was managed at home as a case of gastroenteritis. On examination, he has normal vital signs and diffuse tenderness over the lower quadrants of his abdomen with sluggish bowel sounds. He has no peritonism. Michael is referred for a surgical consult.

A venous blood gas (VBG) demonstrates the following:

pH **7.1** (7.3–7.4)
HCO_3 **7** (22–32) mmol/L
Na **127** (135–145) mmol/L
K+ 3.5 (3.3–4.9) mmol/L
Glucose **30** (3.0–7.7) mmol/L

A Point of care (POC) blood ketone (β-hydroxy butyrate) level is elevated at **5.0** mmol/L (N < 0.6 mmol/L). Michael is diagnosed with moderate DKA likely due to first presentation of type 1 diabetes mellitus (T1 DM) and is started on an intravenous insulin infusion and intravenous fluids. As the acidosis and ketones resolve,

S. Vijayanand (✉)
Bendigo Health, Monash Children's Hospital, Clayton, VIC, Australia

C. F. Lynch et al. (eds.), *The Art of Paediatric Medicine Beyond the Evidence Base*,
https://doi.org/10.1007/978-981-96-7234-9_31

Michael's abdominal pain also improves. Over the next 24 hours, the abdominal pain completely resolves, and Michael is switched to subcutaneous insulin injections.

3 Discussion

DKA is an acute medical emergency with metabolic decompensation (blood glucose >11 mmol/L, venous pH <7.3 or bicarbonate <18 mmol/L and β-hydroxy butyrate ≥3 mmol/L) [1]. The severity of DKA is related to the acidosis and graded as:

(a) mild (pH < 7.3 or serum bicarbonate <18 mmol/L).
(b) moderate (pH < 7.2 or serum bicarbonate <10 mmol/L).
(c) severe (pH < 7.1 or serum bicarbonate <5 mmol/L).

It is often preceded by osmotic symptoms (polyuria and polydipsia) and weight loss in children with a new diagnosis of T1 DM. In a patient with known T1 DM, DKA is precipitated by either non-adherence to the insulin regimen or intercurrent illness.

Abdominal pain mimicking an acute abdomen is a common symptom in DKA, usually associated with nausea and vomiting. It is however prudent to rule out an intra-abdominal cause such as appendicitis or pancreatitis as the cause for the abdominal pain. The underlying mechanism for abdominal pain in DKA is not well understood, however is likely multifactorial and includes metabolic, neural and humoral processes. Hyperglycaemia and ketone bodies cause decreased gastrointestinal motility, gastroparesis and impaired gallbladder contractility. Other reported factors for abdominal pain are rapid expansion of the hepatic capsule due to fatty liver and bowel ischaemia due to volume depletion and metabolic acidosis [2, 3].

There is a paucity of data describing the prevalence of abdominal pain in children presenting with DKA. The abdominal pain and guarding may be striking but is usually generalised rather than localised. Other clinical features potentially assisting in differentiating abdominal pain in DKA from an acute surgical abdomen include:

(a) osmotic symptoms such as polyuria and polydipsia. These symptoms precede the abdominal pain and may be misinterpreted as urinary frequency.
(b) deep (as opposed to shallow), rapid respiration.
(c) severe dehydration.
(d) pain improving as the ketoacidosis improves [4].

4 Other Gems

- Starvation ketosis is a physiological response to carbohydrate unavailability and as opposed to DKA, glucose levels are not elevated.
- In rural and remote centres, urinary ketones can be measured when blood ketones are not available.

References

1. Glaser, N., Fritsch, M., Priyambada, L., Rewers, A., Cherubini, V., Estrada, S., Wolfsdorf, J. I., & Codner, E. (2022). ISPAD clinical practice consensus guidelines 2022: Diabetic ketoacidosis and hyperglycemic hyperosmolar state. *Pediatric Diabetes, 23*(7), 835–856. https://doi.org/10.1111/pedi.13406. PMID: 36250645.
2. Qian, X., et al. (2021). A case of persistent severe abdominal pain caused by type 1 diabetic ketoacidosis. *Journal of Clinical and Translational Endocrinology: Case Reports, 19*, 100077.
3. Tavares Bello, C., et al. (2018). Abdominal pain in diabetic ketoacidosis: Beyond the obvious. *Journal of Endocrinology and Metabolism, North America, 8*(2–3), 43–46.
4. Valerio, D. (1976). Acute diabetic abdomen in childhood. *The Lancet, 307*(7950), 66–68.

Manage the Patient, Not the Numbers

Paul Monagle

1 Clinical Pearl

Children frequently have blood tests for minor/unclear reasons. Numerical "abnormalities" may be found, however these can be safely ignored if the child is clinically well.

2 Clinical Case

Jarod is a 5-year-old well boy with no significant past history or family history from a stable socioeconomic background, who was taken to his General Practitioner (GP) for a routine check and had some blood tests done. The full blood examination (FBE) showed a normal haemoglobin and total white cell count, with a platelet count of **500** $\times 10^9$/L (reference range 150–400 $\times 10^9$/L) and a neutrophil count of 1.4 $\times 10^9$/L (reference range 1.5–8.5 $\times 10^9$/L). His mother was concerned about these abnormal results, and as a result, a follow up FBE was performed 1 week later which showed similar findings. Despite Jarod remaining well, he underwent weekly FBE blood tests for the next month and was eventually referred to a paediatrician for further investigation. He was seen by a paediatrician 6 months later having remained clinically well, and a repeat FBE at that time was completely normal. The family were reassured and discharged from paediatric care.

P. Monagle (✉)
Department of Paediatrics, University of Melbourne, Parkville, VIC, Australia

Clinical Haematology, Royal Children's Hospital, Parkville, VIC, Australia

Haematology Research, Murdoch Children's Research Institute, Parkville, VIC, Australia

C. F. Lynch et al. (eds.), *The Art of Paediatric Medicine Beyond the Evidence Base*,
https://doi.org/10.1007/978-981-96-7234-9_32

3 Discussion

Clinically well children, with normal growth and development, do not need "routine" blood tests and bloods should only be taken for a specific indication. These include:

(a) Clinical signs or symptoms.
(b) Follow up of a previous diagnosis.
(c) A specific family history that is important to detect during childhood.
(d) Screening for specific at-risk populations such as migrant/refugee health assessments.

Invariably "routine" blood tests without a clear indication will have at least one parameter "abnormal" (outside of the reference range), and this often causes anxiety and further unnecessary investigations.

Important facts to remember include:

1. Most reference ranges represent 95% of the population, which means by definition 2.5% of tests will be lower and 2.5% higher than the limits of the range and yet be physiologically normal for that child (Fig. 1).
2. There is a significant difference between being "outside of the reference range" and being pathological. This varies per parameter tested, and clinicians need to understand the tests they order and the clinical significance of the findings. For example, slightly elevated platelet counts (greater than 400 but $<550 \times 10^9$/L) are common in children secondary to transient infection or inflammation and rarely need follow up tests if the child remains clinically well or there is no significant family history [1]. If the child has persistent fever, lymphadenopathy or rashes then earlier follow up may be required.

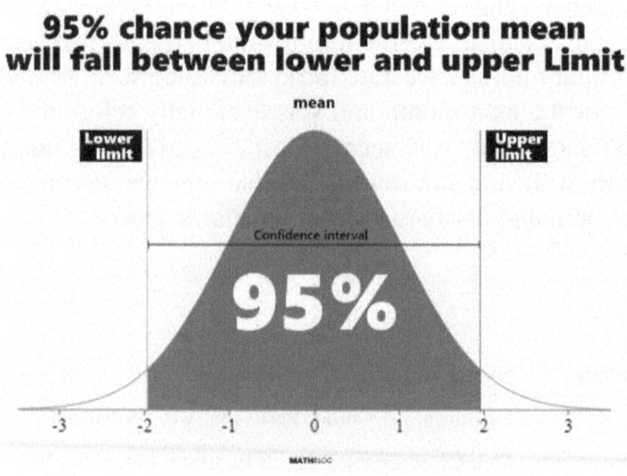

Fig. 1 Graphical representation of a "normal" reference range

3. Children frequently develop mild abnormalities of the FBE secondary to viral infections. Mild abnormalities in children are also common due to sampling errors as blood drawing can be difficult. In clinically well children, repeat testing if required (pending parameter and degree of abnormality) can be delayed 4–6 weeks or even longer to allow abnormalities to normalise [2]. Early retesting frequently increases anxiety and increases trauma for the child. For example, mild neutropenia is frequent in children. While it *may* be an early sign of leukaemia, such children are unwell (recurrent viral symptoms, lethargy, bone pain, pallor, bruising) and if the child is unwell then an early repeat test is justified. However, a neutrophil count of >1.0 is never clinically problematic (that is, it does not increase infection risk). As a result, if the child is clinically well, waiting 4–6 weeks to allow recovery and normalisation is much more useful. Failure to recover in that timeframe may then warrant further follow up.

4 Other Gems

- For most parameters, the reference range changes with age (and may be analyser and reagent specific), and clinicians must check the result is being reported with an age-specific range. There may also be ethnic differences, for example benign ethnic neutropenia.

References

1. Stockklausner, C., Duffert, C. M., Cario, H., Knöfler, R., Streif, W., & Kulozik, A. E. (2021). THROM KID-Plus Studiengruppe der Gesellschaft für Thrombose- und Hämostaseforschung (GTH) and of Gesellschaft für Pädiatrische Onkologie und Hämatologie (GPOH). Thrombocytosis in children and adolescents-classification, diagnostic approach, and clinical management. *Annals of Hematology, 100*(7), 1647–1665. https://doi.org/10.1007/s00277-021-04485-0. Epub 2021 Mar 12. PMID: 33712866; PMCID: PMC8195939.
2. Katsaras, G., Koutsi, S., Psaroulaki, E., Gouni, D., & Tsitsani, P. (2024). Neutropenia in childhood – A narrative review and practical diagnostic approach. *Hematology Reports, 16*(2), 375–389. https://doi.org/10.3390/hematolrep16020038. PMID: 38921186; PMCID: PMC11203312.

A Pinch of Salt

Nina Dhaliwal and Dushan Jayaweera

1 Clinical Pearl

Maintain a high index of suspicion for poisoning in children with unexplained clinical features or pathology.

2 Clinical Case

A 5-year-old girl, Isabella, was brought in by ambulance to a tertiary paediatric emergency department (ED) with an altered conscious state. Isabella was floppy and unresponsive. On initial assessment in ED, her airway was patent, her respiratory rate was **32/min** (normal range for age: 20–30/min) with SpO2 100% on room air, and a clear chest on auscultation. Assessment of circulation revealed a heart rate of **70 beats/min** (normal range for age: 80–120 beats/min), and blood pressure of **130/60 mmHg** (normal systolic blood pressure range for age: 90–110 mmHg). Isabella appeared profoundly dehydrated and mottled. She was unresponsive with a Glasgow Coma Scale (GCS) of **8** and had global hyperreflexia and clonus. A blood sugar level was 6.6 mmol/L, and temperature of 36 degrees Celsius. Electrocardiogram demonstrated sinus rhythm.

N. Dhaliwal (✉)
Emergency Department and Toxicology Department, Nepean Hospital, Kingswood, NSW, Australia

Poisons Information Centre, Melbourne, VIC, Australia

D. Jayaweera
Blacktown and Westmead Hospital Emergency Department, Western Sydney LDH Toxicology Unit, NSW Poison Information Center, South Wales, Australia

C. F. Lynch et al. (eds.), *The Art of Paediatric Medicine Beyond the Evidence Base*,
https://doi.org/10.1007/978-981-96-7234-9_33

Isabella was accompanied by her mother who stated that her daughter had been unwell for 7–10 days. She had reduced oral intake for 7 days and had been less active than usual. In the preceding 48 hours, she had no urine output with multiple episodes of vomiting. Isabella had been taken to her general practitioner the day prior and was found to be febrile with a temperature of 38 degrees Celsius with no focal infective symptoms. In the last 24 hours, there had been a significant deterioration in her conscious state and Isabella was unable to ambulate and had become unresponsive.

Isabella's past medical history is significant for severe global developmental delay and she is non-verbal. She is usually able to mobilise independently. She has a short stature with failure to thrive. Isabella is not taking any regular medications.

An emergency physician's examination concluded that Isabella was hypertensive, bradycardic, with severe dehydration. She was afebrile. Neurological assessment demonstrated no lateralising signs and normal pupils. Isabella had no obvious meningism and had no evidence of head injury on external examination. There were tremors, global hypertonia and hyperreflexia with bilateral clonus.

Isabella received up to 30 mL/kg of 0.9% sodium chloride boluses, as well as broad spectrum intravenous antibiotics and antivirals to treat potential central nervous system infections or sepsis. Isabella appeared slightly more alert after initial treatment.

An initial venous blood gas was as below. Concerningly, it revealed severe hypernatraemia.

pH (7.35–7.45)	**7.32**
Na (133–143 mmol/L)	**198**
K (3.5–5.5 mmol/L)	**2.1**
Cl (96–109 mmol/L)	**171**
Bicarb (22–26 mmol/L)	**16**
Urea (2.5–6.5 mmol/L)	**8.5**
Creatinine (25–60 umol/L)	49
Lactate (0.5–2.2 mmol/L)	0.9

Computed tomography of her brain showed no intracranial abnormality nor oedema. She had a normal white cell count and inflammatory markers.

Further history revealed that Isabella had been consuming cooking salt and cooking products with a high sodium content, such as soy and oyster sauces regularly.

A final diagnosis of severe hypernatremia secondary to exogenous salt intake and severe dehydration from reduced intake of water was made.

The trend of investigations are listed in Table 1.

Isabella subsequently developed seizures on day 1 and 2 of admission and was treated with midazolam and levetiracetam. Management was challenging with initial rapid correction of her serum sodium level. The trend of her serum sodium is shown in Fig. 1.

Table 1 Isabella's blood tests over the first 5 days of admission

	Admission	24 h	48 h	5 days
Na (133–143 mmol/L)	**198**	**147**	**146**	142
K (3.5–5.5 mmol/L)	**2.1**	3.5	3.6	3.8
Cl (96–109 mmol/L)	**168**	**139**	**124**	107
pH (7.35–7.45)	**7.32**	7.38	7.44	
Urea (2.5–6.5 mmol/L)	**8.5**	5.3	4.4	3.6
Creatinine (25–60 umol/L)	49	48	45	38
Urine osmolality (50–1400 mmol/L)	888	447		
Urine sodium	494	487	440	
Serum osmolality (272–295 mmol/L)	**301**			

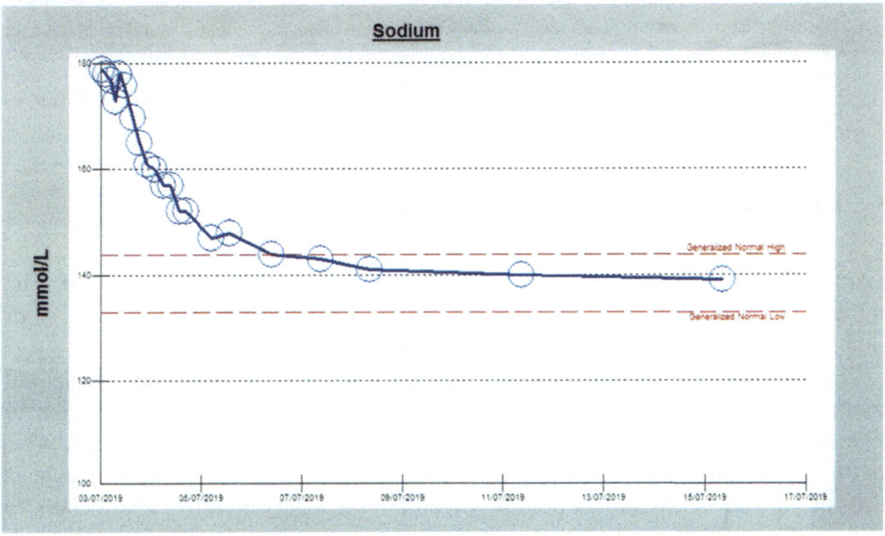

Fig. 1 Trend in serum sodium over 2 weeks

Magnetic resonance imaging (MRI) of brain performed on day 5 of admission revealed supratentorial extrapontine myelinolysis due to severe hypernatremia, characterised by diffusion restriction in certain areas of the brain (Fig. 2).

Isabella made a slow recovery in the paediatric intensive care unit. She completed a 3-week inpatient stay and was discharged to the rehabilitation ward. The child protection unit was involved given suspected neglect.

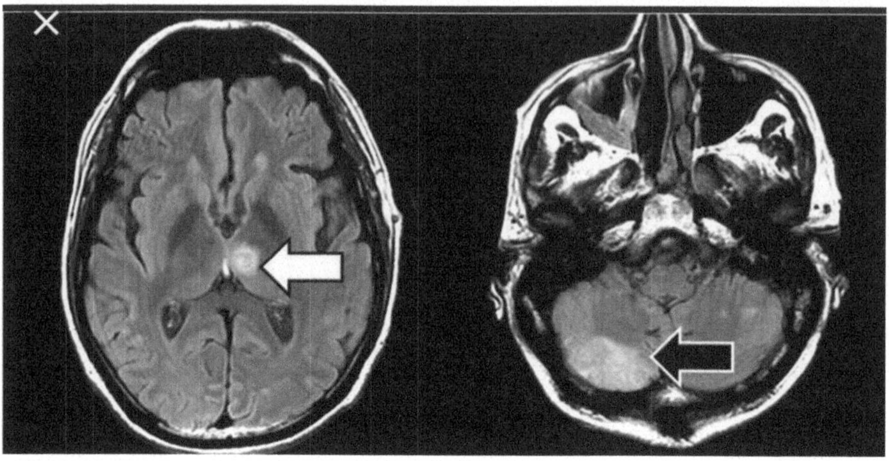

Fig. 2 MRI brain demonstrating right cerebellar (black arrow) and left subcortical (white arrow) areas of myelinolysis

3 Discussion

Extreme hypernatraemia (Na >190 mmol/L) in children is rarely described. The highest ever reported serum sodium concentration was 255 mmol/L, in a case of fatal salt poisoning in an otherwise well 20-year-old [1].

Demyelinating syndromes are a rare complication of hypernatremia [2]. Central pontine myelinolysis can also occur as a complication of rapid overcorrection of severe and prolonged hyponatraemia [3]. It is characterised by concentrated, symmetrical, non-inflammatory demyelination within the central basis pontis. In at least 10% of patients with central pontine myelinolysis, demyelination also occurs in extrapontine regions, including the midbrain, thalamus, basal nuclei, and cerebellum [3]. An MRI is the imaging modality of choice. Characteristically, T2 weighted MRI images demonstrate hyperintense or bright areas where demyelination has occurred and has been caused by relatively increased water content in these regions [3]. This was evident on this patient's MRI images as shown above.

Severe hypernatremia is defined as a serum sodium level >170 mmol/L. It can cause acute brain shrinkage with risk of rupture of blood vessels, haemorrhage, demyelination and permanent neurological injury [4]. In patients with demyelination, death is common with maximal recovery taking several months. Most patients require a prolonged period of rehabilitation [3], as this patient did.

Management of hypernatremia is challenging with risk of rapid correction and its complications [5]. Hypernatremia is a life-threatening medical emergency warranting expert management to prevent complications of hypernatremia and its rapid correction [6]. Guidelines recommend commencing intravenous treatment early with IV sodium chloride 0.9% + glucose 5% to aim for a rate of correction of less than 0.5 mmol/L/hour, and 10–12 mmol/L per day to prevent cerebral oedema [4].

However, there is a paucity of evidence for management of extreme hypernatremia with severe neurological symptoms such as this patient.

It is important to maintain a high index of suspicion of poisoning in children, particularly in those with unexplained clinical features. Children are curious and often have access to household poisons and medications at home. A 10-year retrospective analysis of children hospitalised with poisoning in Australia demonstrated that over 70% of cases were due to pharmaceuticals, particularly simple analgesics found in most homes [7]. Severe outcomes, such as those associated with this case, were rare [7]. Children with developmental delay are at increased risk of poisoning, and a history of poisoning may not be immediately evident. It is therefore important to explore the social circumstances and be mindful of the possibility of intentional or accidental poisoning resulting in the clinical presentation.

References

1. Ofran, Y., et al. (2004). Fatal voluntary salt intake resulting in the highest ever documented sodium plasma level in adults (255 mmol L−1): A disorder linked to female gender and psychiatric disorders. *Journal of Internal Medicine, 256*(6), 525–528. https://doi.org/10.1111/j.1365-2796.2004.01411.x
2. Varanda, S., et al. (2016). Central pontine myelinolysis caused by hypernatremia. *Journal of the Neurological Sciences, 370*, 274–276. https://doi.org/10.1016/j.jns.2016.10.001
3. Central pontine myelinolysis: Overview, pathophysiology, causes (2022) *eMedicine* [Preprint]. Available at: https://emedicine.medscape.com/article/1174329-overview?form=fpf#a3
4. The Royal Children's Hospital Melbourne. (2012). *Clinical Practice Guidelines: Hypernatraemia*. [online] Rch.org.au. Available at: https://www.rch.org.au/clinicalguide/guideline_index/hypernatraemia/
5. Arambewela, M. H., Somasundaram, N. P., & Garusinghe, C. (2016). Extreme hypernatremia as a probable cause of fatal arrhythmia: A case report. *Journal of Medical Case Reports, 10*(1). https://doi.org/10.1186/s13256-016-1062-9
6. Casavant, M. J., & Fitch, J. A. (2003). Fatal hypernatremia from saltwater used as an emetic. *Journal of Toxicology: Clinical Toxicology, 41*(6), 861–863. https://doi.org/10.1081/clt-120025352
7. Arbaeen, A., Noghrehchi, F., Wheate, N. J., & Cairns, R. (2023). Hospitalised poisonings in Australian children: A 10-year retrospective study. *Clinical Toxicology (Philadelphia, Pa.), 61*(3), 153–161. https://doi.org/10.1080/15563650.2022.2147538. [online].

Too Hot to Play: Heat Stroke in Children

Nathan Forsyth and Tom Solan

1 Clinical Pearl

Immediate cooling is crucial in paediatric heat stroke to prevent irreversible systemic damage.

2 Clinical Case

Ben, a 5-year-old boy, was brought to the emergency department on a scorching summer afternoon after collapsing at an outdoor family gathering. His parents reported he had been playing in direct sunlight for over 4 h with minimal water intake. Initially energetic, Ben grew lethargic, disoriented, and then suddenly fainted. On arrival, his core temperature measured 40.5 °C, his skin was dry and flushed, and he was minimally responsive. Recognising these as classic signs of severe heat stroke, emergency cooling and hydration measures were immediately initiated to stabilise his condition and prevent further deterioration.

3 Discussion

Heat stroke is a severe form of heat-related illness (HRI) that develops when the body's thermoregulatory mechanisms fail, leading to a dangerous rise in core temperature. Paediatric patients like Ben are especially vulnerable due to their higher surface area-to-mass ratio and immature thermoregulatory systems, which result in

N. Forsyth · T. Solan (✉)
Emergency Department, The Royal Chidren's Hospital, Melbourne, VIC, Australia

C. F. Lynch et al. (eds.), *The Art of Paediatric Medicine Beyond the Evidence Base*,
https://doi.org/10.1007/978-981-96-7234-9_34

faster heat absorption and less efficient cooling. Ben's prolonged exposure to sunlight with minimal hydration created ideal conditions for heat stroke—a stark reminder of how quickly this condition can develop in children under extreme heat.

Paediatric heat stroke is typically categorised into two types:

1. **Non-Exertional (Classic) Heat Stroke**: This type, which Ben exhibited, occurs due to passive environmental exposure and affects young children who cannot independently escape hot environments or manage their hydration. Hot, confined spaces or unshaded outdoor settings, as seen in Ben's case, are frequent culprits [1].
2. **Exertional Heat Stroke**: More common among older children and adolescents, exertional heat stroke occurs during vigorous physical activity, especially without adequate hydration. Although Ben's case was non-exertional, it underscores the similar risk factors associated with high temperatures and inadequate hydration [1, 2].

Ben's presentation was typical of severe paediatric heat stroke, with core temperature exceeding 40 °C, altered mental status, and an absence of sweating—all of which required urgent intervention. His case highlights the primary clinical features:

- **Hyperthermia**: Ben's high core temperature, if untreated, could rapidly progress to irreversible systemic and neurological damage [3].
- **Altered Mental Status**: Ben's increasing lethargy and confusion indicated neurological involvement from heat stress, which could have escalated to seizures or coma without intervention. This underscores the urgency of recognising mental status changes early in paediatric heat stroke [3].
- **Absence of Sweating**: Unlike in milder heat exhaustion cases, Ben's dry, flushed skin indicated a complete breakdown of thermoregulatory mechanisms—a critical sign differentiating heat stroke from less severe heat-related illnesses.

In emergency settings, rectal temperature measurement provides the most reliable core temperature assessment. Placing an indwelling urinary catheter (IDC) aids in accurately measuring fluid balance, which is critical for guiding hydration and preventing complications from fluid overload or dehydration. Additional blood tests, including electrolytes, offer essential insights for managing systemic effects and guiding further treatment [1].

Key abnormalities are summarised in Table 1.

Sodium (Na+)

Patients often present with hyponatremia ($Na+ < 135$ mmol/L), commonly due to dehydration or inappropriate fluid resuscitation. Severe hyponatremia can exacerbate neurological symptoms, including confusion and seizures, necessitating careful fluid management to avoid further sodium dilution.

Potassium (K+)

Hyperkalemia ($K+ > 5.5$ mmol/L) is a frequent finding, stemming from cellular breakdown and rhabdomyolysis associated with heatstroke. This is critical to monitor due to the risk of life-threatening arrhythmias. Conversely, hypokalemia

Table 1 Key blood test abnormalities in heat stroke; ++ often abnormal, + sometimes abnormal

Blood test	Low	High
Na+	++	
K+	+	++
Ca++	++	
PO4-		++
UEC		++
LFT		++
Lactate		++
CK		++
Coags		++

(K+ < 3.5 mmol/L) may also be seen if excessive losses occur due to sweating or gastrointestinal symptoms.

Calcium (Ca2+) and Phosphorus (PO4-)
Hypocalcemia (Ca2+ < 2.1 mmol/L) and hyperphosphatemia (PO4- > 1.5 mmol/L) are common in cases with rhabdomyolysis and renal dysfunction. Low calcium may worsen neuromuscular symptoms, including tetany or seizures.

Renal Function (Urea and Creatinine)
Dehydration and muscle breakdown can elevate urea (> 8 mmol/L) and creatinine (> 62 μmol/L), indicating renal impairment. These levels help monitor for acute kidney injury (AKI) and guide fluid resuscitation.

Liver Function Tests (LFTs)
Elevated levels of aspartate aminotransferase (AST) and alanine aminotransferase (ALT) often indicate hepatic stress or damage. Severe heat stroke can induce transaminitis, a marker of multiorgan dysfunction, with AST/ALT levels potentially exceeding 500 U/L.

Lactate
Elevated lactate levels (> 2 mmol/L) are indicative of anaerobic metabolism due to inadequate tissue perfusion. Persistent lactic acidosis may suggest impending organ failure and necessitates urgent intervention.

Creatine Kinase (CK)
Markedly high CK levels (> 1000 U/L) are common due to rhabdomyolysis, especially in exertional heatstroke. Elevated CK serves as an indicator of muscle injury and risk of renal complications, necessitating aggressive hydration.

Coagulation Profile
Coagulopathy can develop, evidenced by prolonged prothrombin time (PT) and activated partial thromboplastin time (aPTT), often due to systemic inflammatory response syndrome (SIRS). Monitoring coagulation is essential for detecting disseminated intravascular coagulation (DIC), a severe complication of heatstroke.

These findings underscore the need for close monitoring in paediatric heatstroke. Early identification of electrolyte and biochemical derangements facilitates targeted management, aiming to correct imbalances and prevent multiorgan failure.

Ben's care highlights several critical interventions:

1. **Cooling Techniques**: Emergency cooling was initiated by spraying Ben with cool water and using fans to increase evaporation, an effective approach for reducing core temperature. In severe cases, placing ice packs in the groin and armpits can help further reduce body heat. Full immersion in cool water, though effective, may be challenging in an emergency setting.
2. **Hydration and Electrolyte Management**: Given Ben's symptoms of dehydration, he received an intravenous bolus of isotonic crystalloid solution (10–20 mL/kg) to stabilise circulation and support organ function. This measure not only rehydrated Ben but also helped maintain his vital signs during the cooling process.
3. **Monitoring and Supportive Care**: Continuous cardiac monitoring was essential for Ben, as electrolyte imbalances can lead to arrhythmias in severe cases of heat stroke. Additionally, an indwelling urinary catheter was considered to monitor fluid balance accurately and assess kidney function, a critical aspect of supportive care in paediatric heat stroke.

Ben's cooling was carefully monitored, and once his core temperature reached approximately 38.5 °C, cooling measures were tapered to prevent rebound hypothermia. If shivering had occurred—a reflex that generates heat counterproductive to cooling—benzodiazepines could be administered to control it, ensuring cooling efforts remained effective.

4 Other Gems

- **Prevention is Key**: Parents should ensure their children remain hydrated by drinking water regularly and avoiding caffeinated or sugary drinks. Outdoor activities should be scheduled during cooler times of the day, while appropriate protective measures, such as lightweight, light-coloured clothing, hats, sunglasses, and sunscreen, should be used to minimise direct sun exposure. Parents should be reminded of the dangers of leaving children in parked cars or other confined spaces where temperatures can rise quickly to dangerous levels. Additionally, they should be able to recognise early symptoms of heat-related illness, such as fatigue, flushed skin, and irritability, and recognise when to promptly initiate cooling and hydration if these signs appear.
- **Children's Thermoregulation Differences**: Ben's case underscores how children's higher body surface area-to-mass ratio and increased metabolic heat production make them particularly susceptible to environmental temperature changes.

- **Need for Rapid Action**: Recognising early signs of heat-related illness, like Ben's lethargy and confusion, can prevent the rapid progression to full-blown heat stroke, underscoring the importance of swift and proactive intervention.
- **Importance of Temperature Monitoring**: In emergency settings, rectal temperature measurement is the most reliable method, especially in young children with suspected heat stroke.
- **Safe Cooling Practices**: Avoiding ice water immersion in children, due to rebound hypothermia risk, is essential. Controlled cooling techniques, paired with IV hydration, provide effective and safe temperature management.

References

1. Forsyth, N., & Solan, T. (2022). It's getting hot in here: Heat stroke in children and young people for paediatric clinicians. *Paediatrics and Child Health.* https://doi.org/10.1016/j.paed.2022.10.004
2. Public Health England. (2019). PHE heatwave mortality monitoring: summer 2018. Available from: https://assets.publishing.service.gov.uk/government/uploads/system/uploads/attachment_data/file/942648/PHE_heatwave_report_2018.pdf
3. Royal College of Emergency Medicine. (2021). Heat-related illness. Available from: https://www.rcemlearning.co.uk/reference/heat-related-illness

Beware the Child with Unequal Leg Length

Stewart Morrison

1 Clinical Pearl

A large apparent leg length difference in young children can represent late presentation hip dysplasia or dislocation, or neuromuscular conditions such as a hemiplegic cerebral palsy.

2 Clinical Case

Eliza, aged 5, always had a funny gait, but her parents attributed this to slowly developing coordination skills. The kindergarten teacher was more concerned, and after assessment Eliza was diagnosed by a physiotherapist as having a leg length difference. Her parents had a 3-centimetre shoe raise made for her, but the problems with her gait persisted, with her grandmother pointing out that she looked like she waddled.

Finally, after seeing their general practitioner, Eliza had a pelvic X-ray which demonstrated left hip dysplasia, with the left hip being completely dislocated (see Fig. 1). As her family had no risk factors, she had not had any ultrasound screening as a child. Notably, there was no family history of hip dysplasia, she was second born, was not breech, she was born at term and had no discernible foot or skin crease issues noted as a baby.

S. Morrison (✉)
The Royal Children's Hospital, Melbourne, VIC, Australia

Alfred Health, Melbourne, VIC, Australia

Epworth Healthcare, Richmond, VIC, Australia

C. F. Lynch et al. (eds.), *The Art of Paediatric Medicine Beyond the Evidence Base*,
https://doi.org/10.1007/978-981-96-7234-9_35

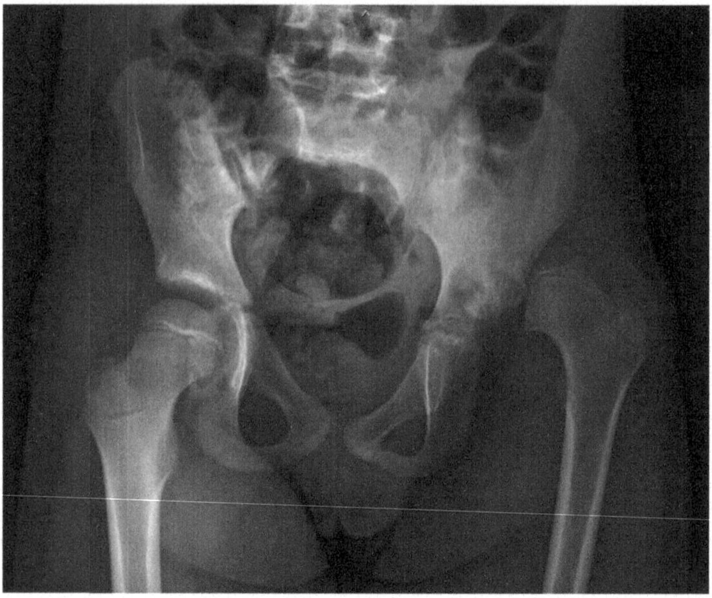

Fig. 1 Pelvic X-ray demonstrating left hip dysplasia and dislocation

Eliza was referred to an orthopaedic surgeon specialising in paediatric hip conditions and underwent reconstructive surgery to realign the hip joint. She returned to school and gymnastics but will require an operation to remove the plates and screws in about a year's time.

3 Discussion

Hip dysplasia has a baseline incidence of 11.5 per 1000 live births. Females make up about 80% of cases, and there is a strong correlation with family history, breech presentation, and some syndromic conditions.

Due to the fact that children with risk factors often undergo screening for hip dysplasia, a large portion of late presentation dysplasia is often in children with none of these risk factors [1]. Late presentation hip dysplasia is far more likely to require surgical management, when compared to cases identified at a younger age [2]. The main signs of a late presentation dislocation include an apparent leg length difference (as the dislocated hip has drifted proximally), restricted (asymmetrical) abduction range, and a Trendelenburg gait, which can be made more obvious by asking the child to hop. In children older than 6 months, the investigation of choice is a standing Pelvic X-ray.

Leg length assessment can be difficult in young children, because of the amount of adipose tissue present, preventing accurate assessment of bony landmarks, and posturing of the child in different positions which can make one leg appear longer than the other. Clinical assessment revealing a 5–10 mm difference can often be attributed to examiner error, but more significant differences in the order of 2 cm or more should be investigated. There are a broad range of differential diagnoses, ranging from the common to the exceedingly rare [3].

In neuromuscular conditions such as cerebral palsy, the child may also posture their leg during gait in a fashion that makes it appear to be shorter, because of knee flexion and/or ankle plantar flexion. Hence in any leg length examination, careful attention should be paid to joint range of motion. Decreased abduction of the hip could indicate hip pathology and signs of a neuromuscular condition include spasticity of the limb, contractures of the knee or ankle, or poor selective motor control.

4 Other Gems

- Standing X-rays are only helpful for assessing limb length if a child can stand with good posture and extended knees. In younger children, clinical assessment may be more accurate.

References

1. Talbot, C., Adam, J., & Paton, R. (2017). Late presentation of developmental dysplasia of the hip: A 15-year observational study. *Bone Joint J., 99*(9), 1250–1255.
2. Johnson, M. D., Kuschel, C., & Donnan, L. (2023). Neonatal clinical examination and selective ultrasound screening are not reliable for the early diagnosis of hip dysplasia: A retrospective cohort study. *Journal of Paediatrics and Child Health, 59*(10), 1146–1151.
3. Stricker, S., & Hunt, T. (2004). Evaluation of leg length discrepancy in children. *Int Pediatr., 19*, 134.

Beware the Child with a Swollen Joint

Jane Munro

1 Clinical Pearl

If a child's joint or joints are swollen, stiff and sore: do not ignore.

2 Clinical Case

A 5-year-old girl presents to her General Practitioner (GP) with 8 weeks of limping. She has had some increasing right lower leg pain, and her mother thinks there is perhaps some swelling around her right knee. Her limp seems worse in the mornings and evenings. She is generally well, with no fevers, no rash, no night pains, and no bruising or bleeding. She has good energy levels, is otherwise mostly playing and participating at childcare normally, although has been a little bit irritable at times. She is eating and sleeping well. She has not had any injury noted to the knee. There have not been any antecedent infections. She has no eye or gut symptoms, no recent medications or travel. There is no history of autoimmune conditions (e.g. arthritis, uveitis, inflammatory bowel disease, psoriasis). She is not taking any medications.

On examination she looks well. She is not dysmorphic and is happy and talkative. Her growth is on the 75th percentiles for both height and weight. She has a limp on the right leg and climbs up onto the bed using her left leg, but is able to put weight through her right side. She has normal joints, except for her right knee which has moderate synovitis and effusion. She also has a 1 cm quadriceps circumference

J. Munro (✉)
Royal Children's Hospital, Murdoch Children's Research Institute, University of Melbourne, Melbourne, VIC, Australia

C. F. Lynch et al. (eds.), *The Art of Paediatric Medicine Beyond the Evidence Base*,
https://doi.org/10.1007/978-981-96-7234-9_36

difference; with right less than the left side. There is no leg length discrepancy. Her oral, skin, nailfold and systems examinations are normal.

She is commenced on regular ibuprofen and blood tests are ordered (FBE, ESR, CRP, ANA, rheumatoid factor, store serum) as well as an X-ray of the right knee. The blood tests show mildly elevated ESR and mildly elevated platelets, but are otherwise normal. The X-ray of the knee demonstrates an effusion and normal bony structures. She is diagnosed as likely Juvenile Idiopathic Arthritis and promptly referred to the local paediatric rheumatologist for urgent assessment. She is seen 2 weeks later and has a joint injection of corticosteroids under nitrous oxide along with an eye review assessing for uveitis, education with a paediatric rheumatology nurse and a physiotherapist.

3 Discussion

Always consider arthritis as a differential diagnosis when assessing a child with a swollen joint or joint pain. After ruling out important acute diagnoses such as septic arthritis or osteomyelitis, including Juvenile Idiopathic Arthritis (JIA) as a potential diagnosis is important.

JIA is the most common inflammatory rheumatic disease of childhood affecting 1–4 per 1000 children making it at least as common as other childhood autoimmune diseases such as Diabetes Mellitus or Inflammatory Bowel Disease [1]. The literature however demonstrates delays in access to care for children and young people with JIA. This is almost always because the clinicians along the child's diagnostic journey have not thought of JIA as a possibility [2]. Many children see a number of different clinicians and have multiple investigations. At the point when someone, be it a GP, physiotherapist, podiatrist, pharmacist, parent, ED doctor, orthopaedic surgeon—whomever it is—thinks of JIA as a diagnosis, there is then a huge acceleration in access to diagnosis and treatment. Unfortunately, the average time to diagnosis in Australia is 10 months [3].

Referring early to a paediatric rheumatologist is critical to facilitate early effective treatment, but the key step is awareness [4]. Early recognition improves outcomes. The good news is that you have all the skills you need to be able to assess and diagnose a child presenting with JIA!

Listen carefully to the history to decide if it is an inflammatory presentation. Mechanical and non-inflammatory musculoskeletal pain presentations are very common, much more common than JIA. Pattern recognition of persistent swelling of a joint(s) and pain in joints associated with stiff joints as JIA is critical. Inflammatory joint pain is associated with an improvement with movement and worsening with rest. On the other hand, non-inflammatory musculoskeletal presentations are characterised by worsening with movement and improvement with rest. There is usually no morning stiffness present.

A careful history and a thorough clinical examination are essential in detecting and confirming arthritis. Children and young people will usually be able to give an excellent history of their symptoms, which can outline whether their joint pain and swelling is located in only one joint or in more joints, and whether it is inflammatory or mechanical joint pain. Ask specifically about recent viral infections and trauma. Understanding whether the child is systemically well (fever, rash, haematological symptoms) is important, particularly for ruling out concerns about septic arthritis or osteomyelitis. Look out for any signs of chronicity, these can be subtle, such as quadriceps wasting or leg length discrepancy.

The use of the paediatric Gait, Arms, Legs and Spine (pGALS) exam can facilitate a quick and easy validated paediatric musculoskeletal exam [5].

There is currently no diagnostic test for Juvenile Arthritis. However, it is diagnosed in those younger than 16 years of age and with arthritis present for longer than 6 weeks. It is a diagnosis of exclusion and it is important to be vigilant to differentiate JIA from other diagnoses, and this may require some investigations to clarify. Fortunately, there are now many very effective treatments for the management of JIA [6–10], although many children continue to have active disease throughout childhood and into adulthood [11].

Please get in touch with your local paediatric rheumatology team if you need to discuss—all the children's hospitals have them.

4 Other Gems

- If you see a child with a persistently swollen joint, think juvenile arthritis.
- Children should not have ongoing limp, so this should be clinically assessed and reviewed.
- It's often incredibly helpful and important to examine all of a child's joints even when they present with a target joint(s) or painful site.

References

1. Petty, R., Laxer, R., Lindsley, C., et al. (2021). *Juvenile idiopathic arthritis: Classification and basic concepts* (8th ed.). Elsevier.
2. Foster, H. E., Marshall, N., Myers, A., Dunkley, P., & Griffiths, I. D. (2003). Outcome in adults with juvenile idiopathic arthritis: A quality of life study. *Arthritis and Rheumatism, 48*(3), 767–775.
3. Juvenile Arthritis Foundation of Australia IMAPACT Study. (2023). https://www.jafa.org.au/wp-content/uploads/2023/11/Impact-Study-8-pager-22-11-2023-web.pdf
4. Sinnappurajar, P., & Chaitow, J. (2023). Juvenile idiopathic arthritis – A new outlook. *Medicine Today, 24*(10), 12–19.

5. Foster, H. E., & Jandial, S. (2013). pGALS – Paediatric gait arms legs and spine: A simple examination of the musculoskeletal system. *Pediatric Rheumatology, 11*, 44.
6. ANZMUSC. (2022). An Australian living guideline for the management of juvenile idiopathic arthritis. [version 0.2]. Available from: https://app.magicapp.org/. Accessed Oct 2023.
7. Onel, K. B., Horton, D. B., Lovell, D. J., et al. (2022). 2021 American College of Rheumatology guideline for the treatment of juvenile idiopathic arthritis: Therapeutic approaches for oligoarthritis, temporomandibular joint arthritis, and systemic juvenile idiopathic arthritis. *Arthritis Care and Research, 74*, 521–537.
8. Onel, K. B., Horton, D. B., Lovell, D. J., et al. (2022). 2021 American College of Rheumatology guideline for the treatment of juvenile idiopathic arthritis: Recommendations for nonpharmacologic therapies, medication monitoring, immunizations, and imaging. *Arthritis Care and Research, 74*, 505–520.
9. Shenoi, S., Horneff, G., Aggarwal, A., et al. (2024). Treatment of non-systemic juvenile idiopathic arthritis. *Nature Reviews Rheumatology, 20*, 170–181. https://doi.org/10.1038/s41584-024-01079-8
10. Tiller, G., Hernandez, B. L., Buckle, J., Allen, R., Munro, J., Gowdie, P., Cox, A., & Akikusa, J. (2024). Three- and five-year outcomes of an inception cohort of Australian children with juvenile idiopathic arthritis. *International Journal of Rheumatic Diseases, 27*(5), e15189.
11. Filipa, O. R., Carolina, Z., João Eurico, F. (2024). A lifelong journey: Long-term perspectives on Juvenile Idiopathic Arthritis, Best Practice & Research Clinical Rheumatology, Volume 38, Issue 3, 101984

Psychotropic Prescribing in Pre-schoolers. First Ask Yourself: How Young Is Too Young?

Mary Burke

1 Clinical Pearl

Psychotropic Prescribing in Pre-schoolers. First ask yourself—how young is too young?

2 Clinical Case

The mother of Daphne, a young girl aged 5 years 10 months, presented to paediatric outpatient clinic requesting prescriptions of clonidine for both her daughter and 4-year-old son who was not brought to the consultation.

Daphne had been seen at the clinic from 26 months of age regarding temperamental outbursts (screaming, head-banging, kicking, biting) and sleep difficulties. There was an associated history of excessive cow's milk intake with mild iron deficiency. Growth and developmental trajectories were normal. At the time of her initial presentation, Daphne's younger brother was aged 12 months and older half-sister 11 years. Both were medically well and typically developing. Neither Daphne nor her younger brother were attending childcare. The paediatrician prescribed Daphne liquid melatonin for sleep difficulties, initially 1 mg nocte, titrating up to 3 mg nocte if necessary. Ferro-liquid 10 ml daily was added for iron deficiency.

Daphne was reviewed at 30 months when her mother queried possible attention deficit hyperactivity disorder (ADHD) given a paternal diagnosis of the condition. The paediatrician established a diagnosis of early onset ADHD with co-morbid sleep disorder. Clonidine 25mcg bd was introduced with recommendations to titrate

M. Burke (✉)
Canberra Health Services, The Canberra Hospital, Garran, ACT, Australia

C. F. Lynch et al. (eds.), *The Art of Paediatric Medicine Beyond the Evidence Base*,
https://doi.org/10.1007/978-981-96-7234-9_37

the evening dose up to 75mcg nocte if necessary. Referrals to playgroup and occupational therapy were arranged.

Daphne was next seen in the clinic 10 days before her third birthday. Her mother described escalating behavioural difficulties with a mixed response to clonidine. She had ceased the morning dose due to excessive daytime sedation and was giving a total of 100 mcg at night. The paediatrician initiated stimulant medication—immediate-release methylphenidate 2.5 mg tds (mane, midi and 1500 hrs), to be titrated up to 5 mg tds. Clonidine was continued at a dose of 100mcg.

Daphne re-presented to the clinic at 40 months of age with her mother reporting escalating aggression by day and frequent night awakenings. She had commenced pre-school and there were no behavioural concerns in that setting. Methylphenidate had been trialled but ceased within weeks due to adverse effects of emesis and emotional lability. Clonidine 100mcg nocte was continued but to little effect. Daphne remained wait-listed for occupational therapy. Given a poor response to methylphenidate, dexamphetamine 2.5 mg tds (mane, midi and 1500 h) was instead prescribed. The dose of Clonidine was increased to 125mcg nocte and adjuvant melatonin 1-2 mg prn recommended for night-time awakenings.

Daphne was next reviewed at 4 years and 9 months. She had made a positive transition to kindergarten and there were no further concerns about her behaviour at home or school. Her mother had discontinued dexamphetamine as it paradoxically increased agitation. There were ongoing concerns of sleep difficulties with frequent night awakenings. The paediatrician ceased clonidine and melatonin and instead prescribed off-label carbamazepine 150 mg nocte.

Over the following 9 months, multiple prescriptions for clonidine were issued for Daphne via phone consultations. Carbamazepine was no longer being prescribed though the timing and reason for its cessation were unclear. During this time, Daphne's younger brother had also been assessed for behavioural and sleep difficulties and commenced on twice daily clonidine at a dose of up to 200mcg daily. He had not been prescribed stimulant medication. The older half-sister, now aged 14, had ceased attending school and assumed a significant caring role in the home.

Daphne was next seen in the clinic at 5 years and 10 months by a subsequent paediatrician. She was progressing well at school and engaging positively in occupational therapy to build emotional regulation skills. She was sleeping through the night with clonidine 100 mcg nocte. Daphne's mother reported her concerns now centred on her 4-year-old son's behaviour and sleep difficulties. She again reported a paternal history of ADHD and additionally disclosed paternal substance misuse and domestic violence. She described her own physical and mental health difficulties. She reported escalating tensions with her pharmacist and GP regarding restricted access to Clonidine supplies for her two children.

An audit of medication dispensing for both children was conducted with the pharmacist and GP and its findings discussed with the mother. A GP review was recommended to address psycho-social supports for Daphne's mother.

3 Discussion

Preschoolers can and do experience psychological problems that interfere with their development across multiple domains and adversely impact their family functioning, participation in childcare and later school readiness. There is an associated increased risk of mental health problems in later childhood [1].

Yet the approach to mental health conditions in childhood—and very young children in particular—has elicited considerable debate over many decades. Use of The Diagnostic and Statistical Manual of Mental Disorders (5th ed.; DSM–5; American Psychiatric Association, 2013) to identify mental health conditions in children has courted particular controversy. In Australia and North America, the DSM is the most widely accepted classification system for mental health disorders. It groups behavioural symptoms into diagnostic categories and draws the official boundaries between 'normal' and 'abnormal' human experiences [2]. In the majority of cases, it does not attempt to describe aetiological factors and has been criticised for decontextualising mental health problems. But children are profoundly dependent and sensitive to their social contexts. Contrary to 'brain-based' theories that frame mental health disorders as diseases of neurobiological and genetic origin, the strongest predictors of childhood mental health are family and environmental factors [2]. Adverse childhood experiences—including exposure to family violence, abuse and neglect, and parental mental illness, substance use and incarceration—are known to be strongly associated with mental health difficulties in later life [3].

In contrast to DSM taxonomy, a clear distinction between normal development and behaviour and mental health problems can be difficult to draw in very young children. There is a high degree of inter- and intra-individual variability and the rapidity of change in childhood developmental trajectories is such that children may fall into or out of diagnostic categories over time [4].

Regardless of these complexities, there has been a steady increase in the number of children diagnosed with mental health conditions over recent decades, in Australia and worldwide. This is matched by an increased use of psychotropic medications—on- and off-label—to treat such conditions [5–7]. More recently, the issue of paediatric psychotropic polypharmacy has garnered attention [8, 9]. Claims of 'psychiatric fads' and 'epidemics' of over-diagnosis and over-treatment of childhood mental health disorders are widespread [10]. Many view the pharmaceutical industry as a key driver of the trend though social media has now arguably assumed this role. Also relevant is the issue of diagnostic 'upcoding' with a diagnosis of autism particularly enabling access to educational, disability and family support funding [11, 12].

Notwithstanding the gravitas of the DSM, there are other ways of understanding psychological distress in very young children, ways that ensure social and contextual factors—particularly parental attunement and child-parent attachment—are acknowledged alongside the child's behavioural symptoms [2]. Adopting such frameworks shape the therapeutic options that follow, opening up a continuum of mental health supports for both child and caregiver using interventions that are trauma-informed and grounded in attachment theory to improve outcomes for children in the short term and potentially life-long. It avoids premature diagnosis and over-reliance on psycho-pharmacological agents that are less effective and have higher rates of adverse effects in the very young. It avoids premature escalation to polypharmacy and possible exponential risks to the developing brain. It accepts the validity of supportive care and surveillance as a first-line approach, to ensure safety, minimise risk and sit with uncertainty, understanding that a definitive diagnosis may unfold over time [13].

4 Other Gems

- Aggressive behaviour (hitting, kicking, biting, etc) is normative in toddlers, peaking around age 2–3, then decreasing as children build social and emotional regulation skills by age 5–6. Children at risk of sustained aggression in the middle years and beyond have recognisable socio-environmental risk factors including family poverty, low maternal education, sole parenthood and parental mental illness. Their families will benefit from evidence-based parent-child interventions such as the Incredible Years, Circle of Security, Tuning into Toddlers and Parent-Child Interactive Therapy, to optimise later outcomes.
- Sleep is a maturational process. The toddler years are characterised by normative changes in sleep—decreasing daytime naps, decreasing night awakenings and decreasing total sleep time. Parent attunement plays an important role during this developmental stage as toddlers do not put themselves to bed independently. There is a sound evidence base for psycho-education and behavioural interventions as first line treatments for sleep difficulties in toddlers and preschoolers. These interventions centre on helping parents create a healthy sleeping space and calm, consistent bedtime routine for their child. There is limited evidence to support the use of pharmacological agents for the treatment of sleep disorders in typically developing children despite their frequent use in clinical practice.
- Normal developmental variations of social behaviour and functioning must factor into any consideration of a diagnosis of ADHD in very young children. Behaviours suggestive of ADHD in older children may be developmentally appropriate in toddlers and preschool children. DSM-5 diagnostic criteria for ADHD are not differentiated for preschool and school-aged children other than to specify that symptoms be assessed relative to developmentally appropriate behaviours. Current evidence continues to support parent behavioural training as a first-line strategy for the treatment of preschool patients with ADHD symptoms.
- Maternal mental illness can have profound and lasting effects on both mothers and infants. Untreated, it hampers mother-infant attachment and infant care. It is associated with detrimental effects on infant brain development which increases the risk of later childhood neuro-developmental and psychiatric disorders. Recognition and management of maternal mental health disorders is a priority to ensure optimal future health outcomes for both mother and child.

References

1. Gleason, M. M., Goldson, E., Yogman, M. W., et al. (2016). Committee on psychosocial aspects of child and family health; section on developmental and behavioral pediatrics. Addressing early childhood emotional and behavioral problems. *Pediatrics, 138*(6), e20163025. https://doi.org/10.1542/peds.2016-3025
2. Price-Robertson, R. (2018). *Diagnosis in child mental health: Exploring the benefits, risks and alternatives*. AIFS.
3. Felitti, V. J., Anda, R. F., Nordenberg, D., Williamson, D. F., Spitz, A. M., Edwards, V., et al. (1998). Relationship of childhood abuse and household dysfunction to many of the leading causes of death in adults. *American Journal of Preventive Medicine, 14*(4), 245–258.
4. Postert, C., Averbeck-Holocher, M., Beyer, T., Müller, J., & Furniss, T. (2008). Five systems of psychiatric classification for preschool children: Do differences in validity, usefulness and reliability make for competitive or complimentary constellations? *Child Psychiatry and Human Development, 40*(1), 25–41.
5. Wood, S. J., Ilomäki, J., Gould, J., et al. (2023). Dispensing of psychotropic medications to Australian children and adolescents before and during the COVID-19 pandemic, 2013–2021: A retrospective cohort study. *Medical Journal of Australia., 219*(1), 18–25.
6. Fanton, J., & Gleason, M. M. (2009). Psychopharmacology and preschoolers: A critical review of current conditions. *Child and Adolescent Psychiatric Clinics of North America, 18*(3), 753–771.
7. Piovani, D., Clavenna, A., & Bonati, M. (2019). Prescription prevalence of psychotropic drugs in children and adolescents: An analysis of international data. *European Journal of Clinical Pharmacology, 75*(10), 1333–1346.
8. O'Brien, M. J., Pauls, A. M., Cates, A. M., Larson, P. D., & Zorn, A. N. (2024). Psychotropic medication use and polypharmacy among children and adolescents initiating intensive behavioral therapy for severe challenging behavior. *J Pediatr, 271*, 114056–114056.
9. Chen, H., Patel, A., Sherer, J., & Aparasu, R. (2011). The definition and prevalence of Pediatric psychotropic polypharmacy. *Psychiatric Services, 62*(12), 1450–1455.
10. Psychiatric Times. (2010). Normality is an endangered species: Psychiatric fads and overdiagnosis [Internet]. Available from: https://www.psychiatrictimes.com/view/normality-endangered-species-psychiatric-fads-and-overdiagnosis
11. Parry, P. I., & Levin, E. C. (2012). Pediatric bipolar disorder in an era of "mindless psychiatry.". *Journal of Trauma & Dissociation, 13*(1), 51–68.
12. Skellern, C., McDowell, M., & Schluter, P. (2005). Diagnosis of autistic spectrum disorders in Queensland: Variations in practice. *Journal of Paediatrics and Child Health, 41*(8), 413–418.
13. Psychiatric Times. (n.d.). A delicate brain: Ethical and practical considerations for the use of medications in very young children [Internet]. Available from: https://www.psychiatrictimes.com/view/delicate-brain-ethical-and-practical-considerations-use-medications-very-young-children

Diagnosing Attention Deficit Hyperactivity Disorder (ADHD) May Be a Challenge

Lionel Lubitz

1 Clinical Pearl

ADHD is one of the most gratifying conditions to treat.

2 Clinical Case

Johnny is a 6-year-old boy brought to your consulting rooms by both his parents who have significant concerns about his behaviour. He is in his first year of school and is struggling. His teachers report that he is very disruptive in the class, distracts the other students, can't sit still and wants to be the "class clown." He has been suspended once this term after an incident with another student involving punching and kicking. Recently he climbed onto the school roof to fetch an errant football. When instructed to "get down", he promptly leapt off the roof and broke his arm.

Johnny is the second child to Sam (a construction worker) and Suzie (a dietician). Their eldest child Ruby, aged 9, is described as a shy, academically gifted child who never causes any trouble. Johnny was a planned pregnancy. Suzie noted he was a "busy baby" even in the womb. He was born full term and thrived in his first year but struggled with sleep and settling. Kindergarten was challenging with high levels of activity and boisterous play. There is no family history of learning difficulties although Sam mentioned he left school aged 16 to pursue an apprenticeship course.

On examination, Johnny is a well grown boy with a normal physical examination. When asked why he is attending the doctor today, Johnny states "It's because

L. Lubitz (✉)
Victorian Childrens Clinic, Malvern, VIC, Australia

C. F. Lynch et al. (eds.), *The Art of Paediatric Medicine Beyond the Evidence Base*,
https://doi.org/10.1007/978-981-96-7234-9_38

I always get into trouble." He behaves immaculately during the consultation and listens intently to his parent's concerns.

3 Discussion

There is no diagnostic test for ADHD. The approach to diagnosis is first and foremost to obtain a comprehensive history from the patient, their parents and their teacher(s).

The best way to do that is to have a consultation in which the parents and child describe the issues while you observe the child in the consultation and perform a (usually normal) physical examination. Asking the child to do a drawing may assist in identifying the difficulties in attending to tasks and executive function challenges. Children are often attuned to their own challenges and differences. The child may display none of the behaviours of concern in the setting of the doctor's office. It is important to look for other diagnoses such as Autism Spectrum Disorder or Generalised Anxiety Disorder.

Ask the parents, child and teachers to complete one of the questionnaires used to see if the DSM criteria are met for ADHD in its various forms. Remember the questionnaires only reflect the observations and prejudices of the person answering the questions. This process is variable and if your strong clinical impression is that the history and presentation fits your perception of ADHD, allow that to be brought into the discussion as part of the clinical assessment of the child.

Cognitive testing is useful as it will identify comorbidities such as various Specific Learning Disorders (dyslexia, dysgraphia, dyscalculia) which are associated with ADHD in a significant number of children. Relatively lower scores in Working Memory and Processing can be helpful in helping to confirm ADHD as the problem. It can be difficult and expensive to get this done and ADHD can still be diagnosed without it.

Once the diagnosis (as uncertain as it should remain) is made, the conversation needs to focus on what interventions are useful. There are generally two main interventions.

The first and essential intervention is for the school to provide an Individualised Education Plan (IEP) to support the student in the classroom.

The second is the use of stimulant medication. The criteria for choosing to use medication are:

1. To ameliorate the significant impact on self-esteem ("I am dumb!").
2. To support major learning difficulties causing academic 'failure' in a child who is regarded as capable.
3. To prevent family and social disruption especially amongst peers.

ADHD is not a life-threatening condition, and some people find it hard to use medication in a 'healthy child'. This needs to be acknowledged in the conversation. The family and child need to be given time to decide and should never feel 'railroaded' into using medication if it goes against their own philosophy.

After two visits the diagnosis and treatment plan can be made as frequent follow-up appointments are rarely helpful.

The final observation is the response to stimulant medication. In ADHD the response is often dramatic, very positive, descriptions like "It was like night and day", "it felt like the lights were switched on", are often used.

ADHD is one of the most gratifying conditions for a clinician to treat and transformative for the young person.

Children and Alcohol

Katrina Harris

1 Clinical Pearl

Fetal Alcohol Spectrum Disorder (FASD) is a neurodevelopmental disorder that is common, disabling, and preventable. Considering FASD as a differential diagnosis can have a significant positive impact on the child and their family.

2 Clinical Case

Suzie is a 6-year-old girl brought to the clinic by her foster carer, Lara. Lara has significant concerns about Suzie's behaviour and development. These include dangerous behaviours such as taking off her seat belt in the car and hitting the driver, aggression to other children, and running away from school and home. Lara has installed security screens on the windows at home to stop Suzie breaking them by throwing objects about. She has installed specialised seatbelts in her car. Suzie is in Prep and frequently absconds. She struggles with socialisation and academic tasks. Suzie has been in foster care for 5 years with the same carer and her two younger siblings. Lara is concerned about Suzie's safety. She is worried that when Suzie turns 7 years old, funding for her current therapies and family supports through the National Disability Insurance Scheme (NDIS) will cease.

Suzie was delivered at 32/40 gestation by vaginal delivery with a birth weight on the 50th centile. Although there was limited antenatal history because of poor

K. Harris (✉)
Developmental Paediatrics, Monash Children's Hospital, Melbourne, VIC, Australia

Department of Paediatrics, Monash University, Melbourne, VIC, Australia

C. F. Lynch et al. (eds.), *The Art of Paediatric Medicine Beyond the Evidence Base*,
https://doi.org/10.1007/978-981-96-7234-9_39

antenatal attendance, confirmed high levels of prenatal alcohol exposure, cannabis and methamphetamines were noted on the birth records. Postnatally, Suzie failed to thrive. There was no report of developmental regression, seizures, or head injury.

Physical examination revealed a very active child who liked to run away. She had good eye contact and was engaging but had little verbal language. It was clear she was strongly bonded with her carer. Her height and weight were on the 50th centile, with head circumference on the 10th. Three sentinel facial features consistent with FASD (fetal alcohol spectrum disorder) were present. Further physical examination was unremarkable, and did not reveal signs of other syndromes or conditions causing developmental delays.

Suzie's development was assessed by paediatric psychology and allied health clinicians. This showed severe delays in understanding and using language, severe delays in motor skills making it hard for her to write, or dress herself, challenges in activities of daily living, and borderline intellectual abilities. She was highly impulsive and inattentive and met criteria for a diagnosis of attention deficit hyperactivity disorder (ADHD).

Investigations included a normal microarray and Fragile X (FRAX), thyroid function tests (TFTs), urinary metabolic screen, and plasma amino acids. Hearing and vision screening were normal.

Suzie's neurodevelopmental challenges could be described as severe language and motor impairments, adaptive function delay, borderline IQ, and ADHD. Suzie's neurodevelopmental skills were around that of a child half her age. In the context of high prenatal alcohol exposure, and exclusion of other causes, the diagnosis of FASD was made.

3 Discussion

FASD is the major cause of preventable developmental disability in the Western world. It is common and under-recognised. Australians consume a high level of alcohol. A study of Australian women revealed 59% consumed some alcohol during pregnancy and 18.5% drank at binge levels before they knew they were pregnant [1]. The global prevalence is around 1%, and higher in vulnerable populations, such as children in care, children in a correctional facility, Aboriginal children or children in special educational settings [2].

Every child with FASD is unique and will have their own array of skills and challenges. Making a diagnosis of FASD allows care providers to shift the focus to the future, rather than further rounds of assessments and uncertainty.

In assessing a child for FASD, it is vital to have a non-judgemental approach. Integrating a standard series of questions about drinking during pregnancy is useful for all prenatal history taking. Relevant questions to ask include the type of alcohol, amount, frequency and during what period of the pregnancy this occurred. Mothers may drink alcohol before they know that they are pregnant. Biological mothers may not be available to speak with, and in these situations reviewing birth records, child protection and medical records, and history for those who may have observed the child's mother drinking alcohol during the pregnancy can be helpful. Moderate and heavy alcohol use is more likely to be associated with FASD. Collaboration with psychology and allied health colleagues enables a broad assessment of the child's skills and impairments.

Examination of the child includes a full examination of growth and development and a general examination looking for other abnormalities. Microcephaly is associated with FASD; head circumference (HC) should be carefully measured, and birth HC reviewed. Cardiac, renal, skeletal and hearing abnormalities are all increased with FASD. The facial phenotype is distinctive with clear guidelines for assessment, however the majority of children with FASD do not have three sentinel facial features, and these are not required for a diagnosis (Table 1).

Phenotypic facial features of FASD include three sentinel features [3]:

1. Short palpebral fissures.
2. Smooth philtrum.
3. Thin upper lip.

FASD is **excluded** as a diagnosis if there is NO alcohol intake confirmed antenatally **or** if <3 sentinel facial features and neurodevelopmental criteria are NOT met. Updated 2025 Australian guidelines are now available on https://fasdhub.org.au/fasd-information/australian-guidelines-for-assessment-and-diagnosis-of-fasd/.

Developmental Age Equivalent (Fig. 1), is a useful concept when considering the child before you. For example, the child while being 10 years chronologically, will have different developmental age equivalents in the different domain/skill sets. This often assists carers in understanding and anticipating the child's behaviour, and in providing developmentally age-appropriate safe environments.

The benefit of providing an early diagnosis (before the age of 6 years but ideally even earlier), is to improve outcomes for the child and the family. Support for the child includes understanding the child's additional needs, targeted early intervention and guiding educational expectations. Ensuring a stable and nurturing living environment and supporting the child's family is crucial for best outcomes. Funding may be available to better enable the child to be maintained in a current stable

Table 1 Australian Guide for the Diagnosis of FASD (2016)

Diagnostic Criteria	FASD with 3 sentinel facial features	FASD with <3 sentinel facial features
Prenatal alcohol exposure	Confirmed or unknown	Confirmed
Neurodevelopmental domains[a]	Severe impairment (>2 standard deviations below the mean) in at least 3 neurodevelopmental domains	Severe impairment in at least 3 neurodevelopmental domains
Sentinel facial features	All three present	Presence of none, one or two

[a]Neurodevelopmental domains include brain structure, motor skills, cognition, language, academic achievement, memory, attention, executive function (impulse control and hyperactivity), affect regulation, adaptive behaviour, social communication

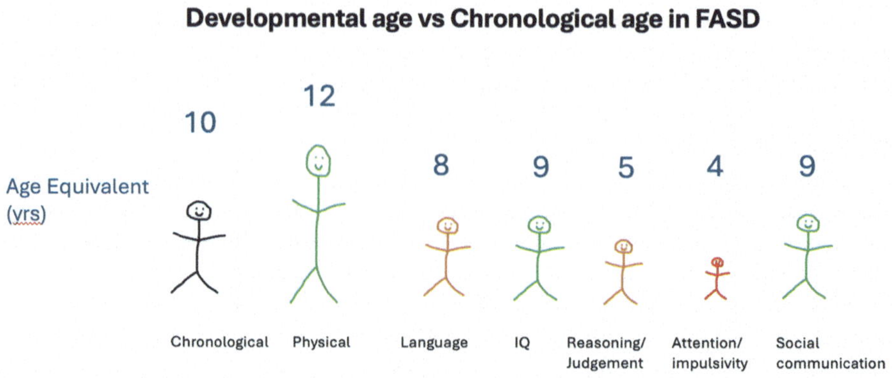

Fig. 1 Developmental Age Equivalent (Drawing by Katrina Harris)

placement. Having realistic developmental age expectations for the child helps family, teachers and carers respond to their child's needs. Diagnosis of a child aims to provide the opportunity to better support the mother to have healthy future pregnancies.

Prevention measures include recognition of FASD at a society level, improved community and individual education regarding the risks of alcohol consumption during pregnancy, targeted interventions for high-risk groups and supported family planning.

As an individual clinician, it is important to integrate an alcohol history into the standard paediatric history-taking, to consider if FASD may be contributing to the child's neurodevelopmental and behavioural challenges, and to support carers and manage symptoms.

4 Other Gems

Consider differential diagnoses and exclude other causes with investigations if indicated:

- Chromosomal abnormality: Microarray and FRAX.
- Structural brain malformation: Magnetic Resonance Imaging (MRI) brain.
- Microcephaly (congenital/acquired): congenital infection (TORCH) screen.
- Thyroid function tests, urine metabolic screen.
- A history of perinatal hypoxia.
- Phenotypes suggestive of specific syndromes e.g. Cornelia de Lange, foetal valproate syndrome.
- Early life trauma/abuse.

Other risk factors that make a diagnosis of FASD more likely include:

- A sibling with FASD.
- Previous Out of Home Care.
- Currently receiving psychiatric care.
- Current or past involvement with Child Protection or Juvenile justice systems.
- Indigenous background.
- Attending special education.

4.1 Resources

- https://everymomentmatters.org.au/resources
- www.nofasd.org.au
- www.fasdhub.org

References

1. Muggli, E., O'Leary, C., Donath, S., et al. (2016). "Did you ever drink more?" A detailed description of pregnant women's drinking patterns. *BMC Public Health, 16*, 683.
2. Lange, S., Probst, C., Gmel, G., Rehm, J., Burd, L., & Popova, S. (2017). Global prevalence of fetal alcohol spectrum disorder among children and youth: A systematic review and meta-analysis. *JAMA Pediatrics, 171*(10), 948–956.
3. Adubato, S. A., & Cohen, D. E. (Eds.). (2011). *Prenatal alcohol use and FASD: A model standard of diagnosis, assessment and multimodal treatment* (pp. 3–28). Susan J Astley.

Don't Forget to Look

Kiri Chan

1 Clinical Pearl

Vulval symptoms are common in prepubertal girls and they need to be carefully examined.

2 Clinical Case

Ally was 7 years old when she presented to the general practitioner (GP) with symptoms of vulval itch. She was initially prescribed treatments like topical antifungal treatments but continued to have symptoms to varying degrees.

By the time she turned 8 years of age she developed recurrent UTIs and urinary incontinence, after previous successful toilet training, and she was referred to a urologist for ongoing assessments, reviews and underwent various treatments.

Eventually at the age of 13 she was offered a procedure to inject Botox into the bladder as her next treatment option. At the time of cystoscopy, she was diagnosed with severe lichen sclerosis (LS), and complete labial fusion with only a pinpoint opening.

She had not been examined for years despite being in contact with multiple health care providers including GPs, paediatricians, urologists and continence nurses.

The severe LS with significant and advanced architectural change was challenging to treat, and it was compounded by compliance difficulties common to this age group. Medical treatment with topical steroid was only partially effective at

K. Chan (✉)
Monash Health /Monash Children's Hospital, Clayton, VIC, Australia

Royal Children's Hospital, Melbourne, VIC, Australia

C. F. Lynch et al. (eds.), *The Art of Paediatric Medicine Beyond the Evidence Base*,
https://doi.org/10.1007/978-981-96-7234-9_40

reducing the fusion, and she will require surgical correction of the architectural loss prior to commencement of sexual activity.

3 Discussion

Prepubertal girls commonly present with vulval discomfort, itch or discharge. Such symptoms can be baffling or concerning for the parents, and the scratching or tugging behaviours they can elicit can attract unwanted attention in the social environment. A gentle examination of the vulval skin conducted in a sensitive manner (or at least assessment of photos taken by the parents, assuming they provide adequate visualisation of the area involved) is always helpful, to inform treatment and response.

Sometimes clinicians shy away from performing a vulval examination in children. It may be perceived to be time-consuming, discomforting or embarrassing to the patient, or clinicians feel inexperienced with interpretation.

However, just like with any other part of the anatomy, if one does not look, one may miss or delay an important diagnosis or miss the opportunity to refer the child to an appropriate specialist.

Examination of the vulva for subtle abnormalities, and particularly the prepubertal vulva, does require some skill which can be obtained with practice. If there is any uncertainty it may be appropriate to refer to a colleague with the expertise, such as a paediatric gynaecologist or dermatologist who is familiar with this area.

Most symptomatic vulval conditions cause significant impairment to quality of life, and it is important to acknowledge and support the patient and their family through these difficulties. Less commonly but importantly, conditions like paediatric vulval lichen sclerosis can cause preventable permanent loss of vulval architecture [1, 2] which may be detrimental to the patient's future physical, psychological and relational wellbeing [3].

Therefore, the patient will benefit from early physical assessment to guide diagnosis, and ongoing assessment if symptoms are not resolving.

4 Other Gems

- Paediatric vulval examination is best undertaken in the frog-leg position, and the perianal area in the left lateral position. However, many children may not be comfortable to adopt these positions, and it may be more acceptable for them to be examined on the parent's knee.
- Consent from the child is essential, and it is very traumatic for a child to be forcibly held down for an examination. Where a child is clearly not consenting to an examination, alternatives may include having the parent assist with positioning

and opening of the labia for visualisation, or even assessment using photographs from the parents as long as they are of an adequate quality.

- It is always worthwhile to examine the remainder of the child's skin to identify other signs of a skin disorder that may affect more than the vulva, or may suggest a diagnosis, for example itchy scaly rashes and nail changes of psoriasis, or eczematous skin rashes, or mouth ulcers characteristic of Bechet's syndrome.
- Candida is a common misdiagnosis for prepubertal girls with vulval symptoms (often without an examination). Candida is exceedingly rare in prepubertal children [4, 5] as they do not have the oestrogenic environment that favours its overgrowth.
- Swab tests for microscopy and culture are reasonable to perform although it is uncommon to yield a single causative pathogen. Internal vaginal swabs including low vaginal swabs are not recommended as they are traumatising. However, a swab can be gently rolled on the external surface of the vulva, or on discharge samples on underwear. Performance of the swab collection may be performed by the parent, which may be more acceptable for the child.
- Vulval biopsy is rarely required in children.
- The principle of examination also applies to other parts of the body!
- Clinical Practice Guidelines are available for further information on this topic [6].

References

1. Chan, K., Terlato, M., Crofts, V., & Grover, S. (2024). Loss of architecture in Pediatric and adolescent patients with Vulval lichen Sclerosus: A retrospective cohort study. *Journal of Lower Genital Tract Disease, 28*(4), S21.
2. Kherlopian, A., & Fischer, G. (2022). Does compliance to topical corticosteroid therapy reduce the risk of development of permanent vulvar structural abnormalities in pediatric vulvar lichen sclerosus? A retrospective cohort study. *Pediatric Dermatology, 39*(1), 22–30.
3. Morrel, B., Van der Avoort, I., Ewing-Graham, P., Damman, J., Schappin, R., Van Zeijl, K., & Voorham, Q. (2023). Long-term consequences of juvenile vulvar lichen sclerosus: A cohort study of adults with a histologically confirmed diagnosis in childhood or adolescence. *Acta Obstetricia et Gynecologica Scandinavica, 102*(11), 1469–1478.
4. Fischer, G. (2010). Chronic vulvitis in pre-pubertal girls. *The Australasian Journal of Dermatology, 51*(2), 118–123. https://doi.org/10.1111/j.1440-0960.2010.00631.x
5. Jaquiery, A., Stylianopoulos, A., Hogg, G., & Grover, S. (1999). Vulvovaginitis: Clinical features, aetiology, and microbiology of the genital tract. *Archives of Disease in Childhood, 81*(1), 64–67.
6. The Royal Children's Hospital. (2022). *Clinical practice guidelines: Vulval and vaginal conditions*. Accessed 21 Jan 2025.

Scratching the Surface

Emer Crowley and Ann Boyapati

1 Clinical Pearl

The most common reason for persistent eczema is failure to use topical corticosteroids at the appropriate strength and for an adequate duration.

2 Clinical Case

A seven-year-old girl, Lyla, attended the Dermatology clinic with her parents with the complaint of worsening pruritic, lichenified plaques in flexural areas, consistent with the diagnosis of atopic dermatitis. Diagnosed with atopic dermatitis at the age of two, her management had involved twice daily emollients and the intermittent application of a topical corticosteroid during flares.

Over the past 3 months, Lyla's eczema had worsened, causing severe itching that disrupted her sleep. Her parents reported teasing at school due to the appearance of the plaques, leading to refusal to wear shorts and T-shirts. They stated that the topical steroids that they had been using were ineffective and requested a different treatment.

Further discussion revealed that her parents had been applying a mild-potency topical steroid sparingly, twice daily. They had been advised by their pharmacist to cease treatment after 2 weeks, due to the potential for side effects.

E. Crowley
St Vincent's Hospital, Fitzroy, VIC, Australia

A. Boyapati (✉)
Department of Dermatology, Monash Health, Clayton, VIC, Australia

C. F. Lynch et al. (eds.), *The Art of Paediatric Medicine Beyond the Evidence Base*,
https://doi.org/10.1007/978-981-96-7234-9_41

The team addressed the family's concerns regarding side effects, explaining the safety and efficacy of topical corticosteroids when used correctly. A potent topical corticosteroid was prescribed twice daily to affected areas, weaning to a moderately potent topical corticosteroid after a period of three to 4 weeks. Lyla's parents were provided with a written action plan to increase the frequency and potency of topical corticosteroids during flares. At a follow up appointment 3 months later, there was significant improvement in both the lesions and Lyla's self-confidence, and she attended the appointment wearing a dress.

3 Discussion

Atopic dermatitis (AD) is a chronic, inflammatory skin condition, characterised by pruritic, scaly plaques and a relapsing course. It is one of the most common non-communicable skin diseases, affecting 15–20% of children worldwide [1].

Treatment begins with optimising and restoring the skin barrier. This involves avoiding common eczema triggers such as heat and irritants, particularly soaps. Dry skin should be managed with the regular application of emollients, and infections can be prevented with the use of bleach baths [2]. This basic management should be continued even in the absence of visible plaques.

Topical corticosteroids (TCS) are a cornerstone in the management of eczema and are highly effective in reducing inflammation and itch. Effective TCS therapy hinges on three key principles: adequate potency, adequate dosage, and adequate application [1].

Flaring and deterioration of AD despite treatment, as seen in the case above, is a very common paediatric presentation. The clinician's natural instinct is to move up the treatment ladder, or to consider alternative treatments. However, a significant proportion of these cases result from non-adherence to management plans. This may be due to inadequate education, incorrect application of topical therapies or delayed use of treatments.

Many instances of non-adherence to TCS treatment regimens can be attributed to steroid phobia. These fears focus on potential side effects such as skin atrophy, or systemic side effects. A study published in the British Journal of Dermatology found that 47.8% of patients did not know the side effects of TCS but were still afraid of their use [3]. In reality, when TCS are used in paediatric eczema according to guidelines, side effects are extremely rare [4].

Conflicting advice from doctors, nurses and pharmacists can increase parental confusion and fear. An example of this is the outdated advice to apply TCS 'sparingly' and for a short duration, which is ubiquitous. However, particularly in cases of severe eczema, TCS should be applied liberally and may need to be used for several weeks to achieve the desired outcome.

This case highlights the importance of exploring parents' concerns and educating on appropriate TCS use. With simple education interventions, under-treatment of eczema can be minimised and, subsequently, unnecessary suffering can be prevented.

4 Other Gems

- Given the prevalence of **steroid phobia**, it is helpful to pre-empt these fears when initiating treatment with TCS. Caregivers can be pre-warned that they may receive advice from health professionals and others to use TCS sparingly and for a short duration, however, they should use TCS as directed.
- To minimise side effects, caregivers should be counselled to be cautious when using TCS in sensitive areas (such as the flexures, face and eyelids), and to cease using TCS once the eczema has cleared. If long term therapy is required, topical calcineurin inhibitors can be utilised.
- In cases where a particular area of eczema repeatedly flares after cessation of TCS, a proactive approach can be used. This involves the regular application of TCS twice a week (for example, on weekends) to chronically affected areas [1]. This preventative approach is effective in maintaining lesion-free skin in many children with atopic dermatitis.
- In cases of persistent eczema despite adequate TCS use, it is important to consider underlying perpetuating factors. These may include concomitant infection [5] or exposure to irritants (such as saliva, which can lead to perioral eczema) [2]. Contact allergy is uncommon, but can occur to ingredients in washes, emollients or even the TCS itself (either the excipients or the corticosteroid molecule) [6].

References

1. Wollenberg, A., Barbarot, S., Bieber, T., et al. (2019). Consensus-based European guidelines for treatment of atopic eczema (atopic dermatitis) in adults and children: Part I. *Journal of the European Academy of Dermatology and Venereology, 33*(7), 1436.
2. Royal Children's Hospital Melbourne. (2022). Clinical practice guidelines: Eczema. [Internet]. Available from: https://www.rch.org.au/clinicalguide/guideline_index/eczema/
3. Aubert-Wastiaux, H., Moret, L., Le Rhun, A., et al. (2011). Topical corticosteroid phobia in atopic dermatitis: A study of its nature, origins and frequency. *The British Journal of Dermatology, 165*(4), 808–814. https://doi.org/10.1111/j.1365-2133.2011.10449.x
4. The Australian College of Dermatologists. (2022). Consensus statement Topical corticosteroids in paediatric eczema [Internet]. Available from: https://www.dermcoll.edu.au/wp-content/uploads/2022/09/ACD-Consensus-Statement-Topical-Corticosteroids-September-2022-.pdf
5. Arkwright, P. D., Motala, C., Subramanian, H., et al. (2013). Management of difficult-to-treat atopic dermatitis. *The Journal of Allergy and Clinical Immunology. In Practice, 1*(2), 142–151. https://doi.org/10.1016/j.jaip.2012.09.002
6. Mehta, A. B., Nadkarni, N. J., Patil, S. P., Godse, K. V., Gautam, M., & Agarwal, S. (2016). Topical corticosteroids in dermatology. *Indian Journal of Dermatology, Venereology and Leprology, 82*(4), 371–378. https://doi.org/10.4103/0378-6323.178903

Keep the Child at the Centre of the Consultation

Charlotte Whitelaw

1 Clinical Pearl

How you conduct consultations can empower children.

2 Clinical Case

Jo brings her 7-year-old son Oliver to see you with concerns that he may have Attention Deficit Hyperactivity Disorder (ADHD). Upon greeting the family in your waiting room, Jo leads Oliver, his 10-year-old brother Oscar and her best friend Caroline into the consulting room. Oliver is engrossed in a game on his iPad and doesn't look up on his way into the room. He sits in the far corner and continues his game. Jo immediately pulls her chair up close to your desk, positioning herself so that your view of Oliver is blocked, and pulls out her list of concerns. She then begins talking about Oliver fighting with his brother, lying, school suspensions, being 'uncontrollable', running away from home, and not making progress with reading. She compares him to his big brother who she describes as 'my good boy' and offers this as proof that 'it's not my parenting'. She then invites Caroline into the conversation to 'back her up' saying Caroline knows how difficult Oliver is. Oscar is listening to proceedings with a smirk. Fifteen minutes into the consultation Oliver is yet to speak or disengage from his iPad.

C. Whitelaw (✉)
FRACP, Hobart, TAS, Australia

C. F. Lynch et al. (eds.), *The Art of Paediatric Medicine Beyond the Evidence Base*,
https://doi.org/10.1007/978-981-96-7234-9_42

3 Discussion

As paediatricians we are the doctor of, and advocate for, the child. Unlike our adult colleagues, fulfilling this role means not just working directly with our patient but also working via parents/carers to achieve change for children.

Best outcomes occur when paediatricians, children and parents come to a shared view of the problem and work with shared purpose towards agreed goals. This often happens easily. Many parents value their child's perspective and allow them to have input into the process. However, some parents do not make space for the child to have a role in consultations. Parents are often understandably anxious to get their views across. Some may not feel the child's view matters. Others may feel the child does not have the ability to be an active participant, particularly if they are young.

How we set up and conduct consultations can help keep the child at the centre of our work; allowing them a role, encouraging their input and making them feel powerful and valued.

- In the waiting room, seek out and address the child first. Make eye contact and speak initially with them. Introduce yourself to the child first and the parents second. Welcome them to *their* appointment and ask them to explain who the grown-ups accompanying them are.
- Give them the choice of who they would like to accompany them into their appointment. If this choice causes obvious stress for the child, you can make a suggestion as to who should come in and seek their agreement. Time alone with you is often sought by parents and this should be offered, as well as time alone with adolescents at some point, but in the first instance, giving the child the choice about who should hear their story is a powerful act and can set the tone for the appointment.
- Clearly state your 'screens-off-during-appointments' rule and make this a condition of entry to your consult room. Extend this boundary to yourself also. Avoid looking at your own computer screen throughout and typing at the same time as you take a history. You will miss crucial information if you are not watching the child play and seeing their interactions with the others present. Give the child your full attention. When it feels right to start history taking, first suggest the child tell you why they have come along. If they are hesitant, you might suggest that they choose which adult should go first to 'tell the story', but that they should 'jump in if Mum/Dad gets it wrong' to encourage active listening and give them power of veto. Check in frequently with the child during adult history giving; "Is that right? What do you think?"
- Upon entering your room, ask the child to choose who sits where. Offer them the seat closest to you. Many may feel more comfortable further away from you; perhaps on their parents' lap, or even under a chair, but the important thing is that you have offered them the prime position.
- Provide opportunities for creative play in your room. Not only will this occupy small children while adults talk and provide hugely helpful information about their developmental skills, the process of creating something (a picture for your

wall perhaps) gives an opportunity for them to be seen, praised and to contribute. Many children who have drawn pictures for me are eager each time they re-enter the room to seek out their previous artwork and to admire that of others; perhaps reassuring proof of their own capacity and also of the fact that many other children have walked this path before them in this space.

- When discussing treatment options, make sure the child is happy with the plan. Explore their concerns. Why don't they like the idea being suggested? It might be a small and modifiable thing. Reassure them that they have power (to a degree) over the course chosen. Give them choices; we could do A or B, which do you think we should try first? When checking in to see how treatment is going at review appointments, ask the child's opinion first and then the parents.

It is heartwarming to see children like Oliver who initially felt shut down and left out of the medical process become helpful and active participants in their own care. This approach may provide role-modelling for parents which may shift how they view and interact with their child. It encourages a strong, warm and respectful alliance between paediatrician and child which will contribute to successful management of all paediatric problems.

The 'Three Magic Wishes' Question Can Open a Window to the Child's Mind

Charlotte Whitelaw

1 Clinical Pearl

Understanding what matters most to the child is important.

2 Clinical Case

You have just spent 50 min with a new 7-year-old patient Sarah and her separated parents. Sarah has previously been reviewed by her general practitioner, a dietician, school counsellor and naturopath. Parental concerns include poor sleep onset and maintenance, picky eating, poo accidents, reluctance to attend school, hair pulling, temper tantrums, poor progress in literacy, fighting with her sister, fatigue, perceived poor weight gain, and skin rashes. The parents hold differing views about the importance of these various problems. Dad is concerned only about the literacy problems. Mum is convinced there is an undiagnosed medical problem leading to Sarah's small size.

You have taken a full history and examined Sarah. Physical examination reveals a well girl with weight and height following the 40th centile. Previous investigation results are all normal. Sarah has been quiet and hard to engage in conversation during the consultation.

You are trying to formulate in your own mind a problem list and a plan for investigations. You are feeling somewhat exhausted by managing these combative parents in the room and overwhelmed by the number of concerns raised.

C. Whitelaw (✉)
FRACP, Hobart, TAS, Australia

C. F. Lynch et al. (eds.), *The Art of Paediatric Medicine Beyond the Evidence Base*,
https://doi.org/10.1007/978-981-96-7234-9_43

You realise that with 5 min left in the consultation you do not yet have a good sense of what matters most to Sarah, so you ask: "Sarah, if I could give you three magic wishes and you could wish anything in the whole world, what would you wish?"

3 Discussion

Perhaps better known in the field of psychology, the three magic wishes question has long been used to gain insight into what matters to children. It is no substitute for spending time alone with the child hearing their story and gaining their trust, but it can be a useful tool for a paediatrician to bring out of their toolbox on occasion.

Answers such as "I wish I didn't have Tommy in my class" or "I wish I didn't have to go to Daddy's house when his girlfriend is there" might reveal underlying concerns that have not yet been explored.

Whether this is done in front of parents or with the child alone requires judgment and depends on the situation. Sensitive answers may be more likely to be given privately. On the other hand, answers given in front of parents can be a powerful message to the parents themselves, as in "I wish Mum and Dad wouldn't fight so much."

Some children will ask for three new material possessions. While useful for birthday shopping planning, this has limited further value. A follow up question such as "OK, what if you couldn't wish for a thing, but you could wish for anything at all to change in your life?" might reveal more of interest.

Another variation on the question can be helpful, when trying to prioritise your management plan, if there are several active issues all worthy of intervention. "If I had a magic wand which could only fix one thing for you, what would you have me fix?" This helps differentiate the child's priorities from yours and those of the parents.

This question may also be of value in older children or teenagers who have chronic health conditions e.g. cystic fibrosis, epilepsy. What matters most to them may surprise you and may not always relate directly to medical issues; for example, "I want to be able to manage at school camp" or "I want to get my driving learner's permit."

Magic wishes are a very familiar concept for all children (and even some adults).

Talk to the Hand: Part 1

Jacinta Coleman

1 Clinical Pearl

"The Hand Model of the Brain" can help children manage anxiety.

2 Clinical Case

An eight-year-old boy, Tom, came in to see me with a long history of avoidant restrictive food intake disorder (ARFID). For several years his parents had tried all sorts of different approaches supported by dietitians, several psychologists, and occupational therapists. As a three-year-old, he had a choking episode and developed a long-standing fear of choking on food. This led to initial restricted food choices but gradually evolved into the development of ARFID. Meal times were a nightmare, with parents alternating between cajoling, bribing and punitive approaches. There was a lot of anxiety in the family system and his mother felt exhausted, overwhelmed and clearly anxious about her son's physical state.

Physically, Tom weighed 21 kg (<10th centile) and measured 121 cm (10th centile). His "baby book" revealed previous growth on the 50th centile for both weight and height. It was clear the restrictive eating patterns were having an impact on his weight and growth trajectory, with failure to grow on his expected percentile. Further physical examination was unremarkable with no overt signs of malnutrition or physiological instability. Pathology investigations revealed significant iron and zinc deficiency but no other abnormalities.

Using the framework of the Hand Model of the Brain (see discussion below), I engaged Tom using characters in a movie which he loved. By creating a playful

J. Coleman (✉)
Head of Unit, Adolescent Medicine, Monash Children's Hospital, Clayton, VIC, Australia

C. F. Lynch et al. (eds.), *The Art of Paediatric Medicine Beyond the Evidence Base*,
https://doi.org/10.1007/978-981-96-7234-9_44

narrative around his inner world, Tom could approach fear-inducing situations more bravely and with a sense of control. He chose a Villain that represented Anxiety, and a Hero who was able to use special powers to detect the tricks the villain was utilising to prevent him from eating his food and growing. We discussed how his Thinking brain was not really doing its job and needed food to help it work more effectively. We talked about his Emotional brain being very easily influenced by the villain who was putting bad thoughts into his head about food. He gave his Thinking brain and his Emotional brain names according to the characters in his favourite movie. We made a plan with his parents to address mealtimes in this new creative and playful way. This enabled some levity to be put back into the situation around mealtimes and it helped Tom's parents feel less anxious. It was a good distraction as they tried to think of various characters and names to give to "the bullies and villains" in his head; the thoughts causing his anxiety and disordered eating. We agreed for him to challenge himself with a new food and that there was to be no pressure. All he had to do was allow the food to sit on his plate and if he felt comfortable, just smell it, touch it, and tolerate it being near him. As his confidence grew and he was able to work through his fear using box breathing techniques and distraction with the game, he gradually felt strong enough to put food in his mouth and taste it. There was no expectation for him to chew it or swallow it unless he felt that his Thinking brain was ready to support him and protect his Emotional brain from the villains. As he was leaving the room he was quite excited to go shopping to choose one item he thought he might be able to manage.

I met with Tom and his parents a few weeks later. Tom came running into the room telling me that he'd been really brave and he had chosen a few new foods to try. Tom allowed them to sit on his plate for a couple of days before giving himself permission to touch them, smell them, and lick them. Meals became less stressful, with an emphasis on curiosity and play rather than coercion or punishment. A few days later, he took the brave step to put some carrot in his mouth and was overwhelmed with disgust as he felt a burst of flavour in his mouth and spat it out. To his credit he tried the carrot again and over the following few weeks, he let himself try a few new foods. He was very pleased to tell me that his Thinking brain had grown muscles and was much stronger! His Thinking brain was able to keep him calm so he could do his deep breathing and could shut down the anxiety and the fear response. He was able to reassure himself that nothing bad was going to happen and that he could do this.

Over the next 6 months, Tommy's parents managed to extend his repertoire to the point where he would go with them to the market and together, they would try and choose a new food and he would help his parents prepare the meal. Celebrating small victories reinforced Tom's confidence and sense of agency. He is now 13 years of age, is back on his height trajectory and will eat a reasonable variety of foods. He is now able to tolerate sleepovers with friends and recently was able to attend school camp. He still has a limited range of foods, but the fear has dissipated. He uses the concept of his Thinking and Emotional brain when he's feeling anxious in other aspects of his life.

3 Discussion

Several years ago, I attended a workshop and discovered a tool which changed my practice in ways I couldn't have imagined. This tool is called the "Hand model of the Brain" and was developed by a neuro-psychiatrist, Dr. Daniel Siegel [1]. It gives a visual representation of the brain. Holding your hand in front of the young person you divide the brain into its component parts: the Thinking brain, the Emotional brain, the Brainstem and the Spinal cord (Fig. 1).

The Thinking brain (cortex) is represented by your fingers and is responsible for thinking, logic and problem solving. It is the "protector" (the Hero in the above case) and guides one to make healthy and safe choices. It helps one to be aware of internal bodily sensations and emotions and it checks in with different parts of the body to see how everything is functioning and what needs attention.

Lying beneath your thinking brain is your Emotional brain (hippocampus and amygdala) and is represented by your thumb. If left unsupported by the Thinking brain, the Emotional brain (the Villain in the above case) is vulnerable and easily influenced by "unwelcome visitors" such as mental health illnesses. These unwelcome guests like to take residence inside one's brain and take over the controls from the Thinking brain. The Emotional brain feels things intensely and is not practical or logical. It doesn't consider consequences, and it acts on impulse. If left in control of influences other than the Thinking brain, it can take one on a wild ride to dangerous places. Folding the hand into a fist represents the protection of the Emotional Brain by the Thinking brain. Without it in place, one is likely to "flip one's lid" and become emotionally dysregulated and irrational. This is demonstrated to the patient by quickly opening the fingers and exposing the thumb.

Beneath the Emotional brain lies the Brainstem which is represented by one's wrist. Here lies the control centre for breathing and one's heart rate. It functions independently but is easily influenced by both the Thinking brain and the Emotional brain. The former will calm down the heart and breathing rates with the support of techniques such as Box breathing [2] and distraction.

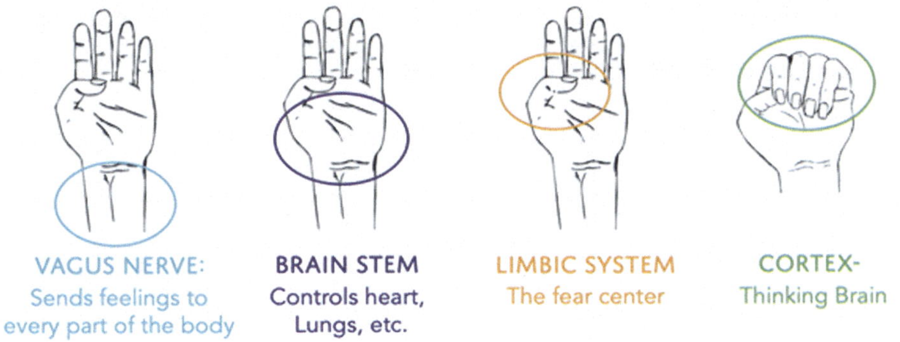

Fig. 1 Hand model of the brain. (Reproduced with permission from the artist Mikayla Maidlow; concept Dr. Dan Siegel)

I have modified the model to consider mental health illnesses as external forces which generate thoughts which may be very bossy, demanding, intimidating, and humiliating. Examples include anorexia nervosa, anxiety, depression, and obsessive compulsive disorder (OCD). Patients with neurodiversity such as Attention Deficit Hyperactivity Disorder (ADHD) and Autism spectrum disorder (ASD) are at increased risk for psychiatric comorbidity [1]. If the Thinking brain is "hiding", "malnourished" or "too exhausted", our Emotional brain becomes vulnerable to these external mental health influences which can be visualised as a bully, a villain, a Prima Donna or as a coercive partner. When it's not being protected and supported by the Thinking brain, our Emotional brain can take us on a wild ride. Tachycardia and rapid breathing herald the onset of a heightened emotional response which can leave one feeling overwhelmed and out of control. The fear response or the "fight/flight" response, can be visualised as "flipping one's lid." The Thinking brain needs to mobilise early to prevent this happening. The Thinking brain, when in control, can recognise that our Emotional brain is being influenced by these "external forces" and it can quickly come to the rescue.

4 Other Gems

- For growth concerns in childhood or adolescence, it is always helpful to review the "baby book" to see the previous growth centiles. Deviation across centiles is cause for concern and requires investigation.

References

1. Siegel, D. (2010). *Mindsight: Transform your brain with the new science of kindness*. Oneworld Publications.
2. Balban, M. Y., Neri, E., Kogon, M. M., Weed, L., Nouriani, B., Jo, B., Holl, G., Zeitzer, J. M., Spiegel, D., & Huberman, A. D. (2023). Brief structured respiration practices enhance mood and reduce physiological arousal. *Cell Reports Medicine, 4*(1), 100895. https://doi.org/10.1016/j.xcrm.2022.100895

Let's Be Aware of Trauma from Our Systems

Jennifer Harrison

1 Clinical Pearl

De-traumatising care is the responsibility of all services.

2 Clinical Case

A 7-year-old boy, Eli, was referred to the local child psychiatry service for urgent concerns about behaviour.

He was born at term and developed as expected (engaging with others at childcare, making eye contact, putting two words together) until age 2 years 6 months when his parents noticed a regression in development. He stopped engaging socially and became withdrawn and silent. Stereotypies, preoccupation with his own play interests and repetitive play were noted.

He was diagnosed with Autism Spectrum Disorder with cognitive and language impairment (Level 3/Level 3) according to the criteria of *The Diagnostic and Statistical Manual of Mental Disorders, Fifth Edition* (DSM-5), and with Attention Deficit Hyperactivity Disorder: Combined Type (ADHD) [1].

No report was given to his migrant, multilingual parents, no psychoeducation about the disorders was provided and no investigations were undertaken.

The child was enrolled in Early Childhood Intervention Services and thereafter in a specialised education setting for autistic children in the parents' health service catchment area. Five years later the child was referred for urgent developmental assessment with regression in mood noted at school, as well as behaviours of concern such as scratching, hitting and absconding. The child was unable to be

J. Harrison (✉)
Alfred ICYAMHWS, Melbourne, VIC, Australia

C. F. Lynch et al. (eds.), *The Art of Paediatric Medicine Beyond the Evidence Base*,
https://doi.org/10.1007/978-981-96-7234-9_45

educated in a shared classroom and required 1:1 supervision in a room removed from peers.

At home he required 1:1 supervision by parents because of risky climbing, aggression, absconding and agitated behaviours. There was a history of multiple pharmacological failures including psychotropics, serotonin reuptake inhibitors (SSRIs) and multiple ADHD medications, usually prescribed by a telehealth doctor, often adjusted without advice.

His parents were resorting to physical restraint and there had been multiple Child Protection notifications without positive support outcomes. The marriage between his parents had deteriorated. Distress was evident in the two younger siblings. The parents felt constantly that they were walking on eggshells, that they were trapped, that nobody could help them. Friends had fallen away, family members overseas did not understand the diagnoses and the parents were isolated except for the school and National Insurance Disability Scheme (NDIS) carers.

"You don't know how traumatised we were by the time we found your service" was the heartbreaking sentiment expressed by the parents.

3 Discussion

Approximately 23.9% of children diagnosed with Autism present with a regressive onset, and for most no underlying cause for this is found [2]. An accurate pre-regression history in this case suggested that the parents delighted in the birth of their first child (and their new life in a new country) and were traumatised by the regression in development they observed, such that they were still seeking a cure with obsessive research into new and unproven treatments.

The parents did not trust the system and would alter the child's medication according to their anxieties for their child. They had no diagnostic reports, had not received psychoeducation about the diagnoses, but had undertaken psychogenomic testing and had researched homeopathic treatments through advice from a non-treating, distant organisation. They had found their way to supports through Australia's NDIS (National Disability Insurance Scheme) but were struggling to organise an appropriately funded package of care.

Both parents exhibited symptoms of Complex Post-Traumatic Stress Syndrome (Complex PTSD). The child was non-verbal and the original diagnoses were apt, though there were now increasing behaviours of concern, anxiety and depressive features. Visual strategies, social stories, and a behaviour plan had not been implemented cohesively across settings. Care team meetings had not been implemented and no holistic medication record was available to share across settings.

Recent research suggests that autistic children are often subject to multiple accumulating traumas with more Adverse Child Events reported and increased risk of abuse including maltreatment by a parent [3]. Adults with autism present with more PTSD, as described in DSM-5, but also with more non-DSM-5 traumas [4]. In 2018, a need was identified to standardise autism assessment across Australia and revised national assessment guidelines were released by the Autism Cooperative Research Council of Australia in 2023 [5].

The case described above is complex and the severity of the disability, family isolation, the presence of co-occurring mental health conditions and an incohesive service system all played a part. Multiple factors contributed to the presenting problems including cultural differences, psychoeducation gaps around the time of diagnosis, the paucity of baseline reports, ongoing grief, burgeoning mental health problems and inconsistencies across settings. The family did not receive timely documentation of diagnoses, and there had been little in the way of advocacy or continuity of care across settings. Both parents expressed suicidal ideation and displayed symptoms of Complex PTSD. The child was voiceless and highly reliant on the system of care.

Such a complex child and family system requires a systemic response and access to mental health services as needed. Prevention and treatment are expensive, lengthy, and require systems to come together in a manner that is beyond siloed work. Narrative parent work, rationalised pharmacotherapy, psychoeducation and allied health systems working together with enhanced communication (including cross-setting behavioural support), enriched family welfare, a disability response from Child Protection which features family case conferencing rather than repetitive notifications, care team coordination meetings, and advocacy were all recommended. The aim of the recommendations was to diminish restrictive practice and enhance quality of life. It was important to consider the child's wellbeing individually, in context, but also as mediated through the wellbeing of the parents.

In follow up, the parents engaged in couple work with their mental health therapist. This work was focussed on strengthening the couple's relationship, complex trauma issues and grief work. The care team was established to work together via ongoing meetings with minutes. The issues that were discussed in care team meetings included:

(a) Role definition across the services (this necessitated some changes being made to the care team membership with additional services added).
(b) Clarity of goals (especially how change is measured and how successes may be small and incremental).

The care team meetings also provided support to the membership by decreasing isolation and boosting morale.

4 Other Gems

- A good beginning to the disability journey for parents and child is essential.
- An approach to management and support that is culturally informed, with ongoing, coordinated care is also essential.
- Trauma needs to be seen from an intersectional perspective.

- Co-occurring health and mental health conditions are the norm in autistic children (and adults).
- Grief work is ongoing but is particularly needed at the time of diagnosis.
- Systems do not operate in isolation and need to be integrated with other systemic approaches.
- Trust in the system takes time, diligence and strength from all parties.
- Staff within the systems of care need to be trained in managing complex cases.
- Services need to be well funded to do this work.
- Access to mental health services when needed is essential.

References

1. American Psychiatric Association. (2013). *Diagnostic and statistical manual of mental health disorders, (DSM-5)* (5th ed.). American Psychiatric Association.
2. Parr, J., Le Couteur, A., Baird, G., Rutter, M., et al. (2011). Early developmental regression in autism Spectrum disorder: Evidence from an international multiplex sample. *Journal of Autism and Developmental Disorders, 41*, 332–340.
3. Gajwani, R., & Minnis, H. (2022). Double jeopardy: Implications for neurodevelopmental conditions and adverse childhood experiences for child health. In *European Child and Adolescent Psychiatry*. Springer.
4. Rumball, F., Happé, F., & Grey, N. (2020). Experience of trauma and PTSD symptoms in autistic adults: Risk of PTSD development following DSM-5 and non-DSM-5 traumatic life events. *Autism Research, 13*, 2122–2132.
5. Goodall, E., et al. (2023). *National guideline for the assessment and diagnosis of autism in Australia*. Brisbane: Autism CRC.

Difficult Behaviour in Children Has Meaning

Niroshini Kennedy

1 Clinical Pearl

Behaviour is communication. When thinking about difficult behaviour in children, take time to listen and understand both the child and the parent/carer.

2 Clinical Case

Sharon is a 9-year-old Aboriginal girl in foster care who was referred for assessment of aggressive and defiant behaviour at home and school. She was born prematurely following limited antenatal care as her mother was fleeing from family violence. Sharon had a prolonged and complicated neonatal period including treatment for chronic lung disease, feeding difficulties and mild cerebral palsy.

Sharon was placed in foster care on discharge from a Neonatal Intensive Care Unit and she had several short-term kinship and foster care placements across different areas of the country. In one of these placements, she was sexually abused by a male cousin. When she was a toddler she had an accidental burn on her torso, requiring a prolonged admission and several surgeries.

Sharon had frequent appointments at a metropolitan children's hospital for follow up of her burns care. On one occasion, when she arrived at the hospital for a routine appointment, she became dysregulated in the waiting room, telling her carers that she was afraid to be in the hospital. She ran away, screaming that she wanted to kill herself and became aggressive and distressed. Following the involvement of the police, ambulance and mental health services, she was admitted to the hospital,

N. Kennedy (✉)
Victorian Aboriginal Health Service and The Royal Children's Hospital Melbourne, Melbourne, VIC, Australia

C. F. Lynch et al. (eds.), *The Art of Paediatric Medicine Beyond the Evidence Base*,
https://doi.org/10.1007/978-981-96-7234-9_46

sedated and assessed by the mental health team. When she arrived at the outpatient clinic for her next appointment, she was defiant, disengaged and shrugging her shoulders to any question asked, whilst scrolling on her phone.

After involving the hospital's Aboriginal Liaison team and many sessions with Sharon focusing on building rapport, trust and understanding her goals, we were able to unpack her fear related to past experiences. She asked me, "Am I a bad person? I get so angry when someone tries to touch me." We were able to explain how that fear response was her body trying to keep her safe due to many negative past experiences. We worked together to make a plan, for example, using the safe space of an Aboriginal family place within the hospital, liaising with the burns team to ensure that Sharon had a consistent clinician for each of her visits, allowing her to visit animal attractions within the hospital, and regulating practices of sensory activities that she enjoyed (trampolining and listening to hip hop music on her headphones) on her way to the hospital. She would carry her possum skin with her for comfort.

Her foster carers expressed anger and disappointment in Sharon's behaviour which they interpreted as wilful and defiant. Advocacy with her statutory child protection team about the importance of stability of placement and support for her foster carers was crucial to help them understand Sharon's behaviour so they could better support her. We planned a 'dry run' visit to practice these steps, to meet the people she would be seeing including her treating Burns team. Giving Sharon some control over her care and helping her understand her own behaviour was the key. It meant that Sharon could continue to access the care that she needed and strengthened the therapeutic relationship with her clinicians and built her own sense of agency and empowerment. Sharon developed a poster which mapped out her own "self-care plan" for hospital visits incorporating her regulating activities, and an outline of her plan for hospital days.

3 Discussion

Childhood is a time of immense promise and potential. But the flipside is that it is a time of immense vulnerability. We know that not all children have a healthy childhood. Some children are vulnerable through the social determinants of health, and some are exposed to stress and toxic stress as a result of illness, prolonged hospitalisations, and traumatic events. Adverse childhood experiences (ACE) can profoundly alter brain architecture and disrupt the neurobiological pathways that affect executive function, emotional regulation, learning, wellbeing and physical health.

When children experience trauma, their brains go from a learning brain to a survival brain. Trauma is biochemically encoded in the brain—prolonged or chronic stress causes adaptations in the homeostatic regulation of neurochemicals which means that the brain is primed and has a more sensitive stress response, through cortisol and adrenaline i.e. fight, flight, freeze. This repetitive stress activation takes an adaptive, or lifesaving process, to one that is maladaptive. I always try to keep that adaptive, survivor child in mind when I see a hypervigilant hyperactive child visiting me for the first time in a clinic. That extra movement and defiance kept the child safe for a long time and it will take some time for me to prove to them that I am a safe person.

Trauma informed care is the term that is used to describe care that takes into account a person's early life experiences and their stress responses, then seeks to provide care in a way that is healing, builds safe therapeutic relationships, is sensitive to the responses of a traumatised person and avoids re-traumatisation.

4 Other Gems

- Take time to build a safe relationship with the child. Slow down, ask permission before you examine.
- Understand the child as an individual.
- Interests and strengths: play, particular skills, habits, temperament.
- Triggers/dislikes/sensory preferences.
- Calming rituals and comfort objects.
- Co-regulation in the therapeutic relationship—don't over-react to bad behaviour in the consulting room. Set safe boundaries and model co-regulation.
- Psychoeducation.
- Asking **"What happened to you?"** rather than "What's wrong with you?" [1].
- Talking therapy is rarely useful as a first step. Bruce Perry talks about the three R's: regulate, relate, and reason. Reasoning with the child is the third step, not the first step [2].

References

1. Perry, B. D., & Winfrey, O. (2021). *What happened to you?: conversations on trauma, resilience, and healing*. First edition. New York, NY: Flatiron Books.
2. Perry, B. D. (2008). Child maltreatment: The role of abuse and neglect in developmental psychopathology. In T. P. Beauchaine & S. P. Hinshaw (Eds.), *Textbook of child and adolescent psychopathology* (pp. 93–128). Wiley.

A Spoonful of Medicine Makes the Sugar Go Down?

Jessica Nguyen and Rupert Hinds

1 Clinical Pearl

Sometimes it's "can't eat" not "won't eat."

2 Clinical Case

A 9-year-old boy, Mateo, was referred to the gastroenterology team after a previous inpatient admission for Avoidant Restrictive Food Intake Disorder (ARFID). He had a background of asthma, eczema and resolved egg allergy. His parents had recently separated in an acrimonious manner. Because of his short stature, he had been the victim of some bullying at school. In the gastroenterology clinic, he mentioned that chunks of meat and bread would sometimes feel like they were getting stuck in his throat. His mother commented that he had always been a slow eater. A gastroscopy was performed which revealed some of the classic features of eosinophilic oesophagitis (EOE)—linear furrows, white dots (see Fig. 1). Biopsies subsequently confirmed EOE with significant eosinophilia found at two levels of the oesophagus. Mateo was managed with topical steroids which resulted in an improvement in his dysphagia. His subsequent gastroscopy revealed normalisation of endoscopic appearance and biopsies.

J. Nguyen · R. Hinds (✉)
Department of Gastroenterology, Monash Children Hospital, Clayton, VIC, Australia

C. F. Lynch et al. (eds.), *The Art of Paediatric Medicine Beyond the Evidence Base*,
https://doi.org/10.1007/978-981-96-7234-9_47

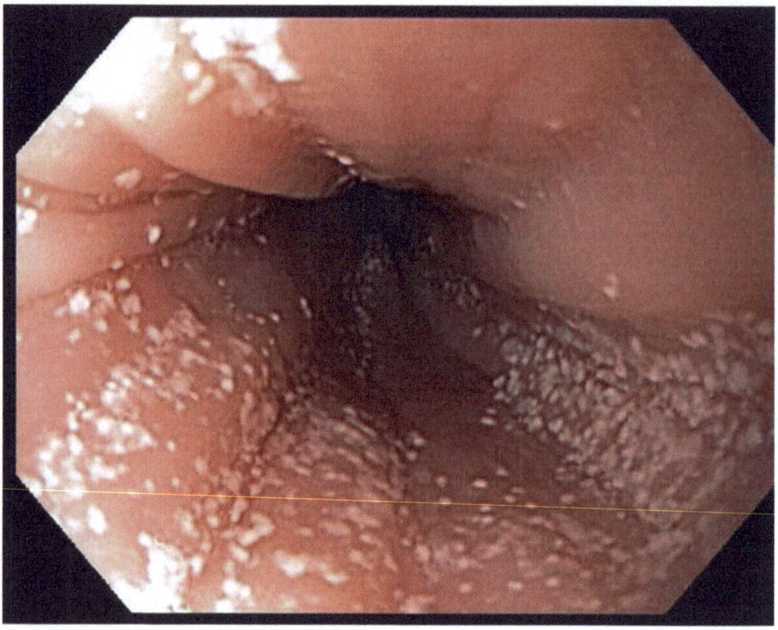

Fig. 1 Endoscopic appearance of EOE

3 Discussion

Eosinophilic oesophagitis (EOE) is a chronic condition leading to oesophageal dysfunction with build-up of eosinophils in the oesophagus. It is more commonly seen in males, patients with an atopic background, a past history of oesophageal atresia or a family history of EOE [1]. The cause of EOE is unclear, however it is believed to be due to exposure to food antigens in genetically susceptible individuals. The incidence and prevalence of EOE is increasing over time [2].

EOE symptoms can vary depending on patient age and severity of inflammation. Toddlers and infants may present with non-specific symptoms such as vomiting, refusing food, or failure to thrive. Children of school age may present with abdominal pain or vomiting. Older children and adolescents may describe dysphagia, heartburn, and food bolus obstruction [3].

In patients with clinical symptoms, the diagnosis of EOE is confirmed on upper gastrointestinal endoscopy with histology of the oesophageal biopsies demonstrating >15 eosinophils per high power field at multiple levels of the oesophagus [4]. Characteristic macroscopic findings, such as rings, white plaques, linear furrows or strictures, are not always seen in patients with EOE, therefore biopsy is critical to confirm the diagnosis. Clinical symptoms may not always correlate with histological findings. Assessment of remission is based on histological appearance on follow-up endoscopies. Allergy testing is usually not helpful in EOE.

Treatment options for EOE in paediatrics include:

(a) Dietary elimination of certain foods.
(b) Proton pump inhibitors (PPIs).
(c) Topical steroids (such as swallowed fluticasone or budesonide) [5].

There are various elimination diets that can be trialled, depending on the patient situation. Clinicians should consider the specific patient and their needs, including referring to a dietician for support if required. In some patients, oral PPIs can be effective to induce remission. Topical steroids are a safe, effective treatment for patients [6]. Long term treatment and follow up is important in EOE to improve symptoms, as well as prevent long term complications such as strictures or food bolus obstructions.

4 Other Gems

- Have a low threshold for investigating for EOE in atopic children, even when there are behavioural concerns with regards to restrictive eating.

References

1. Jorge, A., Salvatore, O., Alexandra, P., et al. (2024). Diagnosis and management of eosinophilic esophagitis in children: An update from the European Society for Paediatric Gastroenterology, Hepatology and Nutrition (ESPGHAN). *Journal of Pediatric Gastroenterology and Nutrition, 79*(2), 394–437.
2. Dellon, E., & Hirano, I. (2018). Epidemiology and natural history of eosinophilic esophagitis. Epidemiology and natural history of eosinophilic esophagitis. *Gastroenterology, 154*(2), 319–332.
3. De Matteis, A., Pagliaro, G., Corleto, V. D., Pacchiarotti, C., Di Giulio, E., Villa, M. P., Parisi, P., Vassallo, F., Ziparo, C., & Di Nardo, G. (2020). Eosinophilic esophagitis in children: Clinical findings and diagnostic approach. *Current Pediatric Reviews, 16*(3), 206–214. https://doi.org/10.2174/1573396315666191004110549
4. Agulló-García, A., Cubero, J. L., Lezaun, A., Boné, J., Guallar, I., & Colás, C. (2020). Clinical and anatomopathological features of eosinophilic oesophagitis in children and adults. *Allergologia et Immunopathologia, 48*(6), 560–567.
5. Sharlin, C. S., Mukkada, V. A., Putnam, P. E., et al. (2023). Treatment of Pediatric eosinophilic esophagitis: Traditional and novel therapies. *Current Gastroenterology Reports, 25*, 289–298. https://doi.org/10.1007/s11894-023-00893-6
6. Hao, L., Lu, Y., Li, T., & Gong, B. (2021). A meta-analysis of efficacy of topical steroids in eosinophilic esophagitis: From the perspective of histologic, clinical, and endoscopic outcome. *Gastroenterología y Hepatología, 44*(4), 251–260.

A B C …. DEFG Airway, Breathing, Circulation…. Don't Ever Forget Genetics

Srinidhi Rao

1 Clinical Pearl

Rapid genomic testing (RGT) in the acute care setting provides a relatively high diagnostic yield. Having this information impacts management decisions and clinical outcomes, with important implications for patient care.

2 Clinical Case

An 8-year-old girl, Mariam, was found by her parents to be unresponsive. Her parents commenced cardiopulmonary resuscitation and called an ambulance for help. Mariam was found to be in ventricular fibrillation and was successfully defibrillated with return to spontaneous circulation. She was transferred to a tertiary institution where she was managed in the intensive care unit with cooling and ventilator support. There was no significant past medical or family history. Mariam had normal cardiac structure and function on echocardiography. Her ECG during the episode and subsequent ECGs are captured below (Figs. 1 and 2).

First ECG

The first ECG demonstrates ventricular fibrillation whilst the second ECG demonstrates sinus rhythm with prolonged QT interval. Mariam made a good recovery and was extubated. She underwent insertion of transvenous implantable cardioverter defibrillator (ICD) implantation in the next few days.

S. Rao (✉)
Monash Children's Hospital, Clayton, VIC, Australia

C. F. Lynch et al. (eds.), *The Art of Paediatric Medicine Beyond the Evidence Base*,
https://doi.org/10.1007/978-981-96-7234-9_48

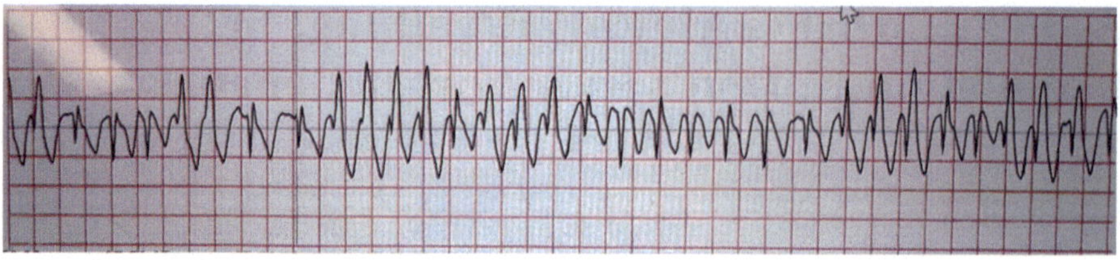

Fig. 1 ECG showing ventricular fibrillation (VF)

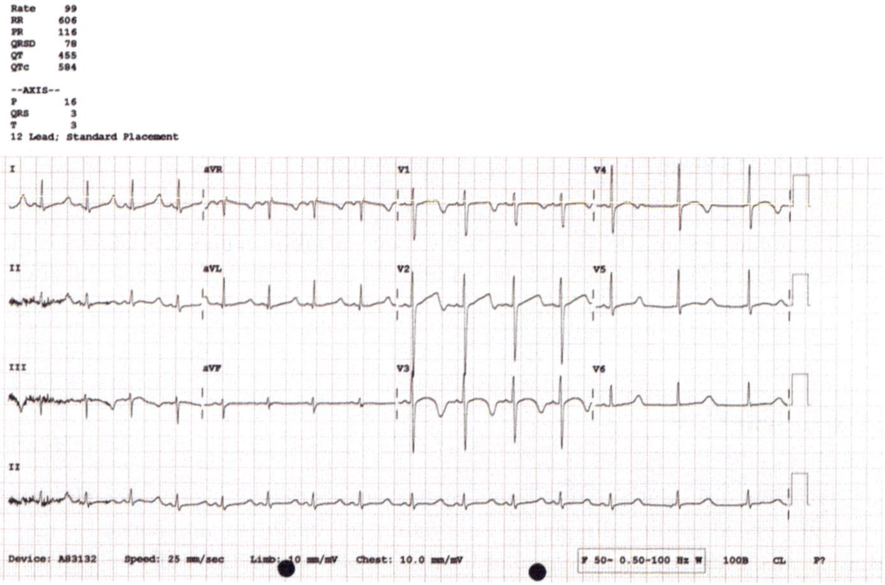

Fig. 2 Subsequent ECG demonstrating prolonged QT interval

The Genetic Team was consulted due to the high probability of long QT syndrome being the cause of her cardiac arrest. Whole genome sequencing was performed for her and her parents as part of acute care genomics flagship.

Long QT syndrome—type 3 was identified due to a de novo mutation in SCN5A c.4453A > G, (pLle1485Val). She was then commenced on nadolol (beta blocker) and mexiletine (effective in LQTS type 3).

Mariam's family were relieved to understand the risk of themselves or their other children having similar events was extremely low.

3 Discussion

Genetics and genetic testing have rapidly evolved in recent years with testing becoming more readily available and results becoming increasingly available in a timely fashion.

From microarray to exome sequencing and now to genome sequencing, testing has evolved with increasing diagnostic yield. Advances in technology, bioinformatics and analytical capabilities have led to the development of rapid genomic testing (RGT), and even ultra-rapid genomic testing (uRGT), where a diagnosis can be made in hours or days, rather than months [1].

Whilst the tests are expensive, complete cost benefit analyses have proven cost effectiveness in the long run. Also, the tests do impact acute and long-term management [2] as demonstrated in the above case.

However, to use the tests effectively, careful patient selection is important and thus it is important to consult clinical geneticists in determining the correct test for a patient.

In addition, even though the tests are conducted in the setting of an acutely ill child, appropriate pre-test and post-test counselling is critical. Psychosocial and ethical aspects need to be considered prior to proceeding with tests.

Careful follow-up of the patients is important as is cascade screening (a systematic process of identification of individuals at risk for a genetic condition) in the presence of significant abnormalities.

References

1. Vears, D. F., Lynch, F., Nisselle, A., Ayres, S., & Stark, Z. (2024). Rapid genomic testing in critically ill patients with genetic conditions: Position statement by the human genetics Society of Australasia. *European Journal of Human Genetics, 32*, 150–154.
2. McDermott, H., Sherlaw-Sturrock, C., Baptista, J., Hartles-Spencer, L., & Naik, S. (2022). Rapid exome sequencing in critically ill children impacts acute and long-term management of patients and their families: A retrospective regional evaluation. *European Journal of Medical Genetics, 65*(9), 104571. https://doi.org/10.1016/j.ejmg.2022.104571

To Block or Not to Block?

Ngai Lam Woo and Srinidhi Rao

1 Clinical Pearl

Adenosine is not always the right treatment option in tachyarrhythmias.

2 Clinical Case

An 11-year-old boy, Sebastian, is brought to Emergency via ambulance after complaining of lethargy, light-headedness, and nausea. He was noted to have a rapid heart rate by his parents at home and mentions that he is known to Paediatric Cardiology for his arrhythmia. His medical notes indicate that he has Wolff-Parkinson-White pattern on his baseline ECG, and that he is not on any medications. Sebastian is hemodynamically stable. His ECG is shown below (Fig. 1).

What treatment options would you consider?

3 Discussion

Wolff-Parkinson-White (WPW) pattern, or pre-excitation, indicates the presence of a congenital accessory pathway bypassing the atrioventricular (AV) node. Most commonly, WPW results in a form of supraventricular tachycardia (SVT) known as

N. L. Woo
The Children's Hospital at Westmead, Westmead, NSW, Australia

S. Rao (✉)
Monash Children's Hospital, Clayton, VIC, Australia

C. F. Lynch et al. (eds.), *The Art of Paediatric Medicine Beyond the Evidence Base*,
https://doi.org/10.1007/978-981-96-7234-9_49

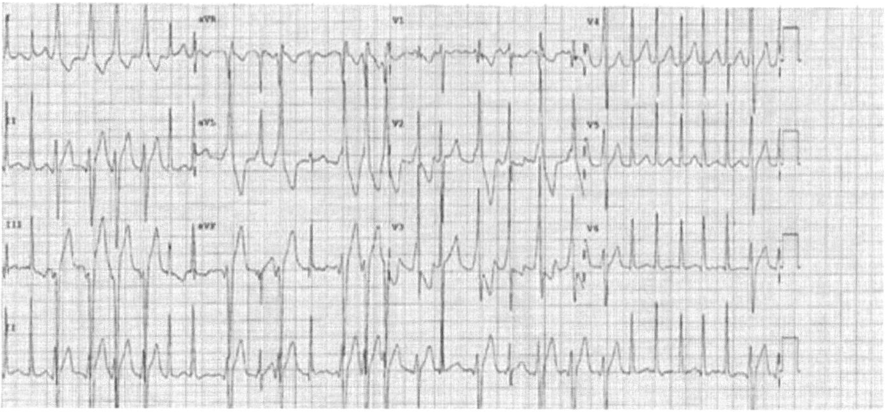

Fig. 1 ECG on presentation to hospital

AV re-entrant tachycardia (AVRT). In AVRT, the accessory pathway creates a "repeating" loop of impulses being sent to the ventricles [1]. This manifests as a regular narrow complex tachycardia and is generally well-tolerated in infants and children.

Atrial fibrillation, as the ECG nicely demonstrates, is an uncommon form of SVT associated with WPW [2]. It is a result of atrial impulses uncontrollably conducting into the ventricles through the accessory pathway. Atrial fibrillation can be life-threatening and is one of the few instances where adenosine is contraindicated [3].

Adenosine acts as an AV nodal blocker and may result in complete conduction through the accessory pathway when used. This will cause the rhythm to progress to ventricular tachycardia (VT) or ventricular fibrillation (VF).

Procainamide and planned electrical cardioversion are the accepted management options for atrial fibrillation in the setting of hemodynamic stability.

In the acutely unstable patient with either form of SVT, electrical cardioversion is the primary modality of treatment.

4 Other Gems

- Atrial fibrillation in the context of WPW is a strong indicator for a prompt referral for an electrophysiology study and ablation of the pathway.
- SVT may not always present as a narrow-complex tachycardia—aberrant conduction through the pathway may present with a rapid and regular broad-complex tachycardia.
- If electric cardioversion is required for SVT, always ensure that it is delivered synchronously—an asynchronous shock during repolarization may precipitate ventricular fibrillation (VF).

References

1. Haxel, C. S., Flyer, J. N., Silver, E. S., et al. (2016). Evaluation and management of the asymptomatic child with Wolff–Parkinson–White. *Current Pediatrics Reports, 4*, 45–52.
2. Centurion, O. A. (2011). Atrial fibrillation in the Wolff-Parkinson-White syndrome. *Journal of Atrial Fibrillation, 4*(1), 287.
3. Chhabra, L., Goyal, A., & Benham, M. D. (2023). Wolff-Parkinson-white syndrome. In: StatPearls [Internet]. Treasure Island (FL): StatPearls Publishing. Available from: https://www.ncbi.nlm.nih.gov/books/NBK554437/

Caution, but Perspective, in Paediatric Bone Lesions

Stewart Morrison

1 Clinical Pearl

Osteochondromas (also known as exostoses) are common. Diligence is important, but overly cautious diagnosis, without perspective, can cause families and children undue stress.

2 Clinical Case

An 11-year-old male, Zayd, bumped his right leg in a football match and noticed a prominent lump on his leg. This was initially treated for a few months by his physiotherapist as Osgood-Schlatter's disease. However, the lump continued to grow, and he attended his general practitioner for an X-ray.

The X-ray reported a solitary osteochondroma (exostosis) of the right proximal tibia. The report concluded that "review by a Paediatric Sarcoma Specialist" could be indicated. Zayd was referred by his general practitioner to a tertiary paediatric centre. However, the use of the word 'sarcoma' worried the family intensely. After receiving the report. Zayd's mother googled extensively about treatment for osteosarcoma and found articles pertaining to the fact that osteochondromas can transform into bone cancers. His family became worried that this tumour could spread, and treatment may arrive too late. After a very stressful 4 days of hearing nothing about a review appointment, Zayd's parents drove him to a Children's Hospital

S. Morrison (✉)
The Royal Children's Hospital, Melbourne, VIC, Australia

Alfred Health, Melbourne, VIC, Australia

Epworth Healthcare, Richmond, VIC, Australia

C. F. Lynch et al. (eds.), *The Art of Paediatric Medicine Beyond the Evidence Base*,
https://doi.org/10.1007/978-981-96-7234-9_50

Emergency Department with an enormous amount of anxiety. They remained in the emergency department overnight before finally meeting a member of the orthopaedic team in the morning and being provided a review appointment in 2 weeks to the appropriate clinic.

During this appointment, Zayd's family learnt that osteochondromas are benign lesions, and reasonably commonly present during an adolescent growth spurt. After learning about the natural history of the lesion, his family were reassured that the chance of malignant transformation was extremely small. After much reassurance and discussion to help them understand, Zayd's family elected to plan surgery for lesion excision, after the current football season had finished at the end of the year.

3 Discussion

Solitary osteochondromas are benign bone tumours that commonly occur in children and adolescents, often manifesting as single cartilage-capped outgrowths near the growth plates of bones, particularly around the knee but can be found throughout the body. These growths typically arise during childhood, get larger more rapidly during the pubertal growth spurt, and cease developing once skeletal growth is complete. This behaviour, coupled with histological and genetic studies as well as the fact they nearly always grow 'away' from the physis, point to a histological origin from physeal cartilage cells [1].

While solitary osteochondromas are isolated occurrences, they can also present as part of multiple hereditary exostoses (MHE), a genetic condition characterised by multiple such growths. This condition can run in families or may present de-novo.

There is a risk of malignant transformation that is variable between studies, but is quoted as between 1% and 2% [2]. Clinical experience may indicate the risk is a lot lower than this, as these studies are often done in tertiary tumour institutions.

Osteochondromas have a very typical radiological appearance (see Fig. 1), either sessile (a gradual 'hill') or pedunculated (a stalk with a bulbous end). In both cases, growth appears to be away from the nearest joint. Signs of a more aggressive process such as sunburst appearance, onion skinning, or immature periosteal reaction, are not seen. CT or MRI imaging is often not required, but may be used in order to identify proximity to local anatomical structures or measure the radiolucent cartilage cap. A thick cartilage cap in an adult may raise concern for malignant transformation, however the cartilage cap can be reasonably thick anyway in the skeletally immature population, with some studies defining up to 30 mm^3 as acceptable [3].

Lesions around the knee (distal femur, proximal tibia) are common areas of presentation because a greater proportion of leg growth happens at the adjacent physes. Medial proximal tibial lesions.

often become symptomatic more quickly than other lesions, due to their irritation of the tendons inserting into the pes anserinus.

Management of osteochondromas depends on the location, the size, and the amount of concern they are giving the patient. Small asymptomatic lesions,

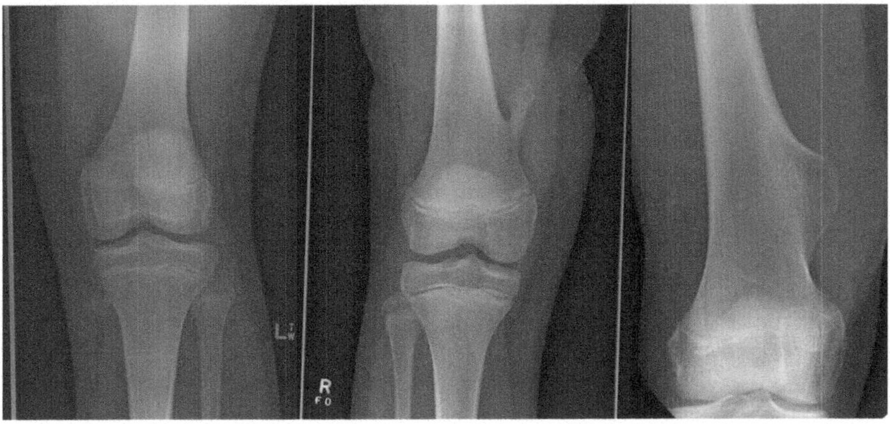

A B C

Fig. 1 (**a**) Proximal Medial Tibial Osteochondroma, (**b**) Distal Femoral Pedunculated Osteochondroma, (**c**) Distal Femoral Sessile Osteochondroma

sometimes identified on x-rays performed for other reasons, may be left alone. Larger lesions, or those causing irritation, can be surgically removed on an elective, non-urgent basis. Restriction of joint motion, or neurovascular compromise due to the mass effect of lesions, is extremely rare, but can happen particularly with proximal fibula lesions, due to their proximity to the common peroneal nerve.

Patients presenting with osteochondromas with completely typical features should be advised that the lesion is likely to increase throughout growth, but then cease to enlarge once skeletal growth is complete. Referral to an orthopaedic service may be warranted in the case of overt parental concern, large lesions, or those causing symptoms.

4 Other Gems

- Malignant tumours of bone in adolescents, such as osteosarcoma and Ewing sarcoma, look very different to osteochondromas.

References

1. Khare, G. N. (2011). An analysis of indications for surgical excision and complications in 116 consecutive cases of osteochondroma. *Musculoskeletal Surgery, 95*(2), 121–125.
2. Righi, A., Pacheco, M., Cocchi, S., et al. (2022). Secondary peripheral chondrosarcoma arising in solitary osteochondroma: Variables influencing prognosis and survival. *Orphanet Journal of Rare Diseases, 17*(1), 74.
3. Bailescu, I., Popescu, M., Sarafoleanu, L. R., et al. (2022). Diagnosis and evolution of the benign tumor osteochondroma. *Experimental and Therapeutic Medicine, 23*(1), 103.

Learning at School Is Everyone's Business: The Paediatrician's Role

Taryn Luitingh and Gehan Roberts

1 Clinical Pearl

A DSM-5 diagnosis is less important than providing understanding and explanation of a child's profile of strengths and vulnerabilities.

2 Clinical Case

Twelve-year-old Tess was referred to our clinic with concerns about learning difficulties, in particular, challenges with reading and comprehension. Tess is the daughter of high achieving parents. There is no family history of learning difficulties, intellectual disability or neurodevelopmental disorders/delays. Tess's parents requested to see a paediatrician due to worries that "Tess is dyslexic", a concern first noticed during the COVID-19 pandemic, a time when Tess was largely engaged in remote learning. Tess's parents observed difficulties with her reading and her ability to understand what she had read. Tess's father supervised her during remote learning and shared how he would often get frustrated when Tess was not able to read stories aloud, often hesitating, making mistakes or making up words. As a result of

T. Luitingh
The Centre of Community Child Health, The Royal Children's Hospital, Parkville, VIC, Australia

G. Roberts (✉)
The Centre of Community Child Health, The Royal Children's Hospital, Parkville, VIC, Australia

Department of Paediatrics, University of Melbourne, Parkville, VIC, Australia

Murdoch Children's Research Institute, Parkville, VIC, Australia

C. F. Lynch et al. (eds.), *The Art of Paediatric Medicine Beyond the Evidence Base*,
https://doi.org/10.1007/978-981-96-7234-9_51

these difficulties, Tess would try to avoid reading and comprehension tasks. When Tess had to discuss or answer questions related to a passage, she would "stare into space" or answer "I don't know." Tess's parents were very keen to get a Specific Learning Disorder (SLD) diagnosis, as they felt this would allow them to access interventions that would "fix the problem."

In our Learning Difficulties Clinic, we rely on a multi-disciplinary assessment and multi-source information to ensure the young person's challenges and experiences are thoroughly understood. We gather information from the child, their parents/carers, schools/tutors, and allied health teams. Members of our clinic team, consisting of a teacher, an educational psychologist and a paediatrician, are involved in aspects of the assessment.

During our time together, we explored Tess's developmental and educational history along with her general health and wellbeing. This was to ensure we identified any other potential co-occurring mental health, developmental, medical conditions and lifestyle factors (diet, sleep, exercise), that may impact her learning and wellbeing. Tess's physical examination was unremarkable, including assessment of hearing and vision. No medical investigations were necessary. We also spent time exploring a detailed family history to gain an insight into the family dynamics as well as any identifying risk factors for learning difficulties.

Tess underwent cognitive and tailored academic assessments with an educational psychologist. This gave insight into the thinking and problem-solving skills Tess uses to tackle academic tasks as well as measuring her academic skills, compared to same age/grade peers. Tess participated in the Wechsler Intelligence Scale for Children Fifth Edition (WISC-V) and the Wechsler Individual Achievement Test Fourth Edition (WIAT-4). The results of these assessments revealed that Tess had subtle relative weaknesses with her literacy skills, compared with her cognitive potential (which was in the average range), with a relative weakness in working memory and processing speed. Her experience of anxiety and lowered self-confidence, however, were particularly evident during the assessment. These likely exacerbated her learning challenges in the classroom. This information was considered in the context of the Diagnostic and Statistical Manual of Mental Disorders, Fifth Edition (DSM-5) criteria for Specific Learning Disorders. Tess did not meet the criteria for an SLD given she had not had a trial of targeted evidence-based support (criterion A); her academic scores were not significantly below that of her same age peers (criterion B); more plausible explanations may include an extended period of remote learning and her anxiety (criterion D).

When constructing Tess's formulation and sharing this with Tess and her parents, we discussed that even though Tess's difficulties did not fulfil SLD criteria, she would still benefit from evidence-based academic interventions. These interventions are likely to help scaffold Tess's learning abilities, increase her self-confidence and reduce her academic task-related anxiety. We highlighted Tess's strengths and added recommendations to incorporate these strengths into her learning experience. The opportunities to utilise these strengths are likely to further build Tess's confidence and increase her school engagement. We also recommended the support of a psychologist to help Tess manage her anxiety. Crucially, we spent time reinforcing the importance of not diminishing Tess's experience of difficulty by deconstructing misconceptions around Tess being "lazy" or it being "her fault because she is not trying." For Tess, advocating for a positive learning environment while incorporating learning and psychology supports is essential for her to thrive and progress successfully along her learning journey.

In addition to providing family feedback, meetings were arranged with Tess's teachers and school wellbeing team to ensure their understanding of Tess's challenges and to discuss suggested recommendations and accommodations so that they could be feasibly implemented. This team-based approach fosters respectful and collegiate interactions between care teams, promoting meaningful and long-term relationships between the health care and education teams.

3 Discussion

Developmental and behavioural concerns encompass the majority of presentations to general paediatricians, and learning difficulties are one of the most common presenting concerns [1]. There are often multifactorial components impacting learning. The paediatrician's role is to identify these contributing factors so that appropriate and effective support can be offered. To achieve identification of co-occurring conditions, we recommend a comprehensive assessment of a child's general health, development, mental health, learning and psychosocial history [2, 3]. This understanding, informing a clear formulation, can guide the implementation of a multipronged approach, with support tailored specifically to the needs of the child.

As was seen in the case study, it is common that families presenting to their paediatrician come with an expectation of a definitive diagnosis that explains the academic difficulty their child is experiencing. Consequently, it is pivotal to take the time to explore a family's understanding of the diagnosis they are seeking, as well as why they are seeking it. For example, *do they believe that a diagnosis will ensure access to services? Does a diagnosis help with acceptance of the struggles their child is experiencing?* We often spend time acknowledging the impact and support needs of the child's learning difficulties, while simultaneously dispelling myths and misinformation around the concept of SLDs.

Due to the complex multifactorial nature of learning difficulties, the support of a multidisciplinary team is essential to gather knowledge and further assess children and their needs [2–4]. Previous research by Mittal et al. found that families who took part in a multidisciplinary assessment better understood their child's difficulties [3]. Within the multidisciplinary team, the paediatrician holds a multifaceted role of investigator, advocate, coordinator of services and provider of a clear management plan. Obtaining collateral history from the child's parents/carers, school and/or external tutors is essential to develop a detailed understanding of the difficulties the child is experiencing, previous assistance and intervention and the response to these interventions. Just as importantly, information gathered should include the child's strengths and interests, promoting a holistic understanding of the child's abilities. Working with teachers and educational psychologists adds vital information about the child's approach to learning and their cognitive and academic profile.

A clear formulation, communicated in lay language to the family, school and the rest of the care team, is essential. It should be made clear whether an SLD diagnosis has been made, and if not, why not, with reference to DSM-5 criteria. The DSM-5 outlines SLD as neurodevelopmental disorders characterised by persistent impairment in at least one of three areas of learning:

- reading (dyslexia)
- written expression (dysgraphia) and/or
- math (dyscalculia)

SLDs are typically diagnosed in early childhood, however, may not be recognised until adulthood.

There are four SLD diagnostic criteria described in the DSM-5 and are summarised as follows [5, 6]:

(a) Difficulties in at least one area of reading, written expression and/or math, for at least 6 months despite targeted support.
(b) Academic skills are considerably below what is expected for the child's age impacting school, work or everyday activities.
(c) Difficulties are present during school-age even if problems experienced are only significant in adulthood.
(d) Learning difficulties are not due to other conditions (e.g. intellectual disability, vision or hearing problems, difficulties with language, neurological conditions etc).

The child's individual profile of vulnerabilities and strengths should form the basis of supportive and tailored recommendations. Incorporating the child's strengths ensures strategies are created to foster self-confidence and self-esteem. Recommendations should be child-centred and take into account what is feasible (e.g. economically and availability of personnel) for both the family and the school to implement. This is imperative to ensure that affordability and practical implementation of the recommendations can be successfully achieved. Furthermore, it should be emphasised to families that the lack of an SLD diagnosis should not restrict access to evidence-based intervention in the school and/or home setting.

Further useful resources for families and schools can be found within the reference section [7–10].

4 Other Gems

- Provide parents reassurance that even if a SLD diagnosis is not made, evidence-based interventions can still be implemented by schools or parent/s to support their child's learning.

- It is important to acknowledge the significant interplay of academic performance with a child's experience of low self-esteem and anxiety that may have evolved during their academic struggles.
- Collateral history is key to discern the functional impact of the child's learning difficulty so that the recommendations are tailored to the child's strength and weakness profile.

References

1. Jongeling, B., & Roberts, G. (2018). Models of care in neurodevelopmental-behavioural paediatrics. *Journal of Paediatrics and Child Health, 54*(10), 1100–1103.
2. Lyon, G. R. (1996). Learning disabilities. *The Future of Children, 6*(1), 54–76.
3. Mittal, R., Sciberras, E., Sewell, J., & Efron, D. (2014). Assessment of children with learning and behavioural problems: Comparison of a multidisciplinary and sole paediatrician model. *Journal of Paediatrics and Child Health, 50*(2), 135–140.
4. Roberts, G., Price, A., & Oberklaid, F. (2012). Paediatrician's role in caring for children with learning difficulties. *Journal of Paediatrics and Child Health, 48*(12), 1086–1090.
5. American Psychiatric Association. (2022). *Diagnostic and statistical manual of mental disorders*, 5th ed. Text Revision (DSM-5-TR) American Psychiatric Association Publishing.
6. American Psychiatric Association. (2024). https://www.psychiatry.org/patients-families/specific-learning-disorder/what-is-specific-learning-disorder. Accessed 13 Nov 2024.
7. SPELDVictoria. (2024). https://speldvic.org.au/. Accessed 13 Nov 2024.
8. AUSPELD. (2024). https://auspeld.org.au/. Accessed 13 Nov 2024.
9. Raising Children's Network. (2024). https://raisingchildren.net.au/school-age/school-learning/learning-difficulties/learning-disabilities-signs-and-support. Accessed 13 Nov 2024.
10. Learning Difficulties Australia (LDA). (2024). https://ldaustralia.org/ors/. Accessed 13 Nov 2024.

Dysphonia in Children: When Should I Be Worried?

Sarah Morrison

1 Clinical Pearl

A hoarse voice in children is often benign but requires a thorough clinical assessment.

2 Clinical Case

Jamie, an 6-year-old boy, developed a hoarse voice which persisted beyond the typical period for laryngitis (more than a mont) , and his GP referred him to see an ENT surgeon due to an ongoing hoarse voice.

3 Discussion

Dysphonia, or a hoarse voice, in children can generate significant anxiety in the family. For most, the cause is benign and very manageable. In saying that, it requires nuance in the clinical assessment to differentiate benign dysphonia from worrisome pathology.

S. Morrison (✉)
Monash Health, Clayton, VIC, Australia

Royal Children's Hospital, Parkville, VIC, Australia

Epworth Richmond Hospital, Richmond, VIC, Australia

Victorian Children's Clinic, Malvern, VIC, Australia

ENT Parkville at MACCS, Parkville, VIC, Australia

C. F. Lynch et al. (eds.), *The Art of Paediatric Medicine Beyond the Evidence Base*,
https://doi.org/10.1007/978-981-96-7234-9_52

Traditional medical training reinforces the message of dysphonia as a sign of airway compromise. Whilst this can be true, especially in the acute setting, it is quite uncommon in a well child in the community. True dysphonia as assessed by speech pathologists occurs in around 5–8% of 5-year-olds [1]. Parental reporting of voice concerns however can be as high as 25%. The disconnect between these numbers may be due to the understanding of what voice and dysphonia mean.

It is relevant to be able to differentiate between dysphonia from articulation errors and prosody (lack of intonation—pitch variation and rhythm of speech). Dysphonia, articulation and prosody all have a large impact on the understandability of speech. The impact of each has a multiplication effect on speech understandability. Ultimately the function of the voice is to communicate clearly, which requires addressing all components of speech.

True dysphonia is described by features such as hoarseness (rough versus smooth), pitch range (low frequency pitch range, limited pitch range), phonation breaks (voice breaks or cracks during speech), and the loss of voice (aphonia). Having some basic descriptors help define the issue and communicate with relevant teams accurately.

Parental anxiety around dysphonia often relates to concern around what is causing the dysphonia, and the potential for serious pathology. Red flags for serious pathology involve symptoms and signs of airway obstruction. This may involve stridor, work of breathing on exertion, new onset snoring. The time frame, persistence of dysphonia and severity of dysphonia are all relevant. Severe low pitch rough voice that has been progressively deteriorating with new onset of stridor is very concerning. This requires assessment by an ENT specialist. The urgency is dependent on the rate of progression of symptoms.

Potential serious pathology includes laryngeal papilloma, also known as juvenile recurrent respiratory papillomatosis (jRRP). jRRP is caused by vertical transmission of HPV (human papillomavirus) [2]. jRRP has almost been eradicated in Australia due to the Gardasil immunization program. However, mothers born outside of Australia may not have been immunized and the children may be at risk.

The acute dysphonia with breathing difficulty is most commonly seen as croup. Croup has a characteristic bark that is generally recognized by caregivers. Other causes of acute dysphonia involve trauma such as fall onto the neck, blow to the neck by an object (blunt or sharp). This is uncommon in prepubertal children as their laryngeal cartilage framework is quite soft and compliant.

The more common scenario is a child with a hoarse voice that fluctuates in severity over a long-time course with no associated difficulty breathing or stridor. In this situation the most likely diagnosis is vocal nodules. Vocal nodules are the cause of between 70–95% of dysphonia seen in paediatric voice clinics at large centres [2–4]. Vocal nodules are a benign thickening of the free edge of the vocal cord. It is thought to be partially due to vocal strain i.e. yelling, making strained noises. Vocal nodules are 3 times more common in boys than girls.

Treatment of vocal nodules, and the majority of paediatric voice concerns, is by speech pathology-delivered voice therapy. The aim of voice therapy is to reduce the strain on the voice (relax the muscles of the voice box), improve voice awareness, and improve the coordination of breath and voice.

In most children, vocal nodules improve with age. This is due to improved emotional regulation and vocal awareness (appropriate volume of voice). As the child proceeds through puberty, the vocal cords lengthen and thicken. This improves the voice. Vocal nodules in boys almost universally resolve in puberty. In girls however, only 2/3 will have their voice concerns resolve in puberty.

Dysphonia in children is relatively common. Serious pathology fortunately is very uncommon. The commonest cause of dysphonia is vocal nodules, which universally improve with age. For any child with dysphonia that is impacting on communication, assessment and therapy by a speech pathologist is the cornerstone of management.

References

1. Deborah, R., & Samayan, K. (2024). Cepstral analysis of voice in school-aged children. *Journal of Voice*. https://doi.org/10.1016/j.jvoice.2024.03.019
2. Yang, F., et al. (2024). Analysis of 1782 Pediatric hoarseness cases: A clinical retrospect study. *Journal of Voice*. https://doi.org/10.1016/j.jvoice.2024.06.024
3. Liu, J., et al. (2022). Vocal nodules in children: Laryngoscopic morphological classification aids prognostic judgment. *Frontiers in Pediatrics, 10*, 941483.
4. De Bodt, M. S., et al. (2007). Evolution of vocal fold nodules from childhood to adolescence. *Journal of Voice, 21*(2), 151–156.

An Online Friend Is a Real-Life Stranger

Janine Rowse and Joanna Tully

1 Clinical Pearl

Children are being sexually harmed through their use of technology. Paediatricians play a key role in protecting children and must ask the questions so children can speak up about a wicked problem hiding in plain sight.

2 Clinical Case

Sally is 12 years old and enjoys sitting in her bedroom playing on her phone. When she receives a message on social media from a guy she does not know who says he is 15, knows a few of her friends, and is really hot, she readily connects with him. They chat for a few days, then he sends her a picture of his genitals, and asks for one back. Sally feels flattered by the attention and sends him pictures of her breasts and some flirty messages. He is complimentary, tells her she is beautiful, that he wants to date her, and asks for a video of her dancing topless. Sally complies, nobody has ever shown this much interest in her, and she so wants him to like her. Soon after sending the video, the boy messages Sally asking her to meet and give him $100, otherwise he will send the pictures and video to all her contacts. Sally is terrified and ashamed. She agrees to meet him that night in the local park. Sally does not tell her parents, fearing they will be angry about the images and take away her phone. When Sally arrives, the "boy" who is an adult male, sexually assaults Sally in the back of his car. Sally does not tell anyone, feeling it is her fault. Sally's mother

J. Rowse · J. Tully (✉)
The Royal Children's and Monash Children's Hospital, Melbourne, VIC, Australia

Department of Forensic Medicine, Monash University, Melbourne, VIC, Australia

C. F. Lynch et al. (eds.), *The Art of Paediatric Medicine Beyond the Evidence Base*,
https://doi.org/10.1007/978-981-96-7234-9_53

grows increasingly concerned about Sally's unexplained school refusal, low mood, and social withdrawal. Sally does not disclose her abuse to anyone until a young doctor in the emergency department asks her directly about her online experiences during a consult for abdominal pain months later.

3 Discussion

Young people are experiencing mental health difficulties at alarming rates, and use of the internet, particularly social media, appears to be a significant factor [1]. As well as familiar social media platforms and apps, children are also accessing platforms designed for adults that are specifically geared toward sexual interactions, including pornography sites and adult dating apps. While the minimum age required to access many social media platforms is 13, age-verification technology is either absent or woefully inadequate. Exposure to sexual content online is commonplace and children as young as 9 or 10 are commonly viewing adult material [2], often violent and sexually graphic. Very high proportions of children interact with unknown contacts online, including via popular apps and gaming sites, and are often encouraged to continue conversations using private messaging, creating relationships with people they view as friends and not strangers [2]. This places children at very high risk of sexual abuse and exploitation, and this can take different forms. These include unwanted exposure to sexual content and language; non-consensual distribution of explicit images that the child has shared; using explicit images to blackmail the child (sextortion); coercing the child into live-streaming sexual acts that are then shared widely (youth-generated child sexual abuse material); and sexually assaulting the child after arranging to meet in person. It has never been easier for predators to contact children. Global data suggests this has reached epidemic proportions, affecting children of all ages, but especially prepubescent children [3]. The downstream harms of online child sexual abuse and exploitation (OCSAE) are significant—with victims more likely to experience feelings of shame, worthlessness, depression, anxiety, post-traumatic stress disorder and relationship difficulties [4]. The persistence of the images in the online space over time leads to unprecedented re-victimisation and perpetual shame [5, 6].

Parents may feel disempowered by relative technological illiteracy or pressured into allowing widely popular apps in the false belief that they are "safe" and that their child will be disadvantaged socially without them. However, in a recent Australian study of sexually assaulted adolescents who met their offender online, a popular social connectivity app was the most common app used to facilitate contact [7]. Parents understand the potential for sexual harm online but express disbelief about it affecting their child, despite the majority of youth-generated child sexual abuse material being produced in a child's bedroom or household bathroom [4]. No app is safe for a child and no child is safe from online exploitation. **It can happen to any child, anytime, anywhere.**

There are additional barriers to reporting technology-facilitated crimes because of the stigma and shame inherent in the child's perceived role in the assault [5]. Children may have lied about their age or fear the reaction of their peers or family, particularly the fear of their device being confiscated. A powerful online disinhibition effect results in an enhanced sense of friendship and trust; many victims feeling profoundly connected to and emotionally dependent on their online 'friend'. OCSAE is a health issue and victims may present to medical providers for a range of reasons. Those of us with an interest in children's health must be familiar with alerting signs, including change in patterns of device use, secrecy, school refusal, and changes in behaviour, activity, and mood [4]. Health professionals play a key role in reducing the stigma associated with negative online experiences, normalising conversations around online harm, and facilitating disclosure, as well as in educating and upskilling parents.

All children and their parents should be routinely asked about online activity and safety, particularly if children present with alerting signs. Conversations should be introduced spontaneously, be open-ended, contextualised, and demonstrate curiosity about the child's cyberlife while explicitly addressing fear of judgment. Talking about the positive aspects of online experiences prior to addressing the negative is good practice, as well as acknowledging how commonplace online harm can be. Structuring conversations to focus on activities and content, patterns of use, online experiences, and specific topics such as image creation and sharing, could be helpful.

The response to a disclosure should be calm and met with firm statements of belief and absence of blame. The child should immediately cease contact with the perpetrator and screenshot all communications. The caregiver may need support to minimise negative responses to the child, particularly blame and threats to remove their device. OCSAE should be reported to the Australian Centre to Counter Child Exploitation (ACCCE). Excellent resources are available through the website of the eSafety commissioner and Emerging Minds, and the office of the eSafety commissioner can work to remove online material, which can be very reassuring. The ACCCE website lists a range of counselling and support services that can assist children and families. Online exploitation of children is an adult responsibility. Healthcare professionals are well placed in their frontline interactions with children to shine a light on a global problem of unprecedented magnitude.

4 Other Gems

- For parents:
  - Primary school-aged children do not need a smartphone, give them a dumb one.
  - No devices in bedrooms or bathrooms.
  - Install parental controls and supervise children online.

    - Do not threaten to confiscate devices, don't blame children for the abuse. Educate, support and help children to be safe online.
    - Create a contract with your child about online use [4, 8].
    - Stay informed about evolving online risks: https://www.esafety.gov.au/

- For children:
    - An online friend is a real-life stranger.
    - "It's OK to say no" to sharing intimate images.
    - Online sexual abuse is never your fault.
- For health professionals:
    - Ask about online experiences, every parent, every child, every consult.
    - Consider online harm when a child presents with an unexplained change in physical or emotional wellbeing.
    - Advocate for digital literacy as a core curriculum subject in schools.

References

1. Bozzola, E., Spina, G., Agostiniani, R., Barni, S., Russo, R., Scarpato, E., Di Mauro, A., Di Stefano, A. V., Caruso, C., Corsello, G., & Staiano, A. (2022). The use of social media in children and adolescents: Scoping review on the potential risks. *International Journal of Environmental Research and Public Health, 19*(16), 9960. https://doi.org/10.3390/ijerph19169960
2. Thorn. (2022). Online Grooming: Examining risky encounters amid everyday digital socialization. Findings from 2021 qualitative and quantitative research among 9–17-year-olds. Thorn. https://info.thorn.org/hubfs/Research/2022_Online_Grooming_Report.pdf. Accessed 14 June 2024
3. ECPAT International and INTERPOL. (2018). Towards a global indicator on unidentified victims in child sexual exploitation material. Summary Report. Interpol. https://ecpat.org/wp-content/uploads/2021/05/TOWARDS-A-GLOBAL-INDICATOR-ON-UNIDENTIFIED-VICTIMS-IN-CHILD-SEXUAL-EXPLOITATION-MATERIAL-Summary-Report.pdf
4. E-Safety Commissioner. (2024). Child sexual abuse online. Australian Government. https://www.esafety.gov.au/key-topics/illegal-restricted-content/child-sexual-abuse-online. Accessed 14 June 2024.
5. Hamilton-Giachritsis, C., Hanson, E., Whittle, H., & Beech, A. (2017). Everyone deserves to be happy and safe – A mixed methods study exploring how online and offline child sexual abuse impact young people and how professionals respond to it. https://bit.ly/2x5fcWY
6. Joleby, M., Lunde, C., Landström, S., & Jonsson, L. S. (2020). "All of me is completely different": Experiences and consequences among victims of technology-assisted child sexual abuse. *Frontiers in Psychology, 11*, 606218. https://doi.org/10.3389/fpsyg.2020.606218
7. Rowse, J., Mullane, S., Bassed, R., & Tully, J. (2022). Technology-facilitated sexual assault in children and adolescents; is there a cause for concern? Fourteen years of experience at a metropolitan forensic paediatric medical service. *Journal of Paediatrics and Child Health, 58*, 409–414.
8. Childnet. (2014). Resources: Family agreement. Childnet International. https://www.childnet.com/resources/family-agreement/. Accessed 14 June 2024.

Part III
Teenagers (13–18 Years)

Adolescence: Opportunities in the Clinical Encounter

Michele Yeo

1 Clinical Pearl

Don't ask and they won't tell.

2 Clinical Case

"I am going in by myself first!" Tayla told her mother as she strolled in and sat herself down, jiggling her right leg. She had pink-streaked hair, a new nose piercing and was dressed in a hoodie and torn jeans. She looked tired. Tayla was an independent 16-year-old teen who had a past history of anorexia nervosa and was being followed up for disordered eating, school avoidance and anxiety. She had just started at an alternative school. She complained of feeling tired and often missed school or fell asleep in classes.

When asked how she found her new school, she replied quickly, somewhat pressured in her speech. "Ok, better than the last. At least the classes are smaller." She was attending sometimes but "too tired" to go at other times. She had made some new friends and told me she would "hang out" with them in the city, at the shopping centre or at a park. When asked further what she did when hanging out, she hesitated and said "window shopping, talking and stuff." Then she stated, "Remember when you asked me about smoking?... I know that it's not great …. but I am smoking weed. Smoking helps me with my anxiety and my sleep."

"I also have a new boyfriend. He goes to my school and I sometimes stay over at his place, so I guess, yeah, I should be on the pill. Mum doesn't know…."

M. Yeo (✉)
Department of Adolescent Medicine, Royal Children's Hospital, Parkville, VIC, Australia

C. F. Lynch et al. (eds.), *The Art of Paediatric Medicine Beyond the Evidence Base*,
https://doi.org/10.1007/978-981-96-7234-9_54

3 Discussion

Tayla was already comfortable speaking to health professionals separately from her parents, having done so since her admission for the eating disorder [1]. Her understanding of confidentiality allowed her to disclose her marijuana use and sexual activity [2]. This had provided the opportunity for further exploration of the context and extent of her marijuana use and possibly the use of other drugs, her understanding of how marijuana had helped her anxiety and sleep in addition to assessing her motivation for changing the pattern of marijuana use. The consultation could also be used to examine her sleep and dietary patterns, provide psychoeducation, discuss consent, provide guidance around safe sex and contraceptive options [3].

Young people rate confidentiality as one of the most important factors in accessing health care [4, 5]. Confidential health care is important in the development of a trusting relationship between a young person and the clinician. It is this that provides the context in which effective assessment and therapeutic interventions can occur. Studies have shown that young people are happy to discuss health issues and mental health concerns with their health professionals, however are reluctant to do so unless it occurs in a confidential setting and only if directly prompted [6, 7]. Routine and opportunistic psychosocial assessment provides a powerful means to promote engagement with the adolescent patient aside from understanding the presence and context of behaviours during this rapidly changing developmental period.

Tayla had previously denied any drug use or other health risk behaviours when asked. Previously she had spoken about her experience with bullying at school and longstanding anxiety that stemmed from this and family conflict. Young people may not disclose sensitive information at the time of being asked, however it has been the routine screening around such issues that provided Tayla the permission to bring up her concerns.

It has been shown that the discussion of sensitive topics has a positive impact on young people's perception of care. They also reported taking a more active role in treatment when sensitive topics were discussed [8].

Understanding and addressing the psychosocial concerns of adolescents is important for promoting their health and wellbeing and each health care visit is a valuable opportunity to influence future health care behaviours.

4 Other Gems

- Time alone with the young person is essential to establishing trust, rapport and giving them an opportunity to participate in conversations, at their own pace.

References

1. Mehus, C. J., Voller, V., Gewirtz O'Brien, J. P., Gower, A. L., McRee, A. L., & Sieving, R. E. (2023). How is time alone introduced? Experiences and preferences of adolescents and parents. *Journal of Adolescent Health, 73*(1), 190–194.
2. Al-Shimari, F., Kahn, N. F., McCarty, C., Parker, E. O., Richardon, L. P., & Shafii, T. (2022). Provider use of time alone with adolescents: Differences by health concern. *Journal of Adolescent Health, 71*(4), 508–511.
3. Rand, C. M., Auinger, P., Klein, J. D., & Weitzman, M. D. (2005). Preventive counselling at adolescent ambulatory visits. *Journal of Adolescent Health, 37*(2), 87–93.
4. Zucker, N. A., Schmitt, C., DeJonkheere, M. J., Nichols, L. P., Plegue, M. A., & Chang, T. (2019). Confidentiality in the doctor-patient relationship. Perspectives of youth ages 14-24 years. *Journal of Pediatrics, 213*, 296–202.
5. Ford, C. A., Millstein, S. G., Halpern-Felsher, B. L., & Irwin, C. (1997). Influence of physician confidentiality assurances on adolescents' willingness to disclose information and seek future health care. A randomised controlled trial. *JAMA, 278*, 1029–1031.
6. Klein, J. D., & Wilson, K. M. (2002). Delivering quality care: Adolescents' discussion of health risks with their providers. *Journal of Adolescent Health, 30*(3), 190–195.
7. Baldridge, S., & Symes, L. (2018). Just between us: An integrative review of confidential care for adolescents. *Journal of Paediatric Health Care, 32*(2), e45–e58.
8. Brown, J. D., & Wissow, L. S. (2009). Discussion of sensitive health topics with youth during primary care visits: Relationship to youth perceptions of care. *Journal of Adolescent Health, 44*(1), 48–54.

Children with Disability Need Teeth Too

Giuliana Antolovich

1 Clinical Pearl

Look beyond the wheelchair and see the child as who they are.

2 Clinical Case

Cassie* is a 16-year-old adolescent with cerebral palsy. Cassie is a wheelchair user and has a severe movement disorder. She has high physical care needs and is reliant on carers to support her daily activities, personal care, and safety. Cassie has a communication disability and complex communication needs.

Cassie was admitted for a dental procedure under general anaesthesia. During the procedure, a number of additional teeth were unexpectedly extracted, including all four of her lower incisors.

Once Cassie was in the recovery room, her parents expressed concern about the removal of her lower teeth. They were "reassured" that it should not be a problem, as "girls like Cassie don't need all of their teeth."

G. Antolovich (✉)
Neurodevelopment and Disability, The Royal Children's Hospital, Melbourne, VIC, Australia

University of Melbourne, Melbourne, VIC, Australia

Murdoch Children's Research Institute, Melbourne, VIC, Australia

C. F. Lynch et al. (eds.), *The Art of Paediatric Medicine Beyond the Evidence Base*,
https://doi.org/10.1007/978-981-96-7234-9_55

3 Discussion

Teeth serve many important functions. The incisors have a narrow edge that help us bite, allowing us to break up food, making chewing easier and swallowing safe—essential to our wellness, nutrition, and enjoyment. The incisors are also the most visible teeth in our mouth and contribute significantly to our appearance and our ability to talk and smile.

In addition to having cerebral palsy, Cassie is also 16-year-old who takes great pride in her appearance—she takes care with her hair, always wears mascara, and has a keen interest in fashion. Cassie has a beautifully expressive face, and this is an important part of how she manages communication with people she does not know well. Drooling is a problem for Cassie, she is embarrassed by it, and being able to keep her mouth closed is important to help control her drooling. Cassie also takes a full oral diet.

This "Pearl" is not really about teeth, it is about "*girls like Cassie*."

Consider ***the experience*** of people with a disability as they navigate health care and health care systems. The literature and lived experience both describe the interface with health as less than ideal. In Australia, people with disability experience premature mortality and higher rates of potentially avoidable deaths, reflecting poor access to routine medical care [1]. Diagnostic overshadowing, failure to provide basic care, and assumptions about quality of life, impact both decision making and access to care for people with disability, with significant outcomes [2]. A survey of physicians in the United States demonstrated that a majority did not feel confident providing care to adults with disability and recognised inequity in access to care [3]. Most of those surveyed also believed that adults with a disability had a worse quality of life than their non-disabled peers [3]. The described experience is not dissimilar for children with a disability**, with many clinicians recognising a gap in their skills to care for this group and the associated risk of poorer outcomes [4].

There are a number of barriers that can interrupt access to medical care for children with a disability. The physical, communication and cognitive impairments are important and can impact engagement, however, other factors can have a more significant bearing on the experience of care. The attitude and beliefs of the doctor***, understanding of diversity, and the language we use can have substantial and important effects.

The physical appearance of a child, especially the presence of a wheelchair, can result in the doctor making assumptions about capacity. Unfortunately, the result is often an automatic *underestimation* of ability, competence, interest and need [4]. The language we commonly use in clinical care can have a further harmful impact. Signifiers such as "developmental delay", "global developmental delay" have the potential to minimise the child to a single dimension. These descriptors do not help us understand a child's individual capability. Likewise, describing a child as "non-verbal" is inherently risky. This implies the child *cannot* communicate and shuts off exploration of alternative communication options. Consideration of the language we use is a critically important part of respectful and inclusive care. An understanding of a child's motor, cognitive and especially communication ability and style, is essential to developing a relationship with that child and family, and necessary to developing a plan of care that meets that child's needs.

Children with more complex and severe disabilities are dependent on others for all daily living supports (such as breathing, feeding, positioning, toileting, and dressing) and may also lack decisional capacity. Nonetheless, they have preferences, and can express their joy, their worries and distress. Our job as doctors is to ensure those preferences are *also* considered and included, so we are *deciding with*, rather than *for* them [5]. It is important to recognise that not all children with a disability lack decisional capacity. We know that adolescents with a disability want and can be supported to make their own health care decisions. The doctor has an obligation to actively explore the capacity for participation in decision making and provide appropriate supports (additional time, visual aids, modified language, assistance from a communication partner) to ensure that involvement.

The "Disability Paradox" describes a recognised tension between the assumption that a person living with a disability has a low-quality life and life satisfaction, versus the lived experience of a good life [6]. This paradox is well described as part of the expressed beliefs that doctors hold [3, 4]. Doctors have their own personal values, which are a key influence in care, especially when the child has a disability [7]. These beliefs and values can have meaningful impacts on care and the relationship with a child and their family. Trust, the care choices offered, and even the prognostic message can be modified by the doctor's values and beliefs [8].

A framework to assess and consider the potential impact of a doctor's beliefs and values on clinical care is important. This is embodied in the ideal of reflexivity—the act of examining our feelings and motivators [9]. The doctor has an obligation to better understand herself and what she brings to the clinical dynamic [10]. She should also be prepared to engage in the emotional and not just the prognostic aspects of care [11].

As doctors, we can change the experience of health care for children with a disability in important and meaningful ways. Each child has a story to tell. Careful consideration of the abilities and needs of a child, ensuring their voice is heard, and making time to reflect on our responses and behaviours, can meaningfully change the experience of a "*girl like Cassie*."

* Cassie's story is an amalgam, drawing on several different children cared for by the author.

** Child/Children will be used to represent both children and adolescents in this chapter.

*** The author is a doctor, and "doctor" is referenced throughout the chapter, but the narrative and experience are relevant to clinicians of all craft groups.

4 Other Gems

- Simply saying “hello” creates an important opportunity to learn about a child’s communication ability and style.
- Practice reflexivity in your clinical care—it will do more than help your patients, it will also help you.

References

1. Reppermund, S., Heintze, T., Srasuebkul, P., Reeve, R., Dean, K., Smith, M., et al. (2019). Health and wellbeing of people with intellectual disability in New South Wales, Australia: A data linkage cohort. *BMJ Open, 9*(9), e031624.
2. Mencap. (2012). Death by indifference https://www.mencap.org.uk/sites/default/files/2016-07/DBIreport.pdf2007 [updated 2012. 1:Report].
3. Iezzoni, L. I., Rao, S. R., Ressalam, J., Bolcic-Jankovic, D., Agaronnik, N. D., Donelan, K., et al. (2021). Physicians’ perceptions of people with disability and their health care. *Health Affairs, 40*(2), 297–306.
4. Ames, S. G., Delaney, R. K., Houtrow, A. J., Delgado-Corcoran, C., Alvey, J., Watt, M. H., et al. (2023). Perceived disability-based discrimination in health care for children with medical complexity. *Pediatrics, 152*(1).
5. Antolovich, G. C., & Kett, J. C. (2024). Deciding with children-beyond disability. In J. Massie & G. L. G. Hall (Eds.), *Deciding with children in Pediatrics. Children’s participation in healthcare decision-making* (1st ed.). Elsevier.
6. Albrecht, G. L., & Devlieger, P. J. (1999). The disability paradox: High quality of life against all odds. *Social Science & Medicine, 48*(8), 977–988.
7. Haward, M. F., Janvier, A., Lorenz, J. M., & Fischhoff, B. (2017). Counseling parents at risk of delivery of an extremely premature infant: Differing strategies. *AJOB Empirical Bioethics, 8*(4), 243–252.
8. Blumenthal-Barby, J. S., Loftis, L., Cummings, C. L., Meadow, W., Lemmon, M., Ubel, P. A., et al. (2016). Should neonatologists give opinions withdrawing life-sustaining treatment? *Pediatrics, 138*(6).
9. Northway, R. (2000). Disability, nursing research and the importance of reflexivity. *Journal of Advanced Nursing, 32*(2), 391–397.
10. Kozlowski, D., Hutchinson, M., Hurley, J., Rowley, J., & Sutherland, J. (2017). The role of emotion in clinical decision making: An integrative literature review. *BMC Medical Education, 17*(1), 255.
11. Antolovich, G., & McDougall, R. (2023). Doctor, isn’t there anything else you can do?: The ethics of information sharing with parents in paediatric care. *Journal of Paediatrics and Child Health*.

Beyond the Neonatal Intensive Care Unit (NICU)

Katrina Harris

1 Clinical Pearl

Clinicians are limited in predicting the future experience of a child and family, or their ability to cope, by the degree of impairment of their child in the Neonatal Intensive Care Unit (NICU). Developmental outcomes after discharge are significantly influenced by factors independent of the NICU experience. Communicating well with families regarding developmental prognosis relies on understanding these broader influences impacting the child and family, and the limitations of our assessments.

2 Clinical Case

Josh was born at term via caesarean section for breech presentation. He required brief resuscitation at birth with intermittent positive pressure ventilation (IPPV) and oxygen. Apgars were 3, 5, 9 at 1, 5 and 10 minutes. He was admitted to neonatal intensive care unit (NICU). Low birth weight of 2.5 kg was noted and examination revealed a submucosal cleft palate. After 48 hours he was transferred to special care nursery (SCN) for feeding establishment. He remained an inpatient for 4 weeks for slow weight gains and slow to establish sucking feeds. A cardiac murmur was noted prior to discharge and confirmed on echocardiogram to be a ventricular septal defect

K. Harris (✉)
Developmental Paediatrics, Monash Children's Hospital, Melbourne, VIC, Australia

Department of Paediatrics, Monash University, Melbourne, VIC, Australia

C. F. Lynch et al. (eds.), *The Art of Paediatric Medicine Beyond the Evidence Base*,
https://doi.org/10.1007/978-981-96-7234-9_56

(VSD). Josh was discharged from the neonatal service to his family and follow up with the Maternal and Child Health Nurse (MCHN).

Josh's neonatal doctor wondered what the future would look like for this child.

The family general practitioner had referred Josh to a general paediatrician for monitoring throughout his childhood. From a medical viewpoint, Josh had a reasonably straightforward childhood. He required a VSD repair in infancy which was successful and he thrived. Developmentally, he was slow to walk and talk. He received early intervention services from the age of 18 months. He walked at 3 years. and used signs to communicate before verbal language developed aged 6 years. Continence was achieved (with support) aged 7 years. He required hearing aids and glasses for hearing and vision impairments. Josh continued to attend mainstream school with many supports following a modified curriculum. At 7 years of age, he had diagnoses of moderate Intellectual disability (ID) due to a known syndromal cause, and Autism Spectrum disorder (ASD). Now as a 16-year-old teenager, he needs help with dressing (buttons, shoelaces) and supervision for showering and toileting. He speaks in sentences, but has trouble with "to and fro" conversation. Socially, he has trouble making friends but plays video games with others at school. Josh is much loved, and an intrinsic part of a large family. Josh describes himself as happy.

3 Discussion

NICU graduates may have a range of outcomes. These may include, but are not be limited to, cognitive impairment ranging from mild to severe intellectual disability (ID), cerebral palsy (CP), autism spectrum disorder (ASD), attention deficit hyperactivity disorder (ADHD), language impairment, specific learning disorder (SLD) and hearing/vision impairments. Patterns of impairment vary across conditions and across individuals. Most children will have deficits; some subtle, some marked in a range of areas.

The experience in NICU impacts the child and family, but is only one factor in a kaleidoscope of life factors. Much work has occurred to reduce the immediate impact of NICU in terms of sensory experiences (e.g. monitoring noise levels, kangaroo care), developmental care practices and minimising pain.

Beyond this, multiple factors influence the child's developmental outcome and include medical, social, cultural and economic forces. Factors within the **child** may include antenatal e.g. toxin exposure (alcohol, fentanyl) and postnatal medical issues e.g. structural neurological deficits (e.g. hypoxic-ischaemic encephalopathy, intraventricular haemorrhage) or medical comorbidities. Factors within the immediate **family** such as parental physical and mental health, and the number and ages of siblings can influence outcome. The family's capacity to respond will be influenced by extended family support, cultural and religious beliefs. **Social** factors include the financial status of the family and whether there is stability of home or care placement. Access to supports and services may depend on where the family lives (ie. less

Table 1 Neurodevelopmental Domains

BRAIN STRUCTURE	LANGUAGE	SOCIAL SKILLS & ADAPTIVE BEHAVIOUR	MOTOR	AFFECT
MEMORY	ATTENTION	COGNITION	EXECUTIVE FUNCTION	ACADEMIC ATTAINMENT

access if living in a regional or isolated area). Avoidance of secondary disability, through surveillance of hearing and vision, is important. Abuse and neglect may also occur.

Families navigate the early years with a degree of anxiety, waiting and watching for expected milestones. Ten domains of neurodevelopment are noted in Table 1. Multiple variables will influence the neurodevelopmental phenotype for any individual [1–6].

It is helpful for neonatal clinicians to understand the process and limitations of developmental assessments. Most assessments are standardised for corrected age. Some examples are the Gross Motor Assessment (GMA), Hammersmith Infant Neurological Exam (HINE) from 3 months of age for motor skills, and the Weschler Preschool and Primary Scale of Intelligence (WPPSI) from 3 years of age for cognition. Some neurodevelopmental domains cannot be formally assessed until later in childhood, such as memory and executive function. The stability of developmental findings depends on the child's age, the aetiology of the impairment, and the type of test. They are not perfect. Patterns of impairment vary across developmental conditions and individuals. The long term experience of the ex-NICU family and their child can be markedly different depending on the child's neurodevelopmental impairment, such as the differences between children with motor and non-motor disabilities. Motor disabilities, such as cerebral palsy, tend to be more visible, measurable, and understandable to the general population. Strong support groups are often available. Non-motor disabilities, such as moderate-severe intellectual disability or ASD, may be invisible at first glance, have impairments that are less easily measured, and are complex for others to understand. Children with intellectual disabilities will have challenges across multiple developmental domains. Milder conditions such as Specific Learning Difficulties (SLD) and Attention Deficit Hyperactivity Disorder (ADHD) are common and manageable.

These are some of the types of questions parents may have for the NICU team.

- Why did this happen?
- Will my child be normal?
- Will my child catch up with the others?
- What can we do to help them get better?
- Will my child have to go to a special school?
- Will my child be able to live independently?
- Who will look after our child once we are gone?

Some of these questions may be asked of the NICU team who have cared for the neonate. Many of these questions are challenging. Medical statistics are less valid in the individual case and can only be used as a guideline when discussing long term outcomes. The "disability paradox" describes the high quality of life experienced by people with disability as compared to a physicians' perception of that life [7–10]. It is very hard to predict what the families will take in at any consultation. Words (especially negative or pejorative words) matter and are often remembered. For example, "The doctor said she/he would never .....walk, talk, go to school..." Medical jargon may be bewildering for parents. Please use the baby's name in any discussion.

A useful framework for the NICU clinician in considering discharge planning is presented in Table 2.

Remember kindness matters. Loving relationships thrive within disability [12]. Hope is vital.

Table 2 How can the NICU clinician help with discharge planning? [2]

How to help the child	How to help the family
Ensure there is general paediatric follow up arranged for all ex-NICU patients prior to discharge.	Anticipate guilt, and address **directly** to remove blame.
Treat the treatable: Prioritise hearing and vision surveillance.	Life will be different from what was expected.
Investigate microcephaly as a marker of future additional needs.	The child's outcome is heavily influenced by factors independent of NICU.
Record information in the file that is uniquely available now and vital for later understanding (prenatal alcohol/toxins).	Reinforce strengths eg. Extended family/participation in routines/community.
Increased pregnancy spacing between children improves outcomes for the child and the parents (>18–24 months) [10, 11]	Facilitate family planning to meet the wishes of parents.

4 Other Gems

- For the NICU clinicians, it is important to reflect that this work is hard. You can't always be right. There are always more sick neonates coming into the system for your care and expertise. Acknowledge uncertainty, seek guidance from your senior colleagues, and support from your team, and take time away when you need to, so you can return with the strength to help the next child and family.

References

1. Hall, I., Strydom, A., Richards, M., Hardy, R., Bernal, J., & Wadsworth, M. (2005). Social outcomes in adulthood of children with intellectual impairment: Evidence from a birth cohort. *Journal of Intellectual Disability Research, 49*(3), 171–182.
2. Guideline for Growth. Health and Developmental Follow-up for Children Born Very Preterm Centre for Research Excellence, MCRI. J Cheong.
3. Allen, L., Leon-Attia, O., Shaham, M., Shefer, S., & Gabis, L. V. (2020). Autism risk linked to prematurity is more accentuated in girls. *PLoS One, 15*(8), e0236994.
4. Crump, C., Sundquist, J., & Sundquist, K. (2021 Sep). Preterm or early term birth and risk of autism. *Pediatrics, 148*(3), e2020032300. https://doi.org/10.1542/peds.2020-032300
5. Spittle, A. J., Thompson, D. K., Olsen, J. E., Kwong, A., & Treyvaud, K. (2021). Predictors of long-term neurodevelopmental outcomes of children born extremely preterm. *Seminars in Perinatology, 45*(8), 151482.
6. Rogers, E. E., & Hintz, S. R. (2016). Early neurodevelopmental outcomes of extremely preterm infants. *Seminars in Perinatology, 40*(8), 497–509.
7. Reppermund, S., Heintze, T., Srasuebkul, P., Reeve, R., Dean, K., Smith, M., et al. (2019). Health and wellbeing of people with intellectual disability in New South Wales, Australia: A data linkage cohort. *BMJ Open, 9*(9), e031624.
8. Lezzoni, L. I., Rao, S. R., Ressalam, J., Bolcic-Jankovic, D., Agaronnik, N. D., Donelan, K., et al. (2021). Physicians' perceptions of people with disability and their health care. *Health Affairs, 40*(2), 297–306.
9. Ames, S. G., Delaney, R. K., Houtrow, A. J., Delgado-Corcoran, C., Alvey, J., Watt, M. H., et al. (2023). Perceived disability-based discrimination in health care for children with medical complexity. *Pediatrics, 152*(1).
10. Dhamrait, G., Fletcher, T., Foo, D., Taylor, C. L., & Pereira, G. (2022). The effects of birth spacing on early childhood development in high-income nations: A systematic review. *Frontiers in Pediatrics, 10*, 851700. https://doi.org/10.3389/fped.2022.851700
11. Zerbo, O., Yoshida, C., Gunderson, E. P., Dorward, K., & Croen, L. A. (2015). Interpregnancy interval and risk of autism spectrum disorders. *Pediatrics, 136*(4), 651–657. https://doi.org/10.1542/peds.2015-1099
12. Albrecht, G. L., & Devlieger, P. J. (1999). The disability paradox: High quality of life against all odds. *Social Science & Medicine, 48*(8), 977–988.

Everyone Blooms

Cyrus Westerland and Jennifer Harrison

1 Clinical Pearl

It is important to support developmental needs and individuation in late adolescence.

2 Clinical Case

A 15-year-old boy, Mason, with previous diagnoses of Autism Spectrum Disorder (ASD) and moderate intellectual disability (ID) was referred to a local child and adolescent mental health team during late high school for increasing meltdowns, aggression, and anxiety symptoms. Mason had tried several medications, including risperidone and fluoxetine, with some benefit. However, the degree of his anxiety and externalising symptoms were becoming increasingly challenging for the young man himself, and also for his family which included his parents and two younger siblings. His ability to function in his specialist school setting was significantly affected, as was his functioning within the family.

A thorough assessment at a newly established service, the Mental Health in Intellectual Disability Initiative-Youth (MHIDI-Y) was commenced. The team, which included a child psychiatrist, psychiatry registrar, and allied health clinicians, met with Mason and all his family members, and liaised with his paediatrician and school. The comprehensive assessment resulted in a dynamic understanding of Mason's strengths and challenges. Across several months, his family and team developed a plan to address his support needs, which involved not only cautious medication trials, but also family support and allied health interventions.

C. Westerland · J. Harrison (✉)
Alfred ICYAMHWS, Melbourne, VIC, Australia

C. F. Lynch et al. (eds.), *The Art of Paediatric Medicine Beyond the Evidence Base*,
https://doi.org/10.1007/978-981-96-7234-9_57

Longer-term work demonstrated the role of preparing this young man for changes to his routine and new situations by using visual and verbal conversations and social stories. Consideration of Mason's sensory profile led to methods of support in challenging situations such as the establishment of a sensory distraction kit.

Working with the multidisciplinary team over several years, it was clear that Mason craved a degree of independence and control, as expected for any adolescent at this stage of life. Supporting him to make choices during this important time of psychological transition ensured that he progressed in his development as a young adult. Anxiety is often a significant driver of fluctuating symptoms such as aggression. With the ongoing support of his family and with significant preparation, Mason has continued to make good progress. This has included several successful international trips (unimaginable to both Mason and his family prior to this intervention). Mason has also transitioned to attending a day program and is working towards overnight stays outside of the family home.

3 Discussion

In the field of dual disability (diagnosis of a neurodevelopmental condition alongside a co-occurring mental illness, such as anxiety), it is very common for young people to present with escalating anxiety, depressive symptoms, or challenging behaviours from mid-adolescence onwards.

Common triggers include the young person becoming aware of the differences in their support needs and the level of their independence compared to peers of the same age, or siblings.

Young people with ID seek to achieve expected milestones, such as working, having a romantic partner, driving or moving out independently, as much as others, but are often not seen as capable.

Experiences of social and educational exclusion are common. Parents and family members typically provide the additional degree of support for these young people. However, the family are also left in a double bind situation where they are acutely aware of the young person's need to separate (often with increased anxiety) whilst they bear the brunt of anger as they seem to stand in the way of an independence that cannot be attained according to a typical adolescent timeline. Each negative incident, for example a significant meltdown, aggression, or absconding, further reinforces this position. In a vicious cycle, such episodes drive heightened concern and monitoring thereby increasing the potential distress or resentment in the adolescent. The young person becomes increasingly aware of the difference between what they are seeking and what is possible.

Whilst medications have a clear role in treating a co-occurring mental illness or in reducing heightened arousal or aggression, this can only go so far. Ensuring that there is a good understanding of the young person's communication profile and sensory needs establishes a solid baseline for carers and treatment teams to consider the young person's developmental stage and appropriate goals for the future. This understanding is integral in considering how best to move forward.

The way that professional teams undertake an assessment and provide support in order to build meaningful daily routines may be somewhat different in other settings. The underlying developmental needs of the young person are similar to neurotypical people, and it is vital that a neurodevelopmental diagnosis does not overshadow curiosity about exploring the hopes and dreams of the adolescent. This is a trap that can be easy to fall into in fast-paced healthcare settings.

4 Other Gems

- Dual disability is a field which allows great creativity and enjoyment in the work itself, and a close and rewarding relationship with young people and families. Spending any time in a multidisciplinary team in this area will build skills in communicating and supporting people in different ways to those taught by standard medical training, yet yields benefits in all areas of practice.
- Many families supporting someone with a neurodevelopmental condition will be exhausted from a lifetime of having to advocate against diagnostic overshadowing in clinical settings. Reading submissions from the 2019 Disability Royal Commission in Victoria [1] will give some insight into the cognitive biases that prevent appropriate diagnosis and treatment in this cohort.
- The role of healthcare-associated trauma should be considered in all patients and families. In dual disability, in particular, there are many who bear the scars of careless and judgemental comments from clinicians. Many young people have unfortunately found emergency departments or clinic waiting rooms to be aggravating and may have upsetting past experiences. These traumas may include prolonged physical restraint or intramuscular sedation to undergo investigations. Greater flexibility in services, such as young people with ID being able to access home-visit pathology services, or work with a Disability Liaison Officer or a disability specialist team (such as the one available at the Centre for Developmental Disability Health in Melbourne) can ensure that further traumatic experiences are avoided.

Reference

1. Victoria. (2019). *Royal Commission into Victoria's mental health system: Interim report summary* Retrieved December 6, 2024, from http://nla.gov.au/nla.obj-2526542615

It Takes a Team to Transition

Stephanie Lee

1 Clinical Pearl

Consider the young person (and often their family, in the case of neurodisability) as part of the care team when transitioning from paediatric to adult medical care.

2 Clinical Case

An 18-year-old girl, Selena, has just moved from a rural to metropolitan locale. She has a complex medical history including cerebral palsy, intellectual disability, epilepsy, and reliance on PEG feeding on a background of neonatal hypoxic ischemic encephalopathy. Selena has limited communication skills and is fully reliant on her parents to meet her daily needs. She attended Year 11 at a specialist school. Whilst living rurally, her medical care was located both locally and with specialists at a metropolitan paediatric hospital (Hospital X). However, her new residence was located closer to another tertiary hospital (Hospital Y). Upon meeting the transition care coordinator at Hospital Y, it became apparent that she was not ready to transfer care. There had been very limited preparation and education on this change for either herself or her parents. A plan was made to "pause" her transfer of care whilst addressing transition education and goals for her and her family.

Unfortunately, shortly after moving, Selena became acutely unwell with aspiration pneumonia. She was admitted to the adult medical ward of Hospital Y due to her age and location. Here, the medical teams met her for the first time. Unfamiliarity with her background and care requirements contributed to a subsequent episode of aspiration. Discussions about advanced care planning were attempted and caused

S. Lee (✉)
Monash Children's Hospital, Clayton, VIC, Australia

C. F. Lynch et al. (eds.), *The Art of Paediatric Medicine Beyond the Evidence Base*,
https://doi.org/10.1007/978-981-96-7234-9_58

great anguish. The overall challenges in communication and coordination of care were highly distressing to the patient and her family.

After this admission, Selena's transition coordinator established transition goals with her family, and provided further education and support. A transition care plan and healthcare "passport" was developed, to which the patient, family, transition care coordinator and specialty clinicians contributed and had access to. A "warm handover" was arranged by her transition coordinator with the patient, her family, GP and paediatric and adult medical specialists.

3 Discussion

Transition is defined as "a purposeful, planned process that addresses the medical, psychosocial and educational/vocational needs of adolescents and young adults with chronic physical and medical conditions as they move from child-centred to adult-oriented healthcare systems" [1]. Transition is a process which results in a safe, coordinated and supportive transfer to adult and community care. Transition is not synonymous with transfer; transition is an active process, whereas transfer is a single event that is part of the transition process.

Advances in care of childhood diseases has led to increased survivorship into adulthood [1]. As a result, an increasing number of patients with chronic health conditions require assistance to bridge the divide from child to adult healthcare services.

Transitioning a young person with chronic disease from paediatric to adult healthcare requires a multidisciplinary team and many hours of coordination. An ideal transition service includes multidisciplinary input from an array of paediatric and adult services and specialities. Transition is a process that takes place over many years, and even though it may be useful to set a target age, there is no "right" time for transition. Ideally however, planning for transition should be started well before transfer of care occurs. A flexible and collaborative approach that takes developmental readiness into account and links to other social transitions (such as leaving school) is ideal.

Most transition programs for chronic disease populations tend to be disease-specific with goals of increasing youth self-directed care and autonomy, and corresponding decrease in parental involvement. However, for young people with complex chronic disease and/or associated neurodisability, transition services need to be holistic and not just focused on a single disease or outcome. Patients who are unable to manage their health needs independently are those most vulnerable during their transition process. They often require substantial ongoing parental/carer involvement and advocacy that is unlikely to decrease over time. Therefore, in these individuals, it is important to also include parents/carers in the transition process.

Key transition outcomes include access to adult healthcare providers and a detailed medical summary and handover from the referring provider [2]. Poor communication and handover between providers have been demonstrated to be a barrier to transition [3]. Paediatric providers usually provide medical information to adult providers in the form of written medical records to the office of the adult provider. However, medical records alone are usually inadequate in relaying information regarding the patient's unique psychosocial or developmental needs. Transition documents should include medical diagnoses and needs, medications, care teams and support people. For those with neurodisability, they should also include enduring power of attorney, advance care plans, communication style methods, normal behaviour and likes/dislikes. Including the young person as part of the care team in a "warm" handover process can familiarise them with their new team, reduce miscommunication and barriers to engagement.

4 Other Gems

- The approach to transition of young people with neurodisability has additional considerations such as enduring power of attorney and advance care planning.
- Although the discussion about transition needs to start early (ideally from the start of adolescence), the stage at which transition occurs is not solely dependent on age, and needs to take into consideration social and developmental readiness.
- Each patient should have an identified transition lead. This can be a medical, nursing or allied health member who is able to span involvement from inpatient to outpatient and community care.
- Educate and prepare the young person and their carers on the cultural and systemic differences between the paediatric and adult healthcare systems.
- Handover documents should include a health summary that the young person and/or their carers can contribute to and have ownership of.
- Consider a "warm handover" that includes the young person, family and care team.

References

1. Blum, R. W., Garell, D., Hodgman, C. H., et al. (1993). Transition from child-centered to adult health-care systems for adolescents with chronic conditions. *Journal of Adolescent Health, 14*(7), 570–576. https://doi.org/10.1016/1054-139x(93)90143-d
2. Betz, C. L., & Smith, K. (2011). Measuring health care transition planning outcomes: Challenges and issues. *International Journal of Child and Adolescent Health, 3*(4), 463–472.
3. Scal, P., & Ireland, M. (2005). Addressing transition to adult health care for adolescents with special health care needs. *Pediatrics, 115*(6), 1607–1612. https://doi.org/10.1542/peds.2004-0458

Too Tired to Teen

Lionel Lubitz

1 Clinical Pearl

Chronic Fatigue Syndrome (CFS) treatment requires hope and patience for the patient and the clinician.

2 Clinical Case

Skyler is a 15-year-old girl who came to the clinic with a 7-month history of fatigue. Earlier in the year she had a viral illness. She was initially ill with fevers, sore throat, whole body aches and fatigue. Her symptoms improved after a week except for the fatigue. Skyler described feeling tired "all the time." She often struggled to get to sleep, then slept 10–11 hours per night but did not awake feeling refreshed. Most days Skyler had a nap in the late afternoon and then missed dinner with the family. Her appetite was poor and she had lost 5 kilograms over the previous 6 months. Her periods were erratic in timing. Skyler described "brain fog" and poor concentration. She had not been able to attend school consistently and her grades were slipping. She often felt dizzy when standing from sitting. She had relinquished all outside activities.

Skyler was a very high achieving year 9 student. She excelled academically, was captain of the women's football team, participated in extracurricular music and drama activities. She lived with her family (mother, father and younger brother) and described a happy family life. She was not in an intimate personal relationship and had many friends. Skyler did not drink alcohol or use recreational drugs.

L. Lubitz (✉)
Victorian Childrens Clinic, Malvern, VIC, Australia

C. F. Lynch et al. (eds.), *The Art of Paediatric Medicine Beyond the Evidence Base*,
https://doi.org/10.1007/978-981-96-7234-9_59

Skyler had been reviewed by her general practitioner (GP) several times. She had visited a naturopath, tried yoga, acupuncture and homeopathic treatments. Skyler stated she was "fed up" and was worried people thought it was "all in her head." She missed her friends and sports. Her mood was low, but she had no acute suicidal ideas or intent.

On examination, Skyler was a slim articulate girl. Her weight was 62 kg, height 164 cm and her BMI was 23.1. Her blood pressure (BP) was 110/60 mmHg lying, 95/60 mmHg standing with a postural heart rate change of 20 beats per minute. Further clinical examination was unremarkable.

Skyler had two questions for the clinician:

1. What's wrong with me?
2. Will I ever get better?

3 Discussion

CFS may severely disrupt the developmental tasks of adolescence and must be treated seriously. It is a challenging condition to manage because it has uncertain diagnostic criteria that change constantly. This includes the Fukuda criteria, the Canadian Criteria, the Oxford Criteria and the Paediatric criteria. The scientific limitations in our understanding of CFS means we need to work in the paradigm of the 'Art of Medicine.'

The impact on the young person's life and the family and educational/social/relationship disruption is profound. The young person, who should be moving into a state of independence and finding where they belong (their tribe outside of the family), is caught in the darkness of their dependency and housebound state. The change from "well-being" to "disabled" has a profound impact on all tasks of adolescence including independence, body image, peer relations and identity. A diagnosis of CFS also attracts stigma from the ill-informed.

The critical start to the management of the patient is to 'believe' them. The way we engage in the consultation and the language we choose is the most significant factor in determining our effectiveness as doctors caring for children/adolescents with CFS. The critical points in eliciting the history are:

(a) onset triggered by a viral illness.
(b) fatigue is not somnolence (somnolence is not a feature of CFS).
(c) post exertional malaise/fatigue is an almost universal symptom.
(d) sleep issues including sleep phase problems and unrefreshing sleep are common.
(e) brain fog is very common.
(f) the presence of somatic symptoms e.g. musculoskeletal/headache.

Clinical examination of the patient is important but often normal. There are no specific diagnostic features but measuring the BP and heart rate to elicit evidence of POTS (Postural Orthostatic Tachycardia Syndrome), muscle deconditioning, nutritional status and mental health are important to explore. Most investigations are normal but are important to exclude other potential causes of the symptoms. FBE, CRP, ESR, U&Es, LFTs, viral serology, coeliac serology, LDH, adrenal function (early morning cortisol/ACTH) are useful blood tests to order. A sleep study may be indicated particularly if somnolence is evident. Holter monitoring to look for POTS is occasionally useful.

Useful management strategies include:

- Your explanation to the young person that you understand their condition and that they have a real and disabling medical problem needs to be clear, concise, developmentally appropriate, accompanied by written information and a suggested approach to managing the condition. Giving them a plan gives them hope.
- Explanation of what CFS is and what it isn't. It is most important to stress that it is real and not something they are just imagining.
- A plan for return to school with a letter for the school.
- Graded exercise with management of "burst and bust" cycle.
- Treat sleep and other symptoms that need medication.

Many parents and children raise the question of alternative therapies such as dietary changes, complementary medicines and other approaches to CFS. My response to that is that I work within a particular context which is the medical model and can help them in that way and I do not have expertise in the alternative medicine area. It is important not to undermine parent's or children's belief systems, but it is also important not to collude with interventions that are at best unhelpful and at worst harmful.

There are a number of medications that can be used to manage the symptoms of CFS:

- Melatonin is helpful for sleep initiation.
- Anti-inflammatories/analgesics can assist with pain but other alternatives to pain treatment such as amitriptyline and pregabalin in small doses may be helpful.
- Anti-migraine medications such as pizotifen may be useful.
- Fluoxetine (an antidepressant) can be useful for mood and motivation as well as acting as a mild stimulant.
- There is no evidence that immunological therapies are useful.
- Naltrexone has been successfully used in adults but in paediatrics it has not been trialled sufficiently.
- Treatment of POTS utilising simple measures such as fluids, extra salt and compression tights as well as medications such as propranolol are sometimes useful [1].
- The use of methylphenidate or dexamphetamine in assisting with brain fog is a controversial area. Small doses of these medications can be helpful and enable the young person to attend school more effectively.

The consequences of not treating this condition are severe disability, long-term disconnection from education, vocation, persistent dependence, failure to develop friendships and intimacy as well as loss of community connections.

In summary, the approach to CFS management is:

- recognise it early and start an intervention program.
- believe the child/adolescent.
- offer a clear explanation to the child and family.
- use medications as needed.
- assist with a rehabilitation approach with graduated return to activities in a very carefully controlled way.
- always maintain optimism of recovery as the prognosis of CFS in childhood is good.

4 Other Gems

- A HEEADSSS screen [2, 3] is important for all adolescents in all settings.

References

1. Zhang, Q., Xu, B., & Du, J. (2020). Update of individualized treatment strategies for postural orthostatic tachycardia syndrome in children. *Frontiers in Neurology, 11*, 525. https://doi.org/10.3389/fneur.2020.00525
2. Goldenring, J., & Cohen, E. (1988). Getting into adolescents heads. *Contemporary Pediatrics, 21*, 75–80.
3. The Royal Children's Hospital. (2025). Engaging with and assessing the adolescent patient clinical practice guideline. https://www.rch.org.au. Accessed January 2025.

Breathing Difficulty During Exercise

Angela McCullagh

1 Clinical Pearl

Difficulty *breathing in* during exercise is not usually due to asthma.

2 Clinical Case

Ava, a 15-year-old girl who had played competitive sport for many years, presented to the respiratory outpatient clinic due to recurrent difficulty breathing during basketball games over the preceding 6 months. Her General Practitioner (GP) had diagnosed her with asthma and prescribed salbutamol to use during sport and, more recently, recommended a trial of inhaled corticosteroids (ICS) as her symptoms were worsening. Although salbutamol appeared to help, her difficulty breathing was occurring multiple times a game and her family were keen for her to be reviewed as asthma treatment was not preventing the problem.

Further history revealed that Ava had difficulty with inspiration, more than exhalation, and that she felt a tightness in her throat rather than her chest when episodes occurred. Her parents reported that she looked like she was struggling to breathe and made a 'wheezing' sound. Some episodes were associated with dizziness and tingling in her hands but no palpitations or chest pain. Symptoms nearly always settled within 5–10 min, after 4 puffs of salbutamol and sitting on the sideline. She was then able to rejoin the game, although often the breathing difficulty returned.

Ava had not experienced episodes as severe as this in any other setting, although did have a milder episode once when taking a test. She had a background of mild generalised anxiety but was otherwise fit and well.

A. McCullagh (✉)
Monash Children's Hospital, Clayton, VIC, Australia

C. F. Lynch et al. (eds.), *The Art of Paediatric Medicine Beyond the Evidence Base*,
https://doi.org/10.1007/978-981-96-7234-9_60

Ava had a normal respiratory examination and normal spirometry, with no evidence of obstruction and no response to bronchodilator (she did not experience any breathing difficulty during testing).

3 Discussion

Difficulty breathing during exercise is a frequent presentation to respiratory outpatient clinics. A careful history is extremely helpful in determining the underlying cause. In an otherwise healthy teenager, the differential diagnosis often lies between exercise-induced asthma and exercise-induced laryngeal obstruction (EILO). The former has a gradual onset/offset, tightness reported in the chest, and breathing difficulty is typically during exhalation, which may be associated with audible wheeze. In EILO, onset and recovery are often rapid, patients appear distressed and describe struggling to get air *in* (+/− out) and experience tightness in the throat, often associated with a stridor and cough [1]. Asking the patient to point to where they feel the discomfort and reproduce any noises is helpful. EILO affects up to 7.5% of the general population [2] and 5% of elite athletes [3, 4] and is broadly defined as inappropriate narrowing of the larynx during high intensity exercise. The condition has previously been referred to as Vocal Cord Dysfunction (VCD) or Paradoxical Vocal Cord Movement (PVCM) as the most common site of obstruction is at the level of the vocal cords, which partially adduct, rather than abduct, during inspiration and may excessively abduct during expiration [5]. It is now recognised that the definition is anatomically broader, as obstruction may also occur at the supraglottis or epiglottis [1, 6]. EILO mainly affects teenagers, with the average age of onset of 14.5 years, and is uncommon in children less than 10 years. It is twice as common in females. The pathogenesis of EILO is not certain, however organic (irritant-induced) and non-organic (psychological or emotional stress) precipitants are recognised [2]. There is a well-described association with asthma, with the incidence of asthma in patients with VCD reported to be as high as 40% [7] and VCD identified in up to 30% of patients with refractory asthma. A prospective study of 52 children in Vancouver referred for poorly controlled exercise-induced asthma found 27% had EILO and not asthma [8].

In a patient with isolated EILO, respiratory examination is normal. Some patients can reproduce the sound that occurs during an episode (inspiratory stridor). Nasal obstruction may be present and contributing to the dysfunctional pattern of breathing. Chest imaging and pulmonary function tests are typically normal. Cardiopulmonary exercise testing may be helpful in reproducing symptoms and elucidating the problem.

In specialist clinics the diagnosis can be made by inducing symptoms and observing laryngeal closure using direct laryngoscopy [9], and currently the 'gold standard' for the diagnosis of EILO is continuous laryngoscopy during high intensity exercise (CLE) [10]. In the paediatric population these tests are typically reserved for cases where standard treatment has failed and diagnostic certainty is required, due to the invasive nature and limited availability of testing.

Management of EILO involves teaching the patient to breathe in a way that prevents the larynx from closing: a 'sniffing' inhalation (3 short sniffs) followed by a slow exhalation via pursed lips. In addition to maintaining airway patency throughout the respiratory cycle, this technique slows the rate of breathing, thus reducing hyperventilation and the symptoms which accompany it. Therapy is tailored to the individual and typically directed by a speech pathologist. Anecdotally this produces a good effect. Other medical and surgical interventions have been proposed, however evidence regarding their benefit is currently lacking [10]. Addressing nasal obstruction, co-existent respiratory pathology such as asthma, and anxiety are also important for success.

4 Other Gems

- Patients/carers are poor at describing respiratory noises. Asking the patient/carer to reproduce the noise or obtaining a recording of the sound allows the clinician to accurately diagnose the likely site of obstruction.

References

1. Roksund, O. D., Heimdal, J. H., Clemson, H., Vollsaeter, M. D., & Halvorsen, T. (2017). Exercise inducible laryngeal obstruction: Diagnostics and management. *Paediatric Respiratory Reviews, 21*, 86–94.
2. Wells, C., Makariou, I., Barker, N., Thevasagayam, R., & Sonnappa, S. (2023). Exercise-induced laryngeal obstruction (EILO) in children and young people: Approaches to assessment and management. *Paediatric Respiratory Reviews, 46*, 37–48.
3. Campisi, E., Shneiderman, J., Owen, B., Moraes, T., & Campisi, P. (2019). Exercise-induced laryngeal obstruction: Quality initiative to improve assessment and management. *International Journal of Pediatric Otorhinolaryngology*, 127.
4. Rundell, K., & Spiering, B. (2003). Inspiratory stridor in elite athletes. *Chest, 123*(2), 468–474.
5. Ibrahim, W. H., Gheriani, H. A., Almohamed, A. A., & Raza, T. (2007). Paradoxical vocal cord motion disorder: Past, present and future. *Postgraduate Medical Journal, 83*(977), 164–172.
6. Roksund, O. D., Matt, R. C., Heimdal, J. H., Olofsson, J., Skadberg, B. T., & Halvorsen, T. (2009). Exercise induced dyspnoea in the young. Larynx as the bottleneck of the airways. *Respiratory Medicine, 103*, 1911–1918.
7. Low, K., Ruane, L., Uddin, N., Finlay, P., Lau, K., Hamza, K., Holmes, P. W., Hamilton, G., & Bardin, P. G. (2017). Abnormal vocal cord movement in patients with and without airway obstruction and asthma symptoms. *Clinical & Experimental Allergy, 47*(2), 200–207.
8. Sear, M., Wensley, D., & West, N. (2005). How accurate is the diagnosis of exercise-induced asthma among Vancouver school children? *Archives of Disease in Childhood, 90*(9), 898–902.
9. Ludovic, G. (2023). Diagnostic work-up of exercise-induced laryngeal obstruction. *European Archives of Otorhinolaryngology, 280*, 1273–1281.
10. Clement, H. H., Olin, J. T., McIntosh, C., Schwellnus, M., Sewry, N., Hull, J. H., & Halvorsen, T. (2022). Exercise-induced laryngeal obstruction (EILO) in athletes: A narrative review by a subgroup of the IOC consensus on 'acute respiratory illness in the athlete'. *British Journal of Sports Medicine, 56*(11), 622–629.

Why Does Nocturnal Enuresis Sometimes Continue into Adolescence?

Michael Harari

1 Clinical Pearl

Nocturnal enuresis (NE), that does not improve spontaneously over time, nor respond to conventional treatment, may well be due to unsuspected overactive bladder (OAB).

2 Clinical Case

A 13-year-old girl, Yasmin was referred with nightly NE from age 4 years. In kinder and early school years she tended to daytime urgency of micturition, with occasional wetting of small amounts. This issue was resolved by age 8. It was thought to be a behavioural issue of "waiting until the last moment." At this stage, she was tried on a bed wetting alarm which "did not wake her." A trial of desmopressin Melt 240mcg sublingual before bed made little or no difference. She had spent long periods under the care of a clinical psychologist who attributed her NE to anxiety, possible Attention Deficit, the birth of two younger siblings and a temporary separation of her parents when she was 10 years old. Her mother wet the bed occasionally until age 7 years. Bladder ultrasound showed no residual post-voiding volume.

At age 13 years, a trial of oxybutynin 5 mg twice daily was initiated for 6 months. There was instant improvement, with nocturnal wetting frequency reduced to about once every 2 weeks. After 2 months the nocturnal wetting disappeared. Oxybutynin was ceased after 6 months with no recurrence at 1 year follow up.

M. Harari (✉)
Department of Pediatrics, Ziv Medical Center, Safed, Israel

C. F. Lynch et al. (eds.), *The Art of Paediatric Medicine Beyond the Evidence Base*,
https://doi.org/10.1007/978-981-96-7234-9_61

3 Discussion

In the 1960s the inherited basis of NE was first suspected epidemiologically, with confirmation by gene linkage analysis coming in the mid-1990s. In the 1980s, the pathophysiology of NE was shown to usually be nocturnal polyuria, and poor arousal to the stimulus of full bladder. This combination was called monosymptomatic nocturnal enuresis (MNE) i.e. night wetting with no daytime urinary symptoms. For MNE, conventional treatments, such as bed wetting alarms or desmopressin (1-deamino-8-D-arginine vasopressin) are usually successful.

Those who also have daytime urinary urgency, frequency, jiggling, or wetting, are regarded as having non-monosymptomatic nocturnal enuresis (NMNE)—mainly caused by the additional problem of an overactive bladder (OAB)—a spasm of the bladder which then empties suddenly, forcefully, and prematurely (i.e. incomplete filling). This group is more resistant to the conventional treatment for NE described above. However, OAB is usually treated successfully with an anticholinergic agent (such as oxybutynin).

Traditionally, those with no daytime symptoms of OAB (i.e. those with MNE) have also been assumed not to have OAB by night and hence are usually not treated with an anticholinergic.

Researchers in Hong Kong investigated what it was about NE in those approaching adolescence, that had led them to be refractory to treatment. They showed that those referred to them with resistant NE, usually had OAB at night, even if they had no daytime symptoms of OAB whatsoever [1, 2].

Overactive bladder may be an unsuspected factor in causing NE to persist into adolescence making it relatively resistant to treatment of NE, even in those without overt daytime bladder overactivity. Hence when an adolescent is referred to me, even with no history of OAB, but having not responded to alarm or desmopressin, I start them on anticholinergic medicine to treat unsuspected bladder overactivity. I have never regretted it.

4 Other Gems

- **Ensure there is no constipation or encopresis**—Constipation or encopresis can cause ongoing wetting by day or night, which will be resistant to the treatments mentioned above. Anticholinergics may also worsen the constipation or encopresis.
- **Arguably, having a past history of an overactive bladder is enough to classify the NE child as non-monosymptomatic NE.** In those with previous overactive bladder, it is acceptable to still classify the child as NMNE and treat with an anticholinergic agent.
- **In any age group, it is sometimes difficult to elicit a history of OAB.** Not all children with OAB have day wetting as their main symptom. Some may have

subtle urgency, or frequency without wetting. Unlike true withholding of urine, those with OAB occasionally (not always) pass small volumes of urine and the sensation of needing to void may even disappear if the child waits a few minutes (because the bladder spasm relaxes and the intravesical pressure drops).

- **In prepubertal girls, consider vaginal reflux as a cause for day wetting (and occasional NE as well).** A careful history of urinary leakage mainly upon getting up from the toilet is suggestive. Typically, there is no urgency of micturition nor jiggling. The manoeuvre of voiding with parted legs and parted labia is both therapeutic and diagnostic. Voiding, while the mother holds up a mirror to the labia of the daughter as she voids, may help instruct the child as to what she needs to do.
- **Combining an anticholinergic agent with desmopressin or alarm may be successful.** I generally try an anticholinergic alone for adolescents or those with NMNE. However, if there is no improvement in NE then one may add desmopressin or an alarm, even if in the past, when used alone, these have not worked.

References

1. Yeung, C. K., Sit, F. K., To LK, et al. (2002). Reduction in nocturnal functional bladder capacity is a common factor in the pathogenesis of refractory nocturnal enuresis. *BJU International, 90*, 302–307.
2. Yeung, C. K., Sreedhar, B., Sihoe, J. D. Y., et al. (2006). Differences in characteristics of nocturnal enuresis between children and adolescents: A critical appraisal from a large epidemiological study. *BJU International, 97*, 1069–1073. https://doi.org/10.1111/j.1464-410X.2006.06074

Don't Ignore Period Pain

Shamitha Kathurusinghe

1 Clinical Pearl

Period pain is a common experience, but it is not necessarily normal.

2 Clinical Case

A 17-year-old girl, Jemima, presents to the general practitioner complaining of severe dysmenorrhea and moderate menstrual bleeding that is disrupting her schooling and ability to participate in netball training.

Further history reveals that Jemima underwent menarche at the age of 13. She has a regular 28-day cycle with five days of bleeding that is usually moderate on day two. Over the last 12 months, Jemima has noticed increasing dysmenorrhea that is now impacting her ability to function despite the use of regular paracetamol and ibuprofen as analgesia. Jemima has severe dysmenorrhoea from day 1 to day 3 of her period and has missed 1–3 days of school each month during her period.

Jemima also gives a history of loose stools with her periods. There are no bladder symptoms. She is sexually active with her 18-year-old boyfriend, using barrier protection. Jemima has sometimes noticed dyspareunia on deep penetration. There is no history of unusual vaginal discharge, and a recently performed Sexually Transmitted Infection (STI) screen was normal. Jemima enjoys school and has a stable family life. She denies any history of smoking, alcohol or recreational drug

S. Kathurusinghe (✉)
Gynaecologist, Laparascopic Surgeon, Royal Women's Hospital Parkville, Eastern Health, Epworth HealthCare, Cabrini Health, Clinical Senior Lecturer (The University of Melbourne), Melbourne, VIC, Australia

C. F. Lynch et al. (eds.), *The Art of Paediatric Medicine Beyond the Evidence Base*,
https://doi.org/10.1007/978-981-96-7234-9_62

use. Her mother had a hysterectomy for pelvic pain and heavy menstrual bleeding (HMB) at the age of 45. An abdominal examination is unremarkable.

The general practitioner organised a pelvic ultrasound, which noted ultrasound findings of adenomyosis. The patient was commenced on a low dose combined oral contraceptive pill along with heat packs and regular simple analgesia following a negative urine pregnancy test. Jemima was given instructions to skip her periods on the combined oral contraceptive pill, which resolved her dysmenorrhoea and moderate menstrual bleeding. Jemima was also referred to pelvic floor physiotherapy for assessment of her dyspareunia symptoms.

3 Discussion

Dysmenorrhoea in adolescents is a common cause of school absenteeism, with a prevalence of 16–93% [1]. Nearly 30% of menstruating adolescents may also experience HMB [2]. While the release of prostaglandins is a key cause of primary dysmenorrhoea, secondary causes such as endometriosis or adenomyosis should be considered in adolescents with severe symptoms [3]. Medical attention may be delayed due to the normalisation of dysmenorrhoea and HMB, leading to a delay in treatment for symptoms that negatively impact education and overall health.

Diagnosing secondary causes of dysmenorrhoea in this age group can be particularly challenging, due to the intrusive nature of investigations such as transvaginal ultrasound or laparoscopic surgery, which are often used in the diagnosis and treatment of endometriosis.

Adenomyosis is a common gynaecological condition previously believed to predominantly occur in multiparous or perimenopausal women. Adenomyosis is typically diagnosed from histology at the time of a hysterectomy, due to the presence of endometrial-like tissue within the uterine myometrium [4]. However, advances in ultrasound and magnetic resonance imaging (MRI) have made it possible to identify adenomyosis in adolescents as young as 12 years old [2]. Heavy menstrual bleeding, or HMB combined with dysmenorrhoea, is significantly associated with ultrasound-confirmed adenomyosis [2, 5]. Endometriosis is another common cause of dysmenorrhoea, and adolescents may experience both endometriosis and adenomyosis concurrently, presenting with symptoms such as dysmenorrhoea, dyspareunia, persistent pelvic pain, and heavy menstrual bleeding [6].

The management of severe dysmenorrhoea in an adolescent patient should include appropriate investigations to exclude secondary causes. A pelvic examination should only be considered on an individual basis. A sexually transmitted infection screen and a pregnancy test should be considered in sexually active adolescents. A pelvic ultrasound that is ideally transvaginal (if sexually active) should be considered to assess the pelvic anatomy if deemed necessary.

Although period pain is a common experience for many, recurring severe dysmenorrhoea may lead to the sequelae of persistent pelvic pain and non-cyclical pain with central sensitisation. Therefore, a person-centred, multidisciplinary management approach is recommended, involving general practitioners, paediatricians, gynaecologists, pain specialists and allied health teams.

Adolescents should be offered lifestyle modifications for symptom management such as regular exercise and complementary strategies, such as zinc sulphate, fish oil and ginger supplements [7]. Non-pharmacological treatments like heat packs, transcutaneous electrical nerve stimulation (TENS), and acupuncture may also be beneficial [2]

Pharmacological management for dysmenorrhoea and HMB can include non-steroidal anti-inflammatory drugs and hormonal treatments such as the combined oral contraceptive [8] or progesterone-only pills, along with long-acting reversible contraceptives such as levonorgestrel intrauterine device (IUD) or progesterone hormonal implants [3].

Patients who continue to have ongoing debilitating symptoms despite 3–6 months of medical treatment may require specialist input for pain management. In select circumstances, following extensive counselling, a patient may require a laparoscopy to diagnose and treat endometriosis, which can be prevalent in up to 75% of adolescents undergoing laparoscopy for persistent pelvic pain [6].

References

1. Gutman, G., Nunez, A. T., Fisher, M. (2022, May). Dysmenorrhea in adolescents. *Current Problems in Pediatric and Adolescent Health Care*, *52*(5), 101186. https://doi.org/10.1016/j.cppeds.2022.101186. Epub 2022 May 4. PMID: 35523674.
2. Vannuccini, S., Meleca, C., Toscano, F., Mertino, P., Pampaloni, F., Fambrini, M., Bruni, V., Petraglia, F. (2024, May). Adenomyosis diagnosis among adolescents and young women with dysmenorrhoea and heavy menstrual bleeding. *Reproductive Biomedicine Online*, *48*(5), 103768. https://doi.org/10.1016/j.rbmo.2023.103768. Epub 2023 Dec 14. PMID: 38432071.
3. Kho KA, Shields JK (2020) Diagnosis and management of primary dysmenorrhea. *JAMA*, *323*(3), 268. https://doi.org/10.1001/jama.2019.16921
4. Chapron, C., Vannuccini, S., Santulli, P., Abrão, M. S., Carmona, F., Fraser, I. S., Gordts, S., Guo, S. W., Just, P. A., Noël, J. C., Pistofidis, G., Van den Bosch, T., & Petraglia, F. (2020, Apr 15). Diagnosing adenomyosis: An integrated clinical and imaging approach. *Human Reproduction Update*, *26*(3), 392–411. doi: https://doi.org/10.1093/humupd/dmz049. PMID: 32097456.
5. Exacoustos, C., Lazzeri, L., Martire, F. G., Russo, C., Martone, S., Centini, G., Piccione, E., Zupi, E. (2022, Feb) Ultrasound findings of Adenomyosis in adolescents: Type and grade of the disease. *Journal of Minimally Invasive Gynecology*, *29*(2), 291–299.e1. https://doi.org/10.1016/j.jmig.2021.08.023. Epub 2021 Aug 28. PMID: 34464760.
6. Shim, J. Y., Laufer, M.R., King, C.R., Lee, T. T. M., Einarsson, J. I., & Tyson, N. 2024, Jan 1. Evaluation and Management of Endometriosis in the adolescent. *Obstetrics and Gynecology*, *143*(1), 44–51. https://doi.org/10.1097/AOG.0000000000005448. Epub 2023 Nov 9. PMID: 37944153.
7. Pattanittum P, Kunyanone N, Brown J, Sangkomkamhang US, Barnes J, Seyfoddin V, Marjoribanks J (2016) Dietary supplements for dysmenorrhoea. *Cochrane Database Syst Rev*, *3*(3), CD002124. https://doi.org/10.1002/14651858.CD002124.pub2
8. Schroll, J.B., Black, A. Y., Farquhar, C., Chen, I. 2023, Jul 31. Combined oral contraceptive pill for primary dysmenorrhoea. *Cochrane Database of Systematic Reviews*, *7*(7), CD002120. https://doi.org/10.1002/14651858.CD002120.pub4. PMID: 37523477; PMCID: PMC10388393.

Act Fast on Acne

Emer Crowley and Ann Boyapati

1 Clinical Pearl

A key aim of acne treatment should be scar prevention. Therefore, early treatment of moderate to severe acne is important.

2 Clinical Case

A 17-year-old girl, Esther, was referred to the Dermatology clinic for management of acne. Her medical history included epilepsy, anxiety and depression.

Esther first developed acne at age 13, however it was initially mild, and she did not seek treatment. At age 14, she was diagnosed with epilepsy and was commenced on carbamazepine. Her acne worsened, likely due to the medication, prompting a visit to her General Practitioner. Initially, she was prescribed topical therapies. Her acne deteriorated, then she was commenced on oral doxycycline.

Over the next two years, Esther's skin gradually worsened, yet doxycycline was continued. Esther was under the impression that she could not take isotretinoin given her psychiatric history.

Upon review at the Dermatology clinic, Esther's acne was classified as severe, with signs of significant scarring. Isotretinoin was commenced, along with cephalexin and a tapering course of oral prednisolone to mitigate the risk of an initial acne flare. Esther's neurologist was contacted to discuss alternative anti-epileptic

E. Crowley
St Vincent's Hospital, Fitzroy, VIC, Australia

A. Boyapati (✉)
Dermatologist, Department of Dermatology, Monash Health, Clayton, VIC, Australia

C. F. Lynch et al. (eds.), *The Art of Paediatric Medicine Beyond the Evidence Base*,
https://doi.org/10.1007/978-981-96-7234-9_63

therapies, and her medication was changed to levetiracetam under their guidance. While taking isotretinoin, she had close follow-up with her psychiatrist and psychologist to monitor her mental health.

Isotretinoin proved very effective, and after eight months of treatment, there were no active acne lesions. Esther reported a significant improvement in her self-esteem and confidence. A year later, she re-presented to the clinic for management of acne scarring, which is currently being treated with a combination of surgical and laser modalities.

3 Discussion

Acne vulgaris is an inflammatory condition affecting the pilosebaceous unit, characterised by the presence of papules, pustules, comedones and cysts [1]. It primarily affects adolescents, with studies demonstrating that approximately 85% of individuals between the ages of 12 and 24 experience some form of acne [2], but symptoms can also continue into adulthood.

While acne is often considered a rite of passage during adolescence, its effects can be profound and long-lasting, impacting not only physical appearance but also emotional and psychological well-being. Acne has a negative effect on self-esteem across all age groups [3] and a meta-analytic review demonstrated a significant association between acne and depression [4]. In a more positive light, the effective treatment of acne results in an improvement in self-confidence and body image [5].

The treatment of acne is generally guided by severity. Mild acne is typically managed with topical therapies, while moderate to severe acne often requires systemic treatment with oral antibiotics, hormonal therapies such as the oral contraceptive pill, or isotretinoin.

Isotretinoin is an orally administered systemic retinoid [6] which has been proven to be the most efficacious treatment for severe acne [7]. Isotretinoin is recommended for severe acne, acne causing scarring, and acne failing standard treatments [1]. Some patients, especially those with severe acne, may experience an initial deterioration in their acne when starting isotretinoin. In patients at risk of this complication, clinicians can prescribe prednisolone and an oral antibiotic to mitigate a flare, as was performed in our case.

Delayed treatment of acne is common and occurs for many reasons, including failure of patients to present early, a preference for conservative treatment and fears of potential side effects. This can result in patients remaining on suboptimal treatments for longer than is necessary [8], allowing the acne to worsen and leading to potentially irreversible scarring.

In our case, the patient's history of anxiety and depression likely caused some degree of apprehension regarding escalation of treatment to isotretinoin. This is likely due to previous theories regarding the association between isotretinoin and depression, which have largely been disproven. In fact, a recent systematic review and meta-analysis suggested that use of isotretinoin improved symptoms of depression, although it acknowledged that further studies are required to confirm this finding [9]. When prescribing isotretinoin, previous psychiatric history should be elucidated, and patients' mental health should be monitored closely during treatment. However, previous episodes of depression are not a contraindication to the medication [6].

Delays in acne treatment can lead to significant scarring, which can be a lasting reminder for many people of their previous skin disease. Treatment options for acne scarring include laser therapy, chemical peels, and microneedling, however, these methods are not always effective and can be both painful and expensive [10]. As such, preventing scarring through timely acne management is critical to minimising psychosocial impacts.

4 Other Gems

- Acne is a common side effect of several medications, including anticonvulsants, some cancer treatments, JAK inhibitors and corticosteroids [11, 12]. The management of drug-induced acne involves stopping the medication where possible and following standard treatment guidelines as for acne vulgaris.
- Many patients with active acne lesions present with concerns regarding scarring. Given treatment of scarring is often difficult, it is prudent to first treat active acne and then give the skin a chance to self-repair, before embarking on scar treatments.
- Hyperandrogenism can increase sebum production and change the sebum lipid profile, leading to the development of acne [13]. Females with acne who also display clinical signs or symptoms of hyperandrogenism, such as hirsutism, menstrual irregularity, infertility or androgenic alopecia, may warrant further endocrinological testing to evaluate for conditions such as polycystic ovarian syndrome [1].

References

1. Reynolds, R. V., Yeung, H., Cheng, C. E., et al. (2024). Guidelines of care for the management of acne vulgaris. *Journal of the American Academy of Dermatology, 90*(5), 1006.e1–1006.e30. https://doi.org/10.1016/j.jaad.2023.12.017
2. Eichenfield, D. Z., Sprague, J., & Eichenfield, L. F. (2021). Management of Acne Vulgaris: A review. *Journal of the American Medical Association, 326*(20), 2055–2067. https://doi.org/10.1001/jama.2021.17633
3. Gallitano, S. M., & Berson, D. S. (2017). How acne bumps cause the blues: The influence of acne vulgaris on self-esteem. *International Journal of Women's Dermatology, 4*(1), 12–17. Published 2017 Dec 6. https://doi.org/10.1016/j.ijwd.2017.10.004
4. Samuels, D. V., Rosenthal, R., Lin, R., Chaudhari, S., & Natsuaki, M. N. (2020). Acne vulgaris and risk of depression and anxiety: A meta-analytic review. *Journal of the American Academy of Dermatology, 83*(2), 532–541. https://doi.org/10.1016/j.jaad.2020.02.040

5. Tan, J. K. (2004). Psychosocial impact of acne vulgaris: Evaluating the evidence. *Skin Therapy Letter, 9*(7), 1–9.
6. Pile, H. D., & Sadiq, N. M. (2020). *Isotretinoin* [Internet]. PubMed. StatPearls Publishing. Available from: https://www.ncbi.nlm.nih.gov/books/NBK525949/.
7. Layton, A. (2009). The use of isotretinoin in acne. *Dermato-Endocrinology, 1*(3), 162–169. https://doi.org/10.4161/derm.1.3.9364
8. Zaenglein, A. L., Pathy, A. L., Schlosser, B. J., & et al. (2020, Jun). Guidelines of care for the management of acne vulgaris [published correction appears] *Journal of the American Academy of Dermatology, 82*(6):1576. doi:https://doi.org/10.1016/j.jaad.2020.02.010. *J Am Acad Dermatol*. 2016;74(5):945–73.e33. https://doi.org/10.1016/j.jaad.2015.12.037.
9. Li, C., Chen, J., Wang, W., Ai, M., Zhang, Q., & Kuang, L. (2019, Mar 15). Use of isotretinoin and risk of depression in patients with acne: A systematic review and meta-analysis [published correction appears] *BMJ Open, 9*(3), e021549corr1. https://doi.org/10.1136/bmjopen-2018-021549corr1. *BMJ Open*. 2019;9(1):e021549. Published 2019 Jan 21. https://doi.org/10.1136/bmjopen-2018-021549.
10. Connolly, D., Vu, H. L., Mariwalla, K., & Saedi, N. (2017). Acne scarring-pathogenesis, evaluation, and treatment options. *The Journal of Clinical and Aesthetic Dermatology, 10*(9), 12–23.
11. Kazandjieva, J., & Tsankov, N. (2017). Drug-induced acne. *Clinics in Dermatology, 35*(2), 156–162. https://doi.org/10.1016/j.clindermatol.2016.10.007
12. Martinez, J., Manjaly, C., Manjaly, P., et al. (2023). Janus kinase inhibitors and adverse events of acne: A systematic review and meta-analysis. *JAMA Dermatology, 159*(12), 1339–1345. https://doi.org/10.1001/jamadermatol.2023.3830
13. Carmina, E., Dreno, B., Lucky, W. A., et al. (2023, Jan 24). Female adult acne and androgen excess: A report from the multidisciplinary androgen excess and PCOS committee [published correction appears] Journal of the Endocrine Society, *7*(3), bvad006. https://doi.org/10.1210/jendso/bvad006. *J Endocr Soc*. 2022;6(3):bvac003. Published 2022 Feb 6. https://doi.org/10.1210/jendso/bvac003.

Reasons for a Racing Heart

Sathyakala Vijayanand

1 Clinical Pearl

Hyperthyroidism is a common thyroid problem in adolescents and can present as anxiety. Performing thyroid function tests can prevent unnecessary delay in the diagnosis.

2 Clinical Case

A 16-year-old boy, Kian, presented to the emergency department (ED) with palpitations while playing basketball. He had recently been reviewed by his general practitioner for anxiety.

On presentation to the emergency department, he was thinly built. Kian's weight was 61 kg (50th centile) and his height was 178 cm (75th centile). His body mass index (BMI) was 19.3 (25th centile). His heart rate was 110 beats per minute at rest (reference range 60–100 bpm) and his blood pressure was 146/68 mmHg (>95th centile for gender and height). He had no goitre or exophthalmos.

His thyroid function tests (TFTs) were as follows:

TSH **< 0.01** (0.4–4.00) mU/L
fT4 **50.4** (9.0–25.0) pmol/L
fT3 **> 30.8** (4.7–7.2) pmol/L
TSH-receptor antibody **15.0** (0–1.8) IU/L.

Kian was diagnosed with autoimmune hyperthyroidism (Grave's disease) and was started on carbimazole 10 mg three times per day. His TFTs normalised after two

S. Vijayanand (✉)
Bendigo Health, Monash Children's Hospital, Clayton, VIC, Australia

C. F. Lynch et al. (eds.), *The Art of Paediatric Medicine Beyond the Evidence Base*,
https://doi.org/10.1007/978-981-96-7234-9_64

years of treatment with carbimazole. His TSH-receptor antibody titre became negative indicating biochemical remission and hence the carbimazole was stopped. His anxiety and palpitations resolved.

3 Discussion

Grave's disease (GD) is an autoimmune condition and accounts for 60–80% of hyperthyroidism in children and adolescents. The second most common cause of hyperthyroidism is Hashitoxicosis (the initial hyperthyroid phase of Hashimoto's thyroiditis). This is also an autoimmune disease but unlike GD, eventually results in hypothyroidism.

Hyperthyroidism presents with heat intolerance, palpitations, weight loss, sweating, restlessness, decreased attention span, anxiety and panic disorder. A prospective study of 35 children and adolescents with Grave's disease and 40 healthy controls, demonstrated that anxiety, depression and inattention were seen more commonly in those with GD [1]. The neuropsychiatric symptoms improved markedly with treatment and normalisation of thyroid function.

Due to signs and symptoms such as diarrhoea, weight loss, palpitations and cardiac murmurs, children may be referred to other specialities before being seen by an endocrinologist. A retrospective study of 76 children (mean age 11.9 years) found that the mean time between symptom onset and diagnosis was 9.6 months and 22.4% of children were seen by a non-endocrinologist. The most commonly referred specialties were cardiology, psychiatry, gastroenterology and ophthalmology. Prior to the diagnosis of GD, 12 patients were diagnosed with attention deficit/hyperactivity disorder resulting in the prescription of psychostimulant medication [2].

Adolescents are sometimes treated with medications for generalised anxiety disorder. This could be prevented by careful comprehensive examination to elicit the findings of tachycardia, fine tremors, exophthalmos, goitre and having a low threshold in performing TFTs.

In addition to unnecessary investigations and treatment, delay in the diagnosis of hyperthyroidism can result in 'thyroid storm', which can be life-threatening. Thyroid storm is an acute emergency which presents with fever, sweating, widened pulse pressure, tachycardia, hypertension and cardiac failure.

4 Other Gems

- Paediatric GD has a myriad of presentations.
- This can impact school performance and general health.

References

1. Hamed, S. A., Attiah, F. A., Abdulhamid, S. K., & Fawzy, M. (2021, Apr 29). Behavioral assessment of children and adolescents with graves' disease: A prospective study. *PLoS One, 16*(4), e0248937. https://doi.org/10.1371/journal.pone.0248937
2. Sims, E. K., Eugster, E. A., & Nebesio, T. D. (2012, Feb). Detours on the road to diagnosis of graves disease. *Clinical Pediatrics (Phila), 51*(2), 160–164. https://doi.org/10.1177/0009922811418823

Not All Depressive Symptoms Are Depression

Tahnee Bridson and Brett McDermott

1 Clinical Pearl

It's all about the developmental trajectory.

2 Clinical Case

Jasper was 15-years-old, an A grade student, completing the third year of high school. He was the dux of the preceding two years at high school, and everyone held similar expectations for the years to come. At an end of year exam, Jasper was observed to be disengaged in the written task. He sat quietly in the classroom, looked somewhat sad and downcast and made only a limited attempt to answer questions on a history exam. Exam questions were across three pages; Jasper did not bother to turn the page. At the end of the exam Jasper could not give any account of his under-performance. Jasper's teacher rang his parents.

Jasper lived with both biological parents (both teachers) and a younger sister. There was no reported adversity experienced by parents, children, or extended family.

The following day Jasper was reviewed by a very experienced general practitioner (GP) who immediately rang a child and adolescent psychiatrist. The GP relayed the history of a very high functioning adolescent who had a strong commitment to his studies and his school, who had a close social group and a range of interests. Both parents attended the GP's appointment and stated that Jasper's behaviour was

T. Bridson
The Australian Centre of Excellence in Youth Mental Health, Parkville, VIC, Australia

B. McDermott (✉)
University of Tasmania, Hobart, Australia

C. F. Lynch et al. (eds.), *The Art of Paediatric Medicine Beyond the Evidence Base*,
https://doi.org/10.1007/978-981-96-7234-9_65

very out of the ordinary. It was the GP's opinion that Jasper appeared depressed. Jasper reported he was sad and had lost interest in activities. There was a two-week history of over-sleeping (very rarely this included school days) and loss of appetite. The GP stated that cognitions were difficult to assess because Jasper seemed to be a little perplexed. Something seemed to be on his mind. He was able to reassure the GP and his parents that there was no current suicidal ideation or planning. The GP administered the Kessler 10 depression screen and Jasper scored in the 'at-risk range for depression'. Physical examination was normal. This experienced GP summarised that over the course of a long career this was a teenager who looked the most like a presentation of adult endogenous depression. Jasper's path to a mental health assessment was rapid if not precipitous.

Intrigued by the unusual nature of the story, Jasper was reviewed the following day by the child psychiatrist. At the appointment time both parents and 15-year-old Jasper were in the waiting room. Jasper was interviewed on his own initially. Walking to the room it was striking that Jasper walked slowly, his head was down, his body appeared stiff with no swinging of the arms and indeed he hardly blinked his eyes. These were some of the endogenous depressive features reported by the perceptive GP. Jasper talked slowly; his speech was somewhat monotonous and lacked amplitude. There was no thought disorder. He was able to relate that for several weeks he felt different, down, dispirited, and unmotivated to engage in usual activities. His ability to feel pleasure was diminished, including interacting with his friends or watching his favourite TV shows or social media activities. He stated there was nothing particular on his mind. There were no strong themes of despair, hopelessness, or helplessness. He was not overly pessimistic although somewhat worried if 'this' persisted. He had not been thinking that life was not worth living, no thoughts of suicide or planning to hurt himself or others. He held no unusual or bizarre thoughts with delusional intensity. There were no unusual perceptions including no evidence of hallucinations. His judgment was not obviously impaired in that he knew something was wrong and had insight into why people were worried. He made his first mistake subtracting 7 from 100 after the third iteration and could not name three prime ministers.

After Jasper was seen, his parents joined the consultation. Their contribution was to validate Jasper's premorbid very high functioning and to emphasise that this change happened quickly over a 2-to-4-week period. They were also able to note Jasper had a normal developmental history, there were no medical illnesses of note, there was no family history of mental illness, and there was no suggestion of issues with drugs and alcohol or youth justice. No adverse childhood experience was noted or suspected. The unusual feature here was Jasper's "developmental discontinuity" with a short time frame for a major change in function. Urgent investigations revealed a diagnosis of a rare intraventricular meningioma. This was sufficient to explain his symptoms and their rapid onset. Following surgery, negotiating various post-operative complications and time, Jasper made a full recovery. He returned to being a very high functioning student with normal mood and cognitions.

3 Discussion

Allow us to now segue into the thought processes of a child and adolescent psychiatrist.

It is important to note that child and adolescent mental health is positioned in a complex reality that is not easily resolved into a medical model or often clarified by medical investigations.

Developmental psychopathology is one method that can be used to help identify the origin of an illness and its likely severity.

It states that invariably infants, children and adolescents are on a developmental trajectory in which their functioning slowly improves over time as they master regulation of feelings and emotions and develop more sophisticated cognitive resources. Often their trajectories have great stability over time and indeed this trajectory can be useful in diagnosis and prognosis. For instance, the autistic child is on a predictable trajectory or 'developmental continuity.' They clearly are developing but are doing so at their own pace. The young adult with Antisocial Personality Disorder often was dysregulated as a young child, developed Oppositional Defiant Disorder in primary school and Conduct Disorder in high school. A rapid deviation of development, as occurred in the case of Jasper where his academic performance changed significantly, is unusual and warrants an explanation. The depressive symptoms were secondary to this. Being deflected from a developmental trajectory (a 'developmental discontinuity') is due to something 'outside the head.' Examples could include severe bullying, or a very frightening adverse childhood experience such a physical or sexual assault. Another could be a major traumatic event such as severe illness or death of a parent. More rare, developmental discontinuities are things that happen 'inside the head' such as the onset of epilepsy, a subdural haematoma, or some other brain insult.

Another framework inherent to child and adolescent mental health is systemic understanding of families as systems. Whilst these can vary between cultures, nevertheless, they are often typified by parents who operate as an executive set, and siblings who are hierarchically less powerful and a step below parents in terms of authority. Families also have boundaries around the family that help to position the influence of grandparents, friends, and acquaintances. Healthy coalitions exist, for example between a parent and child who have a love of sport. Mental health presentations especially child anxiety, depression or disruptive behaviour can arise from alterations in normal family dynamics and be elicited following a systemic analysis. There were no obvious systemic structural or dynamic issues that seemed relevant to Jasper's presentation.

The potential learning from Jasper's presentation is not that rare things happen, and we should aggressively investigate any young person who appears depressed with neuroimaging. Rather, we should understand that all child and adolescent mental health presentations are in the context of the individual's developmental trajectory. The aetiology of many child and adolescent mental health conditions is strongly related to their experience of adverse childhood experiences (ACEs) (1). The number of ACEs, their severity and timing are all relevant. Of adverse child experiences, sexual abuse is arguably the most damaging. Abuse that is repetitive and very early in life during critical periods of brain development usually predicts worse outcomes. Later poor mental health is not a certainty, and it is likely that protection is a complex interaction of genes, temperament, and post-abuse parenting experience. Nevertheless, research is consistent that ACEs confer a non-specific vulnerability to a range of adverse mental health outcomes including depression (2). In Jasper's case, there was no history of ACEs and nothing to suggest he was on a continuum to depression. The rapid onset of his condition suggested the need for an explanation that was either a sudden acute psychologically traumatic event or a rare underlying biological process, hence the decision to undertake a range of tests including neuroimaging.

4 Other Gems

- As is this psychiatrist's practice, middle to older teenagers are seen by themselves first. This approach is to reinforce individuation of a young person who will soon be taking more direct charge of their own health and medical needs. It also allows a young person to interact in a style which is not influenced by the presence of a parent and provide information which they might otherwise withhold.

References

1. Landa-Blanco, M., Vásquez, G., Portillo, G., Sproviero, F., & Echenique, Y. (2024). The impact of adverse childhood experiences on mental health, sexual risk behaviors, and alcohol consumption in adulthood. *Frontiers in Psychiatry, 15*, 1352824. https://doi.org/10.3389/fpsyt.2024.1352824. PMID: 38659462; PMCID: PMC11039929.
2. Emerging Minds. (2025). *ACEs and their health impact*. http://emergingminds.com.au. Accessed January 2025.

Weaning SSRI Medications Thoughtfully

Sari Hayllar

1 Clinical Pearl

"Brain zaps" may be part of a withdrawal syndrome from weaning selective serotonin reuptake inhibitor (SSRI) medications.

2 Clinical Case

A 16-year-old girl, Michelle, came to discuss weaning her current SSRI which had been prescribed for significant depressive symptoms. Michelle had been treated for 18 months with escitalopram 20 mg after developing depressive symptoms in the context of school bullying and family issues. She found it beneficial but did not like its "numbing" effects. Her weaning schedule involved decreasing the dose to 10 mg daily for 1 month, then decreasing to 5 mg for a further month and then 5 mg second daily. Throughout this entire period, she experienced unpleasant "electric shock-like" feelings multiple times per day. Michelle did not have other classic symptoms of withdrawal such as nausea, headache or insomnia. She was compliant with the weaning plan. Physical examination was normal with no neurological signs. Michelle raised the question of "electric zaps" from information she had noted on her social media.

The clinician was unfamiliar with this concept and consulted widely with peers regarding potential alternative diagnoses and/or weaning schedules and withdrawal symptoms. Colleagues shared insights and guidelines with lively discussion about the problems. The clinician reported back to the patient and a new weaning process was successfully undertaken.

S. Hayllar (✉)
Consultant Paediatrician, West Gippsland Healthcare, Warragul, VIC, Australia

C. F. Lynch et al. (eds.), *The Art of Paediatric Medicine Beyond the Evidence Base*,
https://doi.org/10.1007/978-981-96-7234-9_66

3 Discussion

The marked increase in prescription of psychotropic medications in young people has mirrored the rise in the rate of mental health diagnoses. Prescribers are not limited to child psychiatrists but increasingly include consultant paediatricians and general practitioners. Australia's SSRI prescription rates give pause for thought as does the off-label use in younger children. Guidelines for use include to "start low, go slow with dose" and utilise single medications. Recommended duration of treatment with SSRIs is 6–12 months but many patients remain on treatment for much longer periods. Guidelines for weaning and potential withdrawal syndromes may not be as well known.

Withdrawal syndrome (pharmacological/physical dependence) is under recognised, particularly as a syndrome that can last years [1]. Electric shock-type symptoms are increasingly recognised as part of the discontinuation/withdrawal syndrome. The symptoms may be confused with relapse of the condition they were prescribed for and therefore medication incorrectly restarted. They may also be difficult to make sense of in our vulnerable non-verbal patients. The symptoms can get increasingly severe as the doses get lower, hence the advice for hyperbolic tapering. Hyperbolic tapering involves reducing each dose by a fixed percentage (for example 10% at lower doses) and utilising compounded formulations to achieve appropriately small doses for those who are experiencing difficulties with withdrawal, with some schedules requiring a year or more to wean. Symptoms may be worse at the later stages, so tapering more slowly at this time can help offset this. The risk is higher the longer the patient has been on the medication. If the symptoms are really unpleasant, a viable option is to consider changing to a medication with a long half-life and this will 'treat' the withdrawal and can be tapered slowly.

This method is more relevant for antidepressants with a higher incidence of withdrawal [2] (e.g. SNRIs such as venlafaxine or the SSRI paroxetine). These medications are generally avoided in paediatric patients but can be considered in exceptional circumstances. An important consideration is that fluoxetine tastes horrible dispersed. Fluoxetine has a very long half-life and if you are using it for withdrawal, this allows patients to take it on alternate days, or even every third day. This minimises the number of days of having the bad taste and this helps with compliance.

It is useful to review social media about medical topics and then tailor one's approach to counselling patients e.g. dispelling or confirming the current information. Reviewing the duration of SSRI treatment should occur regularly with patients/families. The process of weaning and the increasing evidence available regarding difficulties of withdrawal is also important to discuss.

4 Other Gems

- "Lexapro brain zaps" is a common topic on social media. Social media-savvy young people often access medical information from social media.
- Younger patients may not articulate this particular side effect and may "act out", leading to a cycle of medication changes or increases.
- Collaboration is a powerful tool. Patients are often our teachers. Our colleagues are a useful resource and are generous with their knowledge and experience.
- Useful public resources can be accessed at the following:

  handyfactsheetcomingofffluoxetineau.pdf (choiceandmedication.org)
  https://www.aspm.org.au/resources/public-resources

References

1. Khan, Y. S., Khoodoruth, M. A. S., Albobali, Y., & Haddad, P. M. (2023). SSRI withdrawal syndrome in children and adolescents: A narrative literature review. *Expert Opinion on Drug Safety, 22*(5), 381–390. https://doi.org/10.1080/14740338.2023.2224557. To link to this article: https://doi.org/10.1080/14740338.2023.2224557
2. Quilichini, J.-B., Revet, A., Garcia, P., Bouquié, R., Hamard, J., & Yrondi, A. (2022). François Montastruc comparative effects of 15 antidepressants on the risk of withdrawal syndrome: A real-world study using the WHO pharmacovigilance database. *Journal of Affective Disorders, 297*, 189–193.

Look Beyond What You See

Katy Sullivan and Trupti Jadhav

1 Clinical Pearl

Psychosocial stressors trigger various systemic symptoms, and a thorough assessment of these triggers is important for appropriate diagnosis and management.

2 Clinical Case

A fourteen-year-old girl, Quinn, presented to the paediatric emergency department with worsening chronic headaches. Whilst an inpatient, she developed bilateral lower limb weakness, sensory symptoms with no definite neurological pattern and reported peripheral visual field deficits. Overall, Quinn's symptoms and examination findings were inconsistent and were suspected to be due to psychosomatic disorder.

Her investigations including MRI brain and spine, blood tests and ophthalmological evaluation were normal.

Detailed psychological assessment revealed significant anxiety/depression due to social stressors including moving out of her family home, disliking her mother's new partner and having no contact with her biological father.

K. Sullivan
Paediatric Registrar, Townsville University Hospital, Douglas, QLD, Australia

T. Jadhav (✉)
Paediatric Neurologist and Epileptologist, Townsville University Hospital, Douglas, QLD, Australia

Honorary Research Fellow, Murdoch Children's Research Institute, Parkville, VIC, Australia

C. F. Lynch et al. (eds.), *The Art of Paediatric Medicine Beyond the Evidence Base*,
https://doi.org/10.1007/978-981-96-7234-9_67

Quinn was referred to neurology where a formal diagnosis of functional neurological disorder was made. She then received brief rehabilitation support to overcome the motor symptoms. Quinn was linked with the child and youth mental health team for outpatient follow up.

Her symptoms have continued especially at times of stress (altered sensation in legs as well as peripheral visual field loss) while motor function has improved.

3 Discussion

Functional Neurological Disorders (FND) are disorders of brain networks that deal with automatic (not voluntary) functions—movement, consciousness and sensation, and are usually polysymptomatic with no definite neurological pattern [1].

Symptoms include seizure-like episodes, movement problems, chronic dizziness, cognitive dysfunction, speech difficulties, problems with vision or hearing, pain (including chronic migraine), extreme slowness, fatigue and numbness [2]. It usually coexists with another neurological disorder.

The symptoms of FND are treatable with correct diagnosis, education and intervention. The attacks are disabling but do not constitute a health emergency as there is no poor outcome expected.

Good communication and education of the parent/caregiver and child about the confirmed diagnosis as well as identifying any comorbid conditions that are contributing (e.g. learning disorders, autism, epilepsy) is crucial [3]. It is also important to stress the potential for reversibility. A new approach to the physiotherapy of functional motor disorders is helpful with the physical symptoms [4].

Psychiatric or psychological assessment and formulation usually reveals a more complex picture than initially apparent. Psychological therapy is the mainstay of treatment of FND.

Ensuring an 'attack' management plan is available for school/home is important so that appropriate techniques continue to be used in the community. Ensuring medical follow up to help families problem solve their approach to ongoing attacks until resolution is also required.

Inpatient rehabilitation is rarely required (and often counterproductive to the main approach to treatment). Many families who have had the diagnosis explained effectively can start to work intuitively on how to develop a return to normal life activities and limit focus on the symptoms with support.

4 Other Gems

- Be aware of a patient with polysymptomatic presentation with no definite neurological pattern.

- Detailed psychosocial evaluation is important to identify causative stressors.
- Early diagnosis of FND is important to avoid unnecessary investigations and to initiate directed psychotherapy.

References

1. Hope, F. N. D. (2012–2021). *What is FND?* https://findhope.org/fnd-guide/. Accessed July 2024.
2. Bennett, K., Diamond, C., Hoeritzauer, I., Gardiner, P., McWhirter, L., Carson, A., & Stone, J. (2021). A practical review of functional neurological disorder (FND) for the general physician. *Clinical Medicine (London, England), 21*(1), 28–36.
3. Vassilopoulos, A., Mohammad, S., Dure, L., & Kozlowska, F. A. D. (2022). Treatment approaches for functional neurological disorders in children. *Current Treatment Options in Neurology, 24*(2), 77–97.
4. Nielsen, G., Stone, J., Matthews, A., et al. (2015). Physiotherapy for functional motor disorders: A consensus recommendation. *Journal of Neurology, Neurosurgery, and Psychiatry, 86*, 1113–1119.

Talk to the Hand: Part 2

Jacinta Coleman

1 Clinical Pearl

A novel approach may help in Anorexia Nervosa.

2 Clinical Case

A 17-year-old young woman, Alice, presented with a history of anorexia nervosa (AN), diagnosed when she was 15-years-old. She required several hospital admissions with cardiovascular instability and loss of weight over this time. Her family had been supported to use Family Based Therapy with her local Community Mental Health team. Alice had achieved weight restoration but felt the eating disorder cognitions had never fully resolved.

Alice was in her final year of school with the attendant stress of impending exams. Her relationship with her boyfriend of 8 months had ended, and she was feeling vulnerable and lonely. Her social media feed was full of other young people "having fun" and she couldn't relate to them. The pull of her eating disorder cognitions had grown stronger, and as a way of having a sense of control over her life, she relented. Her demise back into AN started with skipping a few meals, followed by hidden exercise. Quite rapidly, her weight began to decline and her menstruation stopped. She was sleeping fitfully, was cold all the time, she was constipated, and fainted at school. Alice was able to see how her anorexic cognitions had taken hold but felt at a loss to know how to get back on track.

J. Coleman (✉)
Head of Unit, Adolescent Medicine, Monash Children's Hospital, Clayton, VIC, Australia

C. F. Lynch et al. (eds.), *The Art of Paediatric Medicine Beyond the Evidence Base*,
https://doi.org/10.1007/978-981-96-7234-9_68

With a team around her, Alice was able to slowly rebuild her confidence. Using the Hand model of the brain [1] as a framework, Alice developed an understanding of how her brain worked on different levels i.e. thinking, feeling and reacting. The anorexia cognitions were considered as a "coercive partner." This partner promised her love, happiness and success if she listened to it and followed its rules. If she swayed from its expectations, there would be abuse, shaming, and intense feelings of guilt for having done "the wrong thing." She was able to externalise the AN, visualise it as a force separate from herself, and could then develop strategies to free herself from this "toxic relationship." With support, encouragement and the use of motivational techniques, which encouraged her to find her own solutions and trust herself to stand up to "the abuser", Alice was able to rebuild her confidence and self-esteem. She identified and utilised alternative strategies to manage her distress that would not impact her physical and mental health. With the support of her multidisciplinary team, she was able to turn her physical health around, improve her relationship with food and exercise, and re-engage with family and friends to address the social isolation she had experienced as AN took hold.

3 Discussion

Family based therapy (FBT) is an evidence-based approach for the management of anorexia nervosa. The initial focus is on using the strengths of the family system to help support the young person with weight restoration. Definitions of relapse in AN as well as definitions of remission or recovery, on which relapse is predicated, vary substantially in the literature [2]. Weight restoration and maintenance, return of menses, symptom burden and ongoing behaviours are all factors to consider. Relapse is high in the first year after treatment. Full recovery occurs when the young person is able to successfully manage the psychological impacts of the illness and function well in all aspects of their life.

Additional support after the initial "dose" of FBT may require a more individual approach. The Hand Model of the Brain can assist young people to use their own strengths to regulate difficult emotions and thoughts. It provides a visual metaphor to help young people understand the brain's structure and function—Thinking brain (logic), Emotional brain (feelings), and the Brainstem. It enables individuals to see when emotions hijack logical thinking, especially during malnourishment or stress, empowering early self-regulation.

This tool, 'The Hand model of the Brain', was developed by neuro-psychiatrist Dr. Daniel Siegel [1] (refer to Part II, "Talk to the Hand: Part 1"). It gives a visual representation of the brain.

The Thinking brain (cortex) is represented by one's fingers overlying one's thumb which is the Emotional brain (amygdala). The Thinking brain is responsible for logic and problem solving. It is the "protector" and guides one to make healthy and safe choices. It helps one to be aware of internal bodily sensations and emotions and it checks in with different parts of the body to see how everything is functioning and what needs attention. If the Thinking brain is 'malnourished' or 'too exhausted', the Emotional brain, as represented by your thumb folded across the palm of your hand, becomes vulnerable to external mental health influences, such as the intrusive thoughts from anxiety, depression, anorexia nervosa or obsessive compulsive disorder. When the Emotional brain is triggered by these thoughts, it sends messages to the Brainstem, represented by the wrist, to set in motion a flight /fight response with hyperventilation and tachycardia, preparing the body to flee from danger. These messages are sent to the body via the vagus nerve. By supporting the use of self soothing techniques such as slow, deep breaths ("Box" breathing), distractions such as creative expression, social support or mindfulness techniques, the Thinking brain can be calmed to re-engage and return to its function as protector. The goal is to strengthen intrinsic motivation and self-efficacy which can help drive long term recovery.

References

1. Siegel, D. (2010). *Mindsight: Transform your brain with the new science of kindness*. Oneworld Publications.
2. Khalsa, S. S., Portnoff, L. C., & McCurdy-McKinnon, D. et al. (2017). What happens after treatment? A systematic review of relapse, remission, and recovery in anorexia nervosa. *Journal of Eating Disorders, 5*, 20. https://doi.org/10.1186/s40337-017-0145-3

Context Is Always Important

Paul Denborough

1 Clinical Pearl

Always search for meaning underlying abnormal behaviour.

2 Clinical Case

A 15-year-old boy, Arjun, was referred to a mental health clinic with aggressive and oppositional behaviour at home and suspension from school. His behaviour had been gradually deteriorating over the previous 12 months. Arjun displayed no respect for rules either at home or school, and a sharp drop off was noted in his academic performance. Essentially, it appeared as if he didn't care about anyone or anything. He was literally doing no schoolwork.

As a routine at the clinic, the first appointment was with the whole family. In this case, the family consisted of his father, step-mother, 17-year-old sister (with Downs syndrome) and Arjun. When the family entered the room there was obvious tension between father and son. Arjun stated clearly, he "didn't want to be there" and said that he would only stay briefly. His father appeared worn out, frustrated and angry.

After first attempting to engage the family, put them at ease, and put words to their frustration, it was important to collect some context. Of obvious significance was the death of the children's mother three years earlier from an aggressive breast cancer. After a while, Arjun was able to express anger towards his father in what happened in the aftermath of her death. Particularly over the last 12 months, he felt that his father had "forgotten" his mother. He no longer visited his previous in-laws or visited the cemetery where his former wife was buried. He felt his father had

P. Denborough (✉)
Consultant Child and Youth Psychiatrist, Alfred ICYAMHWS, Melbourne, VIC, Australia

C. F. Lynch et al. (eds.), *The Art of Paediatric Medicine Beyond the Evidence Base*,
https://doi.org/10.1007/978-981-96-7234-9_69

moved on too quickly and was disrespecting his mother's memory. The father said this was the first time he had heard this. Rather than get defensive, he stated that his first wife was the "love of his life" and that her death absolutely devastated him. The only way he knew how to cope was to focus on the kids and the future and not "look back" as this was too traumatic. He had become furious with his son, as despite his best efforts to move the family forward, his son's behaviour was dragging them further into misery.

The therapist was able to point out that the two were expressing their grief in different ways and there had been a terrible misunderstanding in how they were supporting each other.

Arjun's step-mother and sister played a vital role by quietly allowing Arjun and his father to express themselves and also not get defensive. It also can't have been easy for the step-mother to hear that another woman had been the love of her new husband's life.

3 Discussion

This case also illustrates the importance of bringing the whole family together and providing a safe place for open communication. Getting the whole family together, bringing curiosity and compassion, as well as seeing the family as the solution to fix the problem rather than the problem to be fixed, seems to lead to the best outcomes.

In these meetings, the therapist is looking for a "pivotal chord" to help the family look at the problem differently and potentially try different solutions. The concept of finding a "dignified way out" is something that is front of mind for the therapist. In this case the "pivotal chord" was obvious but looking for this in other cases and opportunities for a dignified way out is often the key to helping teenagers with behavioural problems.

4 Other Gems

- Participation by the whole family may reveal important clues to the underlying issues.
- Being able to "sit with" the family whilst they discuss sensitive and challenging emotions requires empathy and the ability to tolerate silence in the consultations.
- Often siblings are "truth tellers" in family sessions which initially focus on one child's behaviours.

Are Big Ears a Big Problem?

Will Alexander

1 Clinical Pearl

Aesthetic surgery in older kids—whose idea is it?

2 Clinical Case

A 12-year-old girl, Bonnie, presents with her mother for consideration of 'prominent ears correction.'

Bonnie is otherwise fit and well, and seems socially well adjusted, articulate, and confident. Her mother commands the consultation and tells you that she herself had 'bat ears' when she was a kid, and 'getting them pinned back was the best thing ever.' Her mother wants to avoid any teasing or bullying for her daughter, but upon further questioning this has not, at least until now, been an issue. However secondary school is looming.

The patient's ears are indeed moderately prominent in the upper two thirds, and somewhat out of proportion to her facial shape.

After a referral to a paediatric plastic surgeon, they are educated in the options available and the risks of surgery to 'correct' her ears but are appropriately asked to book a review appointment in a year or two, once they have had some more time to consider their options.

W. Alexander (✉)
Consultant Surgeon, Royal Children's Hospital, St Vincent's Private and Public Hospital, Monash Health, Epworth Freemasons, Victorian Hand Surgery Associates, Parkville, VIC, Australia

C. F. Lynch et al. (eds.), *The Art of Paediatric Medicine Beyond the Evidence Base*,
https://doi.org/10.1007/978-981-96-7234-9_70

3 Discussion

Many surgeons consider this kind of intervention to be 'de-stigmatising' rather than 'aesthetic.' There is certainly a role for surgeons to help children feel strong, confident, and happy within their bodies, but that can often be achieved just as effectively through a series of empowering consultations, as through the surgical pathway. Clear communication, allowing time, and patient education are key. Many paediatric hospitals have access to psychology support, specialising in body image, and this can be an invaluable resource in some instances.

Two of the most common referrals for aesthetic/de-stigmatising surgery in children are for prominent ears, and gynaecomastia. I will address, in broad brush strokes, these conditions separately.

The ears are 85% of adult size by the age of three, and fully grown by ~12 years of age [1]. Just like our faces, they are both different between individuals, and between left and right sides. The common reasons for prominence are underdevelopment of the anti-helical fold, and/or overdevelopment of the conchal bowl [2]. Ear cartilage can occasionally be moulded in the neonatal period, but after that, the cartilage will not 'correct' with time [3].

Otoplasty ('pinning of the ears') is a common procedure with reliable results and a low complication profile; but obviously is not a lifesaving nor function-improving surgery, so should not be undertaken lightly. It is performed as a day procedure, under general anaesthetic. There is typically a short incision behind the ear, and the anti-helical fold can be reconstructed with permanent sutures, with the conchal bowl reduced by partial excision or suturing of it to the mastoid periosteum. Patients need to be compliant with wearing a headband for around six weeks post-operatively, at least for sleeping/sport, and thus performing this operation on a child who hasn't personally consented to it is ill-advised [4].

Gynaecomastia is slightly more complex as there can be underlying endocrinological causes. Once these have been excluded, a similar period of consultation, education, and surgical planning is undertaken. It should be noted that gynaecomastia is proliferation of glandular tissue, and not purely excessive subcutaneous fat [4, 5]. It is very common, and I believe somewhat under-referred. Many of these boys avoid situations where they are physically exposed (beach, swimming, team sports with communal change rooms), as well as certain clothing. Our role as paediatric doctors is to 'keep as many doors open' for these children and, for that reason, surgery can often be warranted in these patients.

Gynaecomastia surgery is targeted to one or both breasts (75% of cases are bilateral), and again has good results and a reasonably low complication profile (which includes seroma, scarring, and asymmetry). It involves a gland excision via a small incision at the areolar margin, with or without concurrent liposuction [6]. Most procedures are day procedures under general anaesthetic, but if more gland is removed some patients will stay overnight with a temporary drain tube. Most surgeons recommend a compression vest for a short period post-operatively.

In summary, when the parents and the child:

- Have been educated thoroughly, and
- Have been given plenty of time to consider their options, and
- Are deemed mature enough to be compliant with post-operative therapy/restrictions,

… AND there is a truly quantifiable anatomic difference to address, then we typically have low hesitation to perform these procedures, as the results are generally good.

4 Other Gems

- A referral to a surgeon does NOT always lead to surgery.
  - Often an empowering conversation from someone who has seen and operated on a lot of prominent ears, for example, is enough for patients.
- The risk profile of these surgeries is relatively low, but given the surgery is not lifesaving nor function-improving, the risk-benefit ratio needs to be carefully balanced.
  - Measuring confidence/psychological distress/bullying/parental overlay is difficult.
- Whilst it is the parent who signs the consent form, the clinician must place an emphasis on the child's desires, particularly in these types of surgeries.
- Time is often our friend in the decision-making process.

References

1. Farkas, L. G., Posnick, J. C., & Hreczko, T. M. (1992). Anthropometric growth study of the ear. Cleft palate-craniofacial. *J Off Publ Am Cleft Palate-Craniofacial Assoc, 29*(4), 324–329. https://doi.org/10.1597/1545-1569_1992_029_0324_agsote_2.3.co_2
2. Janis, J. E., Rohrich, R. J., & Gutowski, K. A. (2005). Otoplasty. *Plastic and Reconstructive Surgery, 115*(4), 60e–72e. https://doi.org/10.1097/01.prs.0000156218.93855.c9
3. Tan, S. T., Abramson, D. L., MacDonald, D. M., & Mulliken, J. B. (1997). Molding therapy for infants with deformational auricular anomalies. *Annals of Plastic Surgery, 38*(3), 263–268. https://doi.org/10.1097/00000637-199703000-00013
4. Janis, J. (2014). *Essentials of plastic surgery* (2nd ed.). Thieme Medical Publishers Inc.
5. Deepinder, F., & Braunstein, G. D. (2011). Gynecomastia: Incidence, causes and treatment. *Expert Review of Endocrinology and Metabolism, 6*(5), 723–730. https://doi.org/10.1586/eem.11.57
6. Simon, B. E., Hoffman, S., & Kahn, S. (1973). Classification and surgical correction of gynecomastia. *Plastic and Reconstructive Surgery, 51*(1), 48–52. https://doi.org/10.1097/00006534-197301000-00009

Part IV
All Ages

The Judicious Use of Silliness

Michael Harari

1 Clinical Pearl

A bit of foolishness, silliness and absurdity are useful adjuncts to the orthodox clinical methods we use when dealing with children.

2 Clinical Case

Janet—aged about 6 years. From a letter written by her mother to Harvey Cushing, biographer of Sir William Osler, Oxford, 1918 [1].

> *He* [Osler] *visited our little Janet twice every day from the middle of October until her death a month later* (from the Spanish Flu), *and these visits she looked forward to with a pathetic eagerness and joy. There would be a little tap, low down on the door which would be pushed open and a crouching figure playing goblin would come in, and in a high-pitched voice would ask if the fairy godmother was at home and could he have a bit of tea. Instantly the sick-room was turned into a fairyland, and in fairy language he would talk about the flowers, the birds, and the dolls who sat at the foot of the bed who were always greeted with, 'Well, all ye loves.' In the course of this he would manage to find out all he wanted to know about the little patient...*
>
> *The most exquisite moment came one cold, raw, November morning when the end was near, and he mysteriously brought out from his inside pocket a beautiful red rose carefully wrapped in paper, and told how he had watched this last rose of summer growing in his garden and how the rose had called out to him as he passed by, that she wished to go along with him to see his little lassie. That evening we all had a fairy tea-party, at a tiny table by the bed, Sir William talking to the rose, his 'little lassie' and her mother in a most exquisite way; and presently he slipped out of the room just as mysteriously as he had entered it, all crouched down on his heels; and the little girl understood that neither fairies nor people*

M. Harari (✉)
Department of Pediatrics, Ziv Medical Center, Safed, Israel

C. F. Lynch et al. (eds.), *The Art of Paediatric Medicine Beyond the Evidence Base*,
https://doi.org/10.1007/978-981-96-7234-9_71

> *could always have the colour of a red rose in their cheeks, or stay as long as they wanted to in one place, but that they nevertheless would be very happy in another home and must not let the people they left behind, particularly their parents, feel badly about it; and the little girl understood and was not unhappy.*

3 Discussion

While the case is touching, it is not enigmatic. However, the approach of the treating physician is not conventional and is worthy of pause and some thought.

Cushing dedicated his biography of Osler (1849–1919) to medical students, who had not known Osler, "*lest it be forgotten who it was that made it possible for them to* (leave the lecture halls and) *work at the bedside …*" Over a hundred years after his death from pneumonia (possibly Spanish Flu), we all remember Osler as the person who laid down the rigid, systematic, bedside clinical method that was inculcated into us. His best-known saying was "Listen to your patient, he is telling you the diagnosis." Yet the snapshot above reveals that with children, even the towering figure of Osler in his 70th year, thought it best to break his own rules.

In examining Janet, he used imaginative play, storytelling, enchanting theatrical devices, distraction, and kindness and through this, he fostered a respectful intimacy with Janet and her mother, thus revealing his humanity. There is no hint of the systematic history-taking that he advocated for use with adults, nor the structured examination from the right side of the bed, starting with the fingertips. Despite the pain of losing his own son a year earlier in the Great War, Osler was able to exhibit humour, playfulness and silliness, and use them judiciously in successfully accompanying Janet on her terminal journey, much to the gratitude of her mother.

Osler gives us an example of coming down to the level of the children in our care and stepping away from being too overtly 'doctorish.' Janet's mother recounts that by playing goblin and talking of fairy godmothers, flowers, birds and the dolls at the foot of the bed, Osler would "manage to find out all he needed to know about the little patient."

Each of us finds our own way to lower a child's guard in the clinical setting—there are endless ways to do this. Clowning, play and distraction are well integrated into modern paediatrics—yet sometimes it seems we have outsourced them to clowns, play therapists and distractors.

I quite enjoy, with a straight face, telling children of a certain age that I have fire coming out of my nose and smoke from my ears. I often proffer my hand as they walk in, and give them a bone rattling, exaggerated hand shake all the while feigning to the parents that it is the child who refuses to let go despite their protestation. I usually share with them what has happened to the few goats that I keep, or tell them why kangaroo mothers have pouches (did you know that they breastfeed their young inside the pouch?) or that the child must do whatever chore I have asked of them after school before thumping their siblings or turning on screens. "Doctor, how did you know?" If I examine their tummy, it is only so that I might guess what they ate for breakfast and if they don't agree with whatever I reveal, I will say it was only because they laughed too much during the examination, when you are not allowed to laugh at all in here. "Didn't you see the sign outside?" After asking a child what their belly button is doing there, I have no shame in telling them that they are wrong and it is only there, screwed in, to stop their bums falling off. I am always keen to know if their teacher at school barks or bites. Before asking a question of a child I might ask them several times to hold on tight so as not to fall off their chair, because the questions are really big ones. I enjoy getting the child's name wrong by crossing some of the syllables in their name with that of their siblings, making a salad of all the names. And so on. The banter is rollicking fun all round.

Yet all this is not in the name of being a comedian, entertainer or unorthodox, but rather about engaging children, gaining their confidence and being a more effective clinician. I imagine Sir William would approve.

4 Other Gems

- *Sit at the level of the child or below.*

  Towering above them is intimidating. A young child sitting on a parent's lap almost looking down at you is less frightening for them. A better physical examination is thus obtained than had they laid down on the examination couch.
- *Talking directly to a child is also engaging and often revealing.*
- *Try whispering to a child who seems not willing to pay attention.*

Reference

1. Cushing, H. (1925). *The life of sir William Osler* (Vol. 2). Oxford University Press.

Assumption Is the Birthplace of Poor Decision Making

Preeti Ramaswamy

1 Clinical Pearl

Be brave and ask the awkward questions when making clinical decisions.

2 Clinical Case

A shy 7-year-old boy, Tanish, presented to my emergency department (ED) on a Saturday afternoon with vomiting. His mother described him as an anxious boy who was due to have a party with 200 guests later that evening and he had been vomiting for the last 6 hours. He was known to vomit when anxious. There were no red flags in the history or examination.

Thoroughly caught up in the narrative, I was determined to get him better so that he could have his moment in the limelight. In the following 3–4 hours, he received ondansetron and even an IV line to rehydrate him, after all he had a benign story, examined well and we were on a deadline!

As time passed and the vomiting did not subside, I decided to do a blood gas… and you guessed it… He had diabetic ketoacidosis (DKA)!

I was horribly embarrassed that I had missed this. My discomfort at having made the incorrect assumption that anxiety explained his vomiting and the resulting delay to diagnosis shaded my clinical management and referral to the endocrinologist. I felt ashamed that I'd missed the diagnosis and delivered poor patient care.

The story unfortunately does not end here…

I heard the next morning from the same endocrinologist that after the initial care in ED, I'd incorrectly documented 'standard' dextrose containing maintenance

P. Ramaswamy (✉)
Monash Medical Centre, Clayton, VIC, Australia

C. F. Lynch et al. (eds.), *The Art of Paediatric Medicine Beyond the Evidence Base*,
https://doi.org/10.1007/978-981-96-7234-9_72

fluids, which were then continued for the next 12 h! This incorrect order was never questioned by the admitting registrar as I was the senior doctor, so the assumption was that I had a good reason for deviating from protocol.

3 Discussion

It is my belief that clinicians come to work every day to do their best for their patients. They make their decisions based on the information that they have. Thus, it is important to ensure that they are getting the accurate data to formulate care plans, whether this is through direct patient interactions or through the interactions with other clinicians.

As an emergency physician, I am firmly in the land of knowing a little about a lot but not really being the master of much. I am constantly humbled by my colleagues who are experts of their domains, and my work is more enjoyable for the learning it involves. I have had numerous instances where I have been given advice that does not resonate with the clinical case I'm faced with. Yet, I have never once regretted querying the plan and seeking the reasoning behind the clinical advice. I am the advocate for the patient, and I've had the privilege of making the assessment and so if the clinical advice does not match, it is important that I articulate my concerns to my colleagues. Is the anomaly in my synthesis of the problem or in my colleague's advice? After all, we are both human, thus inherently fallible and dependent on each other to deliver optimal care.

What is "obvious" to one clinician may not be "obvious" to another. When a plan falls through it is not infrequent that I find an incorrect assumption at the basis of it; an assumption associated with knowledge, consent, communication or attitude. This is of particular importance when one is the senior clinician giving advice or instructions. We must foster a culture which involves exploring reasoning and confirming instructions, as these provide the first line of defence against avoidable and undesirable outcomes.

I am curious about what stops us asking the question; is it a fear of looking stupid? Is it fear of seeming disrespectful? Is it a concern that the question will challenge the status quo? Most importantly should the reasons matter? Are we not bound to action by the ethical pillar of "non- maleficence" which obliges us to privilege patient interests in our decision making?

Most of us have experienced these situations. Whether it concerns how people in a patient cubicle are related or the gender of an individual or receiving advice from senior colleagues that seems incongruous to the clinical scenario, these encounters are ripe for poor decision-making when based on assumptions.

In conclusion, it is prudent to be brave and ask the "awkward" question when it involves the care of a patient. Furthermore, the questions when posed in a professional manner and birthed from genuine curiosity, are more likely to be well received and yield the best results. It is important to foster a culture which asks questions, as only then, as clinicians, can we learn from one another and deliver the best patient care.

The Do's, Don'ts, and Don't Knows

Michael Fishman and Joshua Nagler

1 Clinical Pearl

Clinical experiences shape how we practice, both consciously and subconsciously. We can learn not only from the medicine of the case, but also from reflecting on our own thought processes.

2 Clinical Case

A previously healthy two-year-old, Sylvana, presents with intermittent fussiness and abdominal pain in the setting of fever and diarrhoea. Her fever curve has been improving over the last few days. Sylvana had two episodes of vomiting on the first day of symptoms but has not had any further episodes since. Her family notes that she is reluctant to walk. She is observed to be non-ill appearing.

Sylvana's vital signs are appropriate for age, and she appears well hydrated. She is difficult to examine due to fear of the examiner, but her abdomen is soft when palpated by the mother without any evidence of focal tenderness or rebound/guarding. Sylvana has no long bone tenderness. No source of infection is identified on examination. A urinalysis was obtained which demonstrated 2+ leukocyte esterase and 30 white blood cells per high powered field, urine culture was pending.

An abdominal ultrasound is negative for intussusception, does not visualise the appendix, but comments on findings reflecting possible gastroenteritis and debris in the bladder. Sylvana was given ondansetron, tolerated oral intake, and was discharged home on a course of cephalexin for presumed urinary tract infection (UTI) while awaiting her urine culture results with close paediatrician follow-up.

M. Fishman · J. Nagler (✉)
Division of Emergency Medicine, Boston Children's Hospital, Boston, MA, USA

C. F. Lynch et al. (eds.), *The Art of Paediatric Medicine Beyond the Evidence Base*,
https://doi.org/10.1007/978-981-96-7234-9_73

Sylvana's parents returned to the Emergency Department with her the following night after she developed multiple episodes of emesis and an inability to tolerate her oral antibiotics. Her vital signs demonstrate tachycardia, tachypnoea, and hypotension for age with a distended and firm abdomen. Given concern for distributive shock physiology in the setting of an acute abdomen, Sylvana underwent emergent laparotomy where operative findings were consistent with perforated appendicitis complicated by diffuse peritonitis and reactive high-grade ileus.

3 Discussion

Acute appendicitis is the most common surgical abdominal emergency in children, though appendicitis in pre-school aged children is uncommon (~5% of all paediatric cases) [1–4]. However, rates of perforation are significantly higher in younger children, with previous studies demonstrating between 60–86% in children ages 0–3 years [1]. This may be due in part to nonspecific presentations, symptom overlap with other more common illnesses (such as gastroenteritis and UTI), and inability of the child to communicate symptoms. Together, these lead to high misdiagnosis rates (up to 60% in 2–12-year-old children and approaching 100% in children younger than 2 years) [2].

Equally important is how it might impact your management moving forward. Are you now more likely to order blood tests or imaging in all toddlers with abdominal pain to avoid missing appendicitis? If an abdominal ultrasound is equivocal for appendicitis, would you pursue further work-up? What if the additional evaluation required sedation or transfer to another facility? It is critical to understand how past cases influence our future medical decision making, both consciously and unconsciously. Peter Croskerry, an expert on diagnostic reasoning, promotes moving "from mindless to mindful practice" including reflection and understanding of our inherent biases and thought processes [5].

- **Do**: Allow clinical cases to make an impression and shape our future practice in some capacity. Connecting learning to lived experience is extremely powerful and what separates real-life practice from textbook medicine [6]. Spend time critically reflecting on your own decision-making process and its influences, particularly in cases with unexpected outcomes.
- **Don't**: Don't let the emotional weight of specific cases and/or outcomes unduly influence your decision-making process and understanding of evidence-based medicine. Cognitive biases can lead to unnecessary over- or under-testing of patients in the future, which can have subsequent impact on patient care and outcomes. Table 1 highlights a few key biases that may be relevant to the case described above and identifies their potential impact on future decision making [7].

Table 1 Examples of biases influencing decision-making

Bias	Definition	Relevance in this case
Availability bias	Overestimating or underestimating the prior probability of disease because of the clinician's recent experiences	More likely to obtain unnecessary appendicitis workup in patients presenting with fever, diarrhoea etc. in the future
Confirmation bias	Seeking evidence that supports an initial impression and ignoring (subconsciously) data that may contradict it	Not fully accounting for refusal to walk as part of the clinical picture as that is more atypical of uncomplicated UTIs
Hindsight bias	Knowing the outcome strongly influences the judgment of clinicians' actions in the diagnostic process	Applying a retrospective lens and say that the patient should have had further work-up for acute appendicitis during the first presentation based on the outcome of the case

- **Don't know**: We often don't know what we don't know. This includes our own thought processes. There are many biases that influence our decision making on a subconscious level. Awareness of heuristics can help mitigate the risk of related errors.

Much of clinical learning comes from the workplace—the patients we interact with and the stories we hear. Deliberate reflection on our clinical experiences can promote growth, minimise errors, and reduce our tendency for challenging cases to become paralysing or overly influential.

The first step is recognising the heuristics (i.e. mental short cuts) and cognitive biases that are implicit in our diagnostic reasoning, and then taking steps to mitigate and scaffold these biases to limit their undesired impact for future patients.

4 Other Gems

- Pyuria does not always mean UTI—make sure to keep the clinical context and broader differential in mind and not perform early diagnostic closure [8, 9].
- Try to distinguish between dysuria and abdominal pain with voiding—dysuria can be consistent with a UTI while the latter may reflect intra-abdominal pathology with increased pain secondary to Valsalva during voiding.
- The most commonly mistaken diagnoses for appendicitis in pre-school children on initial evaluation are gastroenteritis and UTI due to notable overlapping features—consider refusal/inability to walk as a potential reason to obtain further workup or monitoring, and always remember the importance of specific return precautions and shared mental model with families [3].

References

1. Bansal, S., Banever, G. T., Karrer, F. M., & Partrick, D. A. (2012). Appendicitis in children less than 5 years old: Influence of age on presentation and outcome. *American Journal of Surgery, 204*(6), 1031–1035. discussion 1035.
2. Almaramhy, H. H. (2017). Acute appendicitis in young children less than 5 years: Review article. *Italian Journal of Pediatrics, 43*(1), 15.
3. Marzuillo, P., Germani, C., Krauss, B. S., & Barbi, E. (2015). Appendicitis in children less than five years old: A challenge for the general practitioner. *World Journal of Clinical Pediatrics, 4*(2), 19–24.
4. Alloo, J., Gerstle, T., Shilyansky, J., & Ein, S. H. (2004). Appendicitis in children less than 3 years of age: A 28-year review. *Pediatric Surgery International, 19*(12), 777–779.
5. Pat, C. (2013). From mindless to mindful practice — Cognitive bias and clinical decision making. *The New England Journal of Medicine, 368*(26), 2445–2448.
6. Charon, R. (2001). The patient-physician relationship. Narrative medicine: A model for empathy, reflection, profession, and trust. *Journal of the American Medical Association, 286*(15), 1897–1902.
7. Scarfone, R. J., & Nagler, J. (2021). Cognitive errors in pediatric emergency medicine. *Pediatric Emergency Care, 37*(2), 96–103.
8. Wise, G. J., & Schlegel, P. N. (2015). Sterile Pyuria. *The New England Journal of Medicine, 372*(11), 1048–1054.
9. Chen, C. Y., Zhao, L. L., Lin, Y. R., Wu, K. H., & Wu, H. P. (2013). Different urinalysis appearances in children with simple and perforated appendicitis. *The American Journal of Emergency Medicine, 31*(11), 1560–1563.

Managing Family Expectations: Uncertainty Is Common in Paediatric Practice

Lionel Lubitz

1 Clinical Pearl

Dealing with uncertainty in paediatrics is a core skill in the art of consultation.

2 Clinical Case

Quotes taken from Google Review:

> Dr X is the best paediatrician in the world.
>
> Dr X is a blessing to our family.
>
> Dr X is an uncaring ignorant person: I wouldn't even send my dog to see them.
>
> One of the worst experiences ever with Dr X. I came out of the appointment crying.

3 Discussion

These hyperbolic reviews are all for Dr. X, a consultant paediatrician working in a private practice. It is unlikely the clinician is a "Jekyll and Hyde" character. It may be that the expectations of the family were mismatched with those of the clinician. It may be that diagnostic uncertainty is present. It may be both.

In paediatrics, there exists a tension between the rational flow of diagnosis, subsequent management and the desired outcome with its (ideally) linear predictable

L. Lubitz (✉)
Victorian Childrens Clinic, Malvern, VIC, Australia

C. F. Lynch et al. (eds.), *The Art of Paediatric Medicine Beyond the Evidence Base*,
https://doi.org/10.1007/978-981-96-7234-9_74

pathway, and the substantial unknowns that can be irrational and unpredictable. The diagnosis may only reveal itself with time as the child grows and develops, or more collateral information becomes available.

Our training encourages confidence, perfectionism, clarity of thought and action, and fear of failure. The fear of being wrong is based on a deep fear of mortality and morbidity that evokes a false need to parade certainty in the face of all the evidence to the contrary. Our world is filled with the opposite, with uncertainty our constant companion, making a level of failure inevitable. This perception of incompetence makes us feel more anxious and incompetent. This is particularly challenging in developmental paediatrics with its comorbidities, diagnostic and management uncertainties. Often over time, a clearer picture of the true nature of the problem emerges.

Authority and infallibility are two important concepts to contemplate. The potential for mistakes, even small inaccuracies, can paralyse our decision making and threaten our sense of authority and infallibility. We are trained to be successful, but success is not always possible. Anxiety is the natural sequel to this pathway.

Care of the child occurs in the context of family. Families come in many different formations.

> Happy families are all alike; every unhappy family is unhappy in its own way. *Tolstoy*

Each family brings its own expectations to the consultation. With the increase in accessibility of medical information in the digital world, the expectations are increased for a successful outcome or "fixing the problem."

We know that being able to engage well with children and families leads to better health outcomes however, the power paradigm persists for two main reasons:

1. The paediatrician holds the bulk of the knowledge and much of the authority and experience.
2. The patient is in a state of vulnerability and weakness. How can you balance that and maintain the patient's 'confidence in your authority'?

The opposite viewpoint to being open, frank, honest and non-authoritarian can be potentially perceived as uncertain and weak. For example, in ADHD and Anxiety disorders, we may believe that our patient will benefit from medication, but we are also aware of the controversies in the community about 'medicating our children.' Adding to this unease, we also have our own potential uncertainty about the management of the problem based on our training and experience. A clinician's level of uncertainty may be enhanced if faced with the threat of medicolegal consequences. Indeed, it may also be a struggle to challenge the certainties presented by 'alternative/complementary health practitioners.'

It is in the Art of the Consultation that resolution lies:

- It is the language of the consultation that holds the key to a successful intervention.
- The capacity to hold the anxiety in the room and allow the decision to occur with the patient/carer feeling that they have control/power, thus enabling them to feel the decision is mutual, not imposed.

We cope with uncertainty using the following guidelines:

1. Trust—trust yourself and your training.
2. Honesty—be open and allow uncertainties into the conversation but watch out that you don't lose the patient's 'faith/trust' in you. This is a delicate balance. The honest space between the doctor and patient/parent will open the bridge to a successful encounter. Self-doubt is inevitable and sharing vulnerabilities and uncertainties can be empowering and may improve the patient/parent's confidence in you.
3. Awareness/Confidence/Empathy—being aware and empathic of the complexities of the issues within the background of your own perceptions, temperament and 'prejudices.'
4. Acceptance—accept that uncertainty, even failure is to some extent inevitable.
5. Allow time during the consultation to enable concerns to be voiced and assist in your decision making.

Love, kindness and hope are probably the most important attributes one can bring to a consultation. Remember:

> People don't care how much you know until they know how much you care. *Roosevelt*

You need to 'hold' yourself and your patient within the uncertainty, with an overt demonstration of care and devotion (a constant challenge).

Travelling Overseas to Visit Family and Friends Is More Dangerous than Disneyland

David A. Foley and Linny K. Phuong

1 Clinical Pearl

Understanding the unique risks associated with travelling to visit friends and relatives is crucial for paediatric healthcare providers to ensure appropriate preventive measures.

2 Clinical Case

A 4-year-old girl, Anushka, was seen by her paediatrician for an acute respiratory tract infection. During the review, Anushka's parents mentioned that they are preparing for her first trip to India to attend a family wedding. Her parents, born in India but now living in Western Australia, plan to stay with family and friends in India and enjoy local cuisine during their visit.

D. A. Foley (✉)
Department of Microbiology, PathWest Laboratory Medicine WA, Nedlands, WA, Australia

Wesfarmers Centre of Vaccines and Infectious Diseases, Telethon Kids Institute, University of Western Australia, Perth, WA, Australia

School of Medicine, University of Western Australia, Perth, WA, Australia

L. K. Phuong
Infection and Immunity Theme, Murdoch Children's Research Institute, Royal Children's Hospital, Parkville, Melbourne, Australia

Department of Paediatrics, University of Melbourne, Melbourne, Australia

C. F. Lynch et al. (eds.), *The Art of Paediatric Medicine Beyond the Evidence Base*,
https://doi.org/10.1007/978-981-96-7234-9_75

3 Discussion

Although high-profile outbreaks, such as those associated with Disneyland [1], have garnered media attention, the infection risks associated with travel to resorts are generally lower than those encountered when visiting friends and relatives (VFR). VFR travel often involves closer interactions with the local community, increased exposure to local food and water sources, and longer duration of stay [2]. This type of travel poses unique health challenges requiring careful risk assessment and preventive measures. Importantly, parents may have a reduced perception of risk due to familiarity with the destination, potentially underestimating the health threats to themselves and their children [2].

- **Foodborne illnesses:** Exposure to foodborne pathogens is a significant risk in VFR travel due to close contact, shared home-cooked meals, street food, and potentially untreated water. Depending on the destination, parents should be advised to ensure the family drinks only bottled or boiled water and to avoid raw or undercooked foods, including fruits and vegetables that may have been washed with contaminated water [3]. Vaccinations for hepatitis A and typhoid fever may be indicated, depending on the region of travel [4].
- **Mosquito-borne illnesses:** Infections such as malaria, chikungunya, Zika, and dengue are prevalent in parts of India [5] and other regions in the world. Preventive measures, including mosquito repellents, bed nets, and wearing long-sleeved clothing, are essential to reduce the risk of mosquito bites [6]. Malaria prophylaxis should be considered based on the specific region of travel and local malaria risk [7].
- **Tuberculosis:** Close contact with friends and relatives in a country with high tuberculosis (TB) incidence poses a risk of TB exposure and infection. Parents should be educated regarding TB symptoms and the importance of timely medical evaluation if symptoms arise after travel. The BCG vaccine, a vaccine that protects against TB, may be indicated for younger children (see Part IV, Chapter "Do All Child Travellers Need BCG Vaccination?").
- **Measles and other routine vaccines:** Ensure immunisations are up to date [4]. If travelling to a measles endemic region, administration of a measles-containing vaccine from 6 months of age is recommended [8].
- **Respiratory virus infections:** Close contact in VFR travel can increase respiratory infection risk. Administering the seasonal influenza vaccination is recommended [4].
- **Other animal risks:** Rabies remains a risk in many countries. It is vital to consider rabies vaccination and to be aware of the importance of seeking urgent medical attention in the case of mammalian bites [4].

The Centers for Disease Control and Prevention Travelers' Health [9] and Travel Health Pro websites [10] provide detailed immunisation recommendations and travel advisories for specific regions, and both are excellent resources for clinicians.

4 Other Gems

- **Diagnosis of fever in returned travelers:** The differential diagnosis of fever in returned travellers is guided by the time from the last travel to the onset of symptoms. A thorough travel and exposure history is crucial for narrowing down potential infectious aetiologies.

References

1. Doll, M. K., & Correira, J. W. (2021). Revisiting the 2014-15 Disneyland measles outbreak and its influence on pediatric vaccinations. *Human Vaccines & Immunotherapeutics, 17*(11), 4210–4215.
2. Heywood, A. E., Zwar, N., Forssman, B. L., Seale, H., Stephens, N., Musto, J., Lane, C., Polkinghorne, B., Sheikh, M., Smith, M., Worth, H., & Macintyre, C. R. (2016). The contribution of travellers visiting friends and relatives to notified infectious diseases in Australia: State-based enhanced surveillance. *Epidemiology and Infection, 144*(16), 3554–3563.
3. Griffith, C. J. (2023). Preventing and managing travel-related foodborne disease. In *Food safety management* (pp. 767–797). Elsevier.
4. Steffen, R., Chen, L. H., & Leggat, P. A. (2023). Travel vaccines-priorities determined by incidence and impact. *Journal of Travel Medicine, 30*, 7.
5. Naik, B. R., Tyagi, B. K., & Xue, R. D. (2023). Mosquito-borne diseases in India over the past 50 years and their global public health implications: A systematic review. *Journal of the American Mosquito Control Association, 39*(4), 258–277.
6. Nasci, R. S., Wirtz, R. A., & Brogdon, W. G. (2016). Protection against mosquitoes, ticks, and other arthropods. In *CDC health information for international travel* (pp. 94–99).
7. Fikadu, M., & Ashenafi, E. (2023). Malaria: An overview. *Infection and Drug Resistance, 16*, 3339–3347.
8. Hyle, E. P., Rao, S. R., Bangs, A. C., Gastanaduy, P., Fiebelkorn, A. P., Hagmann, S. H. F., Walker, A. T., Walensky, R. P., Ryan, E. T., & LaRocque, R. C. (2020). Clinical practices for measles-mumps-rubella vaccination among US pediatric international travelers. *JAMA Pediatrics, 174, (2)*, e194515.
9. Center for Disease Control Travelers' Health. https://wwwnc.cdc.gov/travel (20th September).
10. National Travel Health Network and Centre Travel Health Pro. https://travelhealthpro.org.uk/ (20th September).

Do All Child Travellers Need BCG Vaccination?

David A. Foley and Linny K. Phuong

1 Clinical Pearl

"All child travellers need BCG vaccination" is not a one-size-fits-all rule. Individual risk assessment is crucial, especially for infants and young children.

2 Clinical Case

Hua, a healthy 18-month-old girl, is preparing for her first trip to China to meet her grandparents. Her parents, concerned about the risk of tuberculosis (TB) exposure during their three-month stay, consulted with their paediatrician about the need for BCG vaccination. Hua has not previously received the BCG vaccine, as it is not part of the routine immunisation schedule in their residential country. There is no known history of TB in the family, and Hua is otherwise healthy with no underlying medical conditions.

D. A. Foley (✉)
Department of Microbiology, PathWest Laboratory Medicine WA, Nedlands, WA, Australia

Wesfarmers Centre of Vaccines and Infectious Diseases, Telethon Kids Institute, University of Western Australia, Perth, WA, Australia

School of Medicine, University of Western Australia, Perth, WA, Australia

L. K. Phuong
Infection and Immunity Theme, Murdoch Children's Research Institute, Royal Children's Hospital, Parkville, Melbourne, Australia

Department of Paediatrics, University of Melbourne, Melbourne, Australia

C. F. Lynch et al. (eds.), *The Art of Paediatric Medicine Beyond the Evidence Base*,
https://doi.org/10.1007/978-981-96-7234-9_76

3 Discussion

The BCG (Bacillus Calmette-Guérin) vaccine is a live, attenuated vaccine [1]. Although it may have some benefits in preventing TB infection, its main protective effect is against severe forms of TB, such as miliary TB and TB meningitis, particularly in children under the age of five years [1]. It is considered to be less effective in older children and adults.

The BCG vaccine is administered as a single intradermal dose. Whilst generally considered safe, it can lead to complications such as abscess formation at the injection site and scarring. Dissemination of the vaccine strain can occur in immunocompromised individuals [1].

BCG vaccination is typically recommended in countries with high TB incidence, defined as >40 cases per 100,000 population annually. The BCG vaccine is recommended for children under five years travelling to a high TB-incidence region for over a month [2]. Due to lower utility, it is generally not recommended for older age groups. The BCG vaccine should be administered at least three months before departure to allow adequate immune response.

Key factors influencing the decision to vaccinate include [2]:

- **Age:** children under five are more likely to develop severe forms of TB.
- **TB incidence at the destination:** higher local TB rates (>40/100,000/year) correlate with increased exposure risk.
- **Duration of stay (>one month):** residence in high-risk areas increases the likelihood of exposure and hence infection.
- **Type of contact with local populations:** staying with friends or family in the community elevates the risk.

Before BCG vaccine administration, a risk assessment for TB exposure and, if indicated, subsequent screening for latent TB using a tuberculin skin test (TST) or TB interferon-gamma release assay should be considered [3].

In Hua's case, vaccination with BCG would be recommended as they are travelling to a high-risk region for a longer duration and staying with family.

4 Other Gems

- **Cross-reaction with tuberculin skin test**: BCG vaccination can cause a positive reaction in the tuberculin skin test, reducing its specificity for TB detection in vaccinated individuals [4].
- **TB Interferon-gamma release assays**: these tests, such as the QuantiFERON Gold, are more specific than the TST; receipt of the BCG does not cause a positive result. Interferon-gamma release assays can be used in children under two years old [5].

- **BCG Vaccination for healthcare workers**: healthcare workers working in settings with high exposure risk to drug-resistant TB may benefit from BCG vaccination [6].
- **Protection against other non-TB Mycobacteria**: BCG vaccination also protects against *Mycobacterium leprae* infection, the causative agent of leprosy. Children under five with household contact with leprosy may be considered for BCG vaccination [7]. In these cases, consultation with an Infectious Diseases physician is recommended.

References

1. Hatherill, M., & Cobelens, F. (2022). Infant BCG vaccination is beneficial, but not sufficient. *The Lancet Global Health, 10*(9), e1220–e1221.
2. Ritz, N., Connell, T. G., & Curtis, N. (2008). To BCG or not to BCG?: Preventing travel-associated tuberculosis in children. *Vaccine, 26*(47), 5905–5910.
3. Ritz, N., Tebruegge, M., Camacho-Badilla, K., Haeusler, G. M., Connell, T. G., & Curtis, N. (2012). To TST or not to TST: Is tuberculin skin testing necessary before BCG immunisation in children? *Vaccine, 30*(8), 1434–1436.
4. Taylor, J. W., Curtis, N., & Denholm, J. (2020). BCG vaccination: An update on current Australian practices. *Australian Journal of General Practice, 49*(10), 651–655.
5. Wendorf, K. A., Lowenthal, P., Feraud, J., Cabanting, N., & Murto, C. (2020). Interferon-γ release assays for tuberculosis infection diagnosis in refugees< 5 years old. *Pediatrics, 146*, 4.
6. Bo, M., & Zotti, C. M. (2016). European policies on tuberculosis prevention in healthcare workers: Which role for BCG? A systematic review. *Human Vaccines & Immunotherapeutics, 12*(11), 2753–2764.
7. Orujyan, D., Narinyan, W., Rangarajan, S., Rangchaikul, P., Prasad, C., Saviola, B., & Venketaraman, V. (2022). Protective efficacy of BCG vaccine against mycobacterium leprae and non-tuberculous mycobacterial infections. *Vaccine, 10*(3), 390.

There Is No Such Thing as a Difficult Parent

Felix Oberender

1 Clinical Pearl

There is no such thing as a difficult parent; only humans who react in a way that demands our understanding, analysis and care.

2 Clinical Case

It's been a long day, and the evening round is grinding along. There is just one more case, but we have been warned, "The parents are really difficult." The mother, we're told, is untrusting and demanding, questioning every test and "shopping for opinions." The father is rarely around. When he does attend, he has not been pleasant, making little effort to hide his impatience and frustration.

The child does alright in the end, but barely. When the case is reviewed, we learn that the mother tried to tell us that "something was off" with her child. It took us a long time to see it, too. The father had to keep things together with two other kids at home and his employer calling him back to work. He felt his partner's anxiety and could not understand what looked like our indifference to it all. Meanwhile, the team understood that the family was stressed and tried to convince them to be patient with our treatment plan. It seemed hard to get them "to come around."

F. Oberender (✉)
Monash Children's Hospital, Melbourne, VIC, Australia

Department of Paediatrics, Monash University, Melbourne, VIC, Australia

C. F. Lynch et al. (eds.), *The Art of Paediatric Medicine Beyond the Evidence Base*,
https://doi.org/10.1007/978-981-96-7234-9_77

3 Discussion

This is a fictional case, but it is based on real stories. There will be few paediatricians who would not have heard, at some point in their careers, a lament about a mother, a father or a carer being difficult. Before we call this what it is, unhelpful and unprofessional, let's also take a moment to examine how it comes about; a venting of frustration, exacerbation and maybe worry. For a moment, perhaps, calling someone "difficult" might also lighten the load of responsibility and provide comfort from worry and uncertainty.

Interestingly, though, we don't label a high inflammatory marker "difficult", or the elevated white cell count "obstructive", or the tachycardia "not understanding." These might surprise us, be unwelcome and make us anxious. Yet they are assessed to guide our thinking and to help us understand. We accept them and work with them to the advantage of our patient. So why should friction between the child's closest environment, their family, and health professionals be any different? Perhaps this "pearl" is still not fully recognised for what it is; it is a **vital sign**.

Ignoring it is dangerous and has long been known to risk providing poorer quality care [1]. In paediatrics, there are many reports of families and carers advocating for their child but "the system" being slow to respond [2, 3].

Being confronted with disagreement, anger or aggression is not easy in our professional or our personal lives. Without training, handling conflict can easily be managed poorly. It is a challenge fundamentally different in nature to dealing with objective clinical data. The complex systems we work in are not designed to measure and act on the multifaceted human responses to stress and the abnormal, though some effort is being made [4]. Families are also not infallible, and their worry may not correlate with the actual severity of a situation [5]. In addition, and not least, we must also manage our own emotional reaction to discord and confrontation [6, 7]. Yet like any other concerning finding, this complicated interplay needs an assessment and a plan. It needs a team and the team to work well. It needs the family and carers to be on the team [8].

There is no such thing as a difficult parent—only humans who react in a way that demands our understanding, analysis and care.

References

1. Meadow, R. (1992). Difficult and unlikeable parents. *Archives of Disease in Childhood, 67*(6), 697–702.
2. Ryan's Rule. *Clinical excellence Queensland | Queensland health*. Accessed 22nd Sep 2024. http://staging.clinicalexcellence.qld.gov.au/priority-areas/safety-and-quality/ryans-rule.
3. *Resources—Clinical Excellence Commission*. Accessed September 22, 2024. https://www.cec.health.nsw.gov.au/kccp-patients-safe/reach/resources.
4. Sever, Z., Schlapbach, L. J., Gilholm, P., et al. (2023). Impact of parental and healthcare professional concern on the diagnosis of pediatric sepsis: A diagnostic accuracy study. *Frontiers in Pediatrics, 11*. https://doi.org/10.3389/fped.2023.1140121

5. Albutt, A., Roland, D., Lawton, R., Conner, M., & O'Hara, J. (2022). Capturing parents' perspectives of child wellness to support identification of acutely unwell children in the emergency department. *Journal of Patient Safety, 18*(5), 410–414. https://doi.org/10.1097/PTS.0000000000000949
6. Heyhoe, J., Birks, Y., Harrison, R., O'Hara, J. K., Cracknell, A., & Lawton, R. (2016). The role of emotion in patient safety: Are we brave enough to scratch beneath the surface? *Journal of the Royal Society of Medicine, 109*(2), 52–58. https://doi.org/10.1177/0141076815620614
7. Croskerry, P., Abbass, A. A., & Wu, A. W. (2008). How doctors feel: Affective issues in patients' safety. *The Lancet, 372*(9645), 1205–1206. https://doi.org/10.1016/S0140-6736(08)61500-7
8. Clay, A. M., & Parsh, B. (2016). Patient- and family-centered care: It's not just for pediatrics anymore. *AMA Journal of Ethics, 18*(1), 40–44. https://doi.org/10.1001/journalofethics.2016.18.1.medu3-1601

oneTEAM: Parents as the Experts of Their Child

Annie Moulden

1 Clinical Pearl

Parents often detect deterioration in their child early. This may be before clinicians detect deterioration and before vital signs change. Parents may not know *what* is wrong, but they absolutely know that *something* is wrong.

2 Clinical Case

A toddler was holidaying with his parents in a small country town in summer when he became unwell.

He developed a fever, began vomiting and was lethargic and drowsy. His parents rang Nurse on Call who suggested they go to the closest Urgent Care Centre. Nursing assessment there indicated that he was tachycardic, tachypnoeic, irritable and not tolerating oral fluids. The nurse deemed he needed Paediatric review, so he was taken by his parents to the closest hospital with a Paediatric service.

By this stage, his parents describe he was making a 'high pitched whimpering noise' and was 'groaning in pain', worse when he was sitting up. 'He was floppy and pale; very sick and exhausted.' He was triaged as a Category 2 patient with the expectation of a medical review in 10 minutes.

Over the next 3 hours, the toddler was treated for presumed gastroenteritis. Despite ongoing drowsiness and poor fluid intake, his vital signs improved a little and he was discharged. His mother clearly voiced her concern to the medical and nursing staff at this decision, as to her eyes he was not improving, and indeed seemed worse.

A. Moulden (✉)
Victorian Childrens Clinic, Malvern, Australia

C. F. Lynch et al. (eds.), *The Art of Paediatric Medicine Beyond the Evidence Base*,
https://doi.org/10.1007/978-981-96-7234-9_78

Following his discharge, the boy continued to deteriorate. His parents took him to another Urgent Care Centre and he was transferred back to the regional hospital in a parlous state. After review by the Paediatric team, he was transferred urgently to a Paediatric Intensive Care Unit (PICU) at a tertiary Children's Hospital where he died the following morning from meningitis.

3 Discussion

This devastating clinical scenario occurred in a high resource country with universal health care. It is a sad and sobering case that highlights the critical importance of parents as the expert of their child and the consequences of not listening to them. Paediatric clinicians are taught this early in our training: **listen to the parents**. So how is it that we continue to have children with poor health outcomes, including death, when parents tell us their voices were not heard?

At a recent inquest into the care of this toddler, the coroner found that his death was preventable [1]. His mother told the coroner:

> …I remember feeling relief that he started vomiting again and pushed [the buzzer] 'cause I thought it would mean that they would no longer be making us leave… … … they're going to keep him and do something… …I said, 'Can this please stop the discharge process?' I don't recall who I said that to, but I said it to a member of staff…and I thought that was enough for them to understand that I was concerned, and they didn't follow-up with, 'Oh why do you want that to stop?' It was more, 'No, he will still be going.

For families to repeatedly seek care, knowing that "something is not right" with their child, and having their concerns minimised or dismissed is a failure in the system, in this case with tragic consequences. Even when the consequences are less severe, confidence in the care team is eroded if parents feel their expertise in their own child is not recognised.

The doctor who assessed the patient told the coroner that 'I wish I had escalated this toddler's care to the Paediatric team.' They further stated that 'a big problem for [the parents] was me not listening to them … I've thought about that a lot.' The impact on doctors (especially junior doctors) of a sentinel event is profound and may also have lifelong consequences both professionally and personally.

For all these reasons, we need to actively invite parents to share their concerns and to listen very carefully to them. oneTEAM is one way of formalising this process. oneTEAM is a process at the Royal Children's Hospital in Melbourne, and involves actively including parents and carers as part of the clinical team by inviting them to share their concerns. During observations and ward rounds, parents are asked 'Do you have any concerns at the moment?' and the response documented on the observation chart. Parents are also able to use the same escalation process as clinical staff and request an urgent medical review or call the Medical Emergency Team.

On a statewide level, a process to allow parents to escalate concerns if they continue to be worried (despite escalation to the local team) is being created because of the advocacy of parents and clinicians. Creating a stronger safety net, that wraps around all levels, will hopefully reduce catastrophic events.

Reference

1. Coroners report State of Victoria COR 2021 007004 *Finding Into Death Following Inquest* Form 37 Rule 63(1) Section 67 of the Coroners Act 2008.

Help Parents Help You

Erin Mills

1 Clinical Pearl

Communicate the expected illness trajectory so the parent can tell you when their child's illness deviates.

2 Clinical Case

Siti, a 3-year-old child, presents to the emergency department (ED) in peak influenza season with 3 days of fever, lethargy, muscle aches and sore throat. An external respiratory swab has returned a positive result for influenza A. The primary reason for the presentation is that her parents want to know if there is anything they can do to make Siti feel better faster. On examination Siti looks miserable but not acutely unwell, with vital signs within normal limits at the time of review. There is some coryza noted, and a red throat, but no clinical signs of dehydration with a normal cardiorespiratory exam. The treating clinician makes a working diagnosis of influenza, without any significant current complications, and talks to her parents about supportive care strategies such as analgesia and rest.

Prior to discharge, the clinician tells her parents how they think the next few days with influenza should look: Siti will likely remain tired and febrile for a couple of days before she will slowly start to get better. They inform the parents that they do not, however, expect Siti to get significantly worse. So if Siti is more lethargic/

E. Mills (✉)
Monash Children's Hospital, Clayton, VIC, Australia

Monash University, Clayton, VIC, Australia

Safer Care Victoria, Melbourne, VIC, Australia

C. F. Lynch et al. (eds.), *The Art of Paediatric Medicine Beyond the Evidence Base*,
https://doi.org/10.1007/978-981-96-7234-9_79

drowsy, drinking less, having increased effort to breathe, or the parent has any other concerns, they should seek medical re-review. Siti's parents are happy with this plan, which is written in the discharge summary, and take her home.

Four days later they re-present to the ED because Siti is febrile again after one day of being fever-free. Siti is also drinking less, more lethargic and is breathing 'harder.' On examination, Siti is febrile, tachycardic and tachypnoeic. There is moderate work of breathing, and coarse crepitations in the left lower zone on auscultation of the chest. Chest X-ray confirms a left lower lobe pneumonia, which has likely developed as a complication of the influenza infection.

Siti's parents comment that although they know waiting times in the ED can be long and staff are extremely busy, they felt empowered and welcome to return for review because they were given such clear discharge advice. This resulted in a good outcome for Siti, who recovered well after her pneumonia was treated.

3 Discussion

Regardless of whether a child is discharged home or remaining in hospital, it is very likely a parent or carer will be by their side for **long periods** of the day. **Families** are increasingly viewed as **key stakeholders** to detect deterioration, and their expertise about their own child can be used to identify early and subtle signs not yet evident to clinicians.Reference 11, 2

Unrecognised deterioration either due to an incorrect working diagnosis or an unidentified complication is one of the most common contributors to preventable harm in hospitals. 3, 4If clinicians communicate their working diagnosis, the alternate diagnoses, expected clinical trajectory and possible complications, families can be used as a resource to alert clinicians to a patient deviating from the expected path.

Sometimes this conversation can be difficult when the diagnosis is uncertain, which is common with some presentations such as fever or abdominal pain, especially early in the illness. Some clinicians feel the need to be 'right' and 'provide the answers' and it can be hard to sit with uncertainty. However honest and clear communication will mean the parents know exactly when to worry and can either escalate care or bring the child back for review.

4 Other Gems

- Presentation to a health practitioner for review of a sick child can be a stressful event, and this can lead to poor retention of information discussed.
- Include expected timelines for recovery and worrying signs to look out for as part of written discharge paperwork given to the patient.
- Also include a follow up plan for families, which may include a review with their general practitioner or re-presentation to a hospital service.

References

1. Albutt, A. K., O'Hara, J. K., Conner, M. T., Fletcher, S. J., & Lawton, R. J. (2017). Is there a role for patients and their relatives in escalating clinical deterioration in hospital? A systematic review. *Health Expectations, 20*(5), 818–825. https://doi.org/10.1111/hex.12496
2. Australian Commission on Safety and Quality in Health Care. (2021). *National Safety and quality health service standards* (2nd ed. – version 2). ACSQHC.
3. Oakley, E. M., Mills, E., Phillips, A., Roberts, A., C, M, Farrell, T., Taylor, K., Watson, L., & Rawnsley, K. (2023). *Improving the safety of Care for Victorian Children*. Safer Care Victoria.
4. Committee on Diagnostic Error in Health Care; Board on Health Care Services; Institute of Medicine; The National Academies of Sciences, Engineering, and Medicine. (2015). In E. P. Balogh, B. T. Miller, & J. R. Ball (Eds.), *Improving diagnosis in health care*. National Academies Press (US). Overview of Diagnostic Error in Health Care. Available from: https://www.ncbi.nlm.nih.gov/books/NBK338594/. Accessed 25th Aug 2024

A Worried Parent Is the Most Important Vital Sign

Erin Mills

1 Clinical Pearl

If a parent is worried, don't just reassure them. Ask yourself "Could I be missing something?" and carefully review the child.

2 Clinical Case

Jackson, a four-year-old boy with a history of Autism Spectrum Disorder (ASD) level two, was brought into the emergency department with his parents. He had been febrile for a couple of hours and his parents felt he 'wasn't quite right.' There were no infective or other localising symptoms on history. The child did not look unwell to the treating registrar. His vital signs were all within normal limits except for a temperature of 38.2 degrees. Thorough examination did not reveal any obvious source of the fever with respiratory, cardiac and abdominal examinations within normal limits.

The registrar initially intended to send this child home, with safety netting advice, but the parents were extremely concerned: *'This is not like him. This is different to the virus infections he has had before. We really think something bad is going on.'*

The registrar listened to these concerns and decided to do some simple investigations: a chest X-ray (CXR), urine dipstick, a full blood examination and a C-reactive

E. Mills (✉)
Monash Children's Hospital, Clayton, VIC, Australia

Monash University, Clayton, VIC, Australia

Safer Care Victoria, Melbourne, VIC, Australia

C. F. Lynch et al. (eds.), *The Art of Paediatric Medicine Beyond the Evidence Base*,
https://doi.org/10.1007/978-981-96-7234-9_80

protein (CRP). The urine and CXR results were normal, but the white cell count at **22** (normal 4–11 × 10^9/L), and CRP **290** (normal <5 mg/L) were significantly elevated. These results made the registrar consider a bacterial infection, though the source was not evident, so a review by a consultant emergency physician was requested.

The consultant reviewed the child, who still looked generally well and had normal vital signs. Again, no focus of infection was apparent on history or examination. The clinician also listened to the ongoing concerns voiced by the parents and decided to request an abdominal ultrasound despite the child having a soft abdomen with no peritonism.

The abdominal ultrasound revealed the child had appendicitis, with perforation. Urgent surgery was required.

The concern from the parents that 'something was different', and a reluctance to take Jackson home, were the only clues to the diagnosis for this child. If the treating clinician had not listened, they almost certainly would have missed the diagnosis and the outcome for this child could have been much more serious.

3 Discussion

Delayed recognition of deterioration is one of the most common contributors to preventable harm in hospitalised children [1]. Parents are well placed (literally right there at the bedside) with the expertise to be able to identify the subtle early signs of deterioration in their child, but clinicians frequently do not include them as a resource in clinical decision making. In Australia, a number of states most health services have established patient and carer-initiated escalation systems. For example, in Queensland, parent advocates have resulted in Ryan's Rule [2] and Aishwarya's CARE call [3] in Western Australia. A system for clinicians assess for parent or carer concerns about clinical deterioration as part of routine vital sign monitoring has also proved successful, with carer concerns being more strongly associated with clinical deterioration in the child than any abnormal vital sign [4].

When patients and families raise concerns, clinicians tend to interpret these as 'complaints' and therefore respond with 'reassurance' or 'de-escalation.' Sometimes clinicians may feel defensive as if their judgement is being questioned and sometimes there may be barriers for junior staff to escalate to senior staff. When parents raise concerns their child is deteriorating, this should instead trigger a red flag in the mind of the clinician: 'What have I missed?', 'Is the diagnosis correct?', 'Has a complication developed?' and lead to a clinical review to answer these questions. A parent who seems 'unhappy' with the care provided and reluctant to go home needs a senior review for a second opinion with a fresh perspective.

4 Other Gems

- The responsibility should be placed on clinicians to proactively seek and respond to the concerns of patients and their families about deterioration. The National Safety and Quality Health Service Standards in Australia dictate that each health service must have a process for patients, carers or families to directly escalate care. Unfortunately, often the patients at highest risk of unrecognised deterioration are the least likely to be aware of these processes and be able to articulate their concerns to the relevant staff member.
- Clinicians should be particularly aware when caring for children with disability. Often parents only seek help if they are very concerned for their child because of the increased challenges of presenting to ED. They may also have expert knowledge of the rare medical or genetic condition of their child.
- Children from cultural and linguistically diverse backgrounds may also be at increased risk.
- Consider how the concerns of parents could be routinely included into handovers and huddles, and design systems within your model of care that include patients and parents in clinical decision making.

References

1. Oakley, E., Moulden, A., Mills, E., Phillips, A., Roberts, M., Farrell, T., Taylor, K., Watson, L., & Rawnsley, K. (2023). *Improving the safety of Care for Victorian Children*. Safer Care Victoria.
2. Barnes, M. (2011). *Inquest into the death of Ryan Charles Saunders*. File no COR 4449/07. Available from https://www.courts.qld.gov.au/__data/assets/pdf_file/0004/107536/cif-saunders-rc-20111007.pdf. Accessed 17th Aug 2024.
3. Department of Health, Western Australia. *Aishwarya's CARE Call*. https://www.healthywa.gov.au. Accessed 1st Feb 2025.
4. Mills, E et al. (2025). Association between caregiver concern for deterioration and critical illness in children presenting to hospital: an observational cohort study. The Lancet Child & Adolescent Health, 9(7), 450–458.

Three Strikes and You're In

Erin Mills

1 Clinical Pearl

If a child has multiple unplanned presentations to hospital within the same illness, arrange review by a senior clinician and have a low threshold to perform investigations and/or admit the child.

2 Clinical Case

A six-year-old boy, Charlie, presented to the emergency department (ED) during peak influenza season. He had been febrile for 24 h and was lethargic with a sore throat and bilateral leg pain. The department was very busy that day, with long patient waiting times and several clinical staff on sick leave. A single set of vital signs was performed by the waiting room nurse, which demonstrated that Charlie had a fever of 39 degrees and was mildly tachycardic and tachypnoeic though not meeting any mandatory alert criteria. There were no cubicles available, so he was reviewed by a senior clinician working in a 'rapid assessment' role in the waiting room. They examined Charlie and determined he likely had influenza, given he had the same symptoms as many other children with influenza in the emergency department that day. His parent was instructed to provide supportive care (rest, hydration, analgesia), and they were discharged home.

E. Mills (✉)
Monash Children's Hospital, Clayton, VIC, Australia

Monash University, Clayton, VIC, Australia

Safer Care Victoria, Melbourne, VIC, Australia

C. F. Lynch et al. (eds.), *The Art of Paediatric Medicine Beyond the Evidence Base*,
https://doi.org/10.1007/978-981-96-7234-9_81

The child's mother was unhappy with the diagnosis and management plan. Charlie was the youngest of four children, who had all had viral infections including influenza previously, and his mother had never felt the need to bring any of her children to the ED before. She felt that this illness was 'different', and she was worried. That night she sat by Charlie, who remained febrile. She noticed he had extra effort to breathe the next morning, and brought him back to the ED.

On the second presentation, Charlie was reviewed by a junior registrar who noted the diagnosis made by the more senior clinician the day before. After a brief review, they reiterated that this was consistent with influenza and discharged the child home to continue the supportive care.

That afternoon, at home, Charlie deteriorated. He was more lethargic; he was waking only briefly for small sips of water and refusing to walk due to leg pains. He did not pass urine for more than 12 hours. His mother considered returning to the ED but given they had been reassured twice that this was 'just influenza' she did not see the benefit in a third visit.

That night, the boy's mother sat by his side again, worrying. The next morning, he was barely responsive and had developed a rash over his entire body. They returned to the ED for a third time.

On his third presentation, Charlie was recognised as being severely unwell and rushed to the resuscitation bay. He had a diagnosis of Group A Streptococcal septic shock. Charlie survived his illness, although required a very long hospital stay with invasive multi-organ support.

3 Discussion

It is uncommon for children to present to the emergency department (ED) twice or more, and children with repeated unplanned presentations within the same illness are more likely to have unrecognised serious or rare illness.

Though sepsis is a leading cause of preventable paediatric morbidity and mortality, and important to recognise and treat early, the diagnosis can be difficult to make. Approximately 20% of paediatric ED presentations are due to fever, though only about 1:1000 children with fever will have sepsis. Invasive bacterial infections are more likely in patients re-presenting to the emergency department and in patients whose parents express concerns that 'this illness is different'.

The Consultative Council for Obstetric and Paediatric Morbidity and Mortality (CCOPMM) reviews themes arising from Victorian infant and child deaths. Based on theming of cases of preventable harm, they have published recommendations that children presenting for the second time in the same illness have a senior clinician review and a low threshold for further investigation. CCOPMM recommends clinicians strongly consider admission for a paediatric patient presenting to hospital for the third time in the same illness.

Repeated unplanned presentations may indicate:

- deterioration
- development of a complication (for example a secondary bacterial infection with viral illness)
- the severity of illness has not been appreciated by clinicians
- diagnostic error
- significant parent or caregiver concern

Re-presentation to a hospital within the same illness is a red flag and needs to be taken seriously.

4 Other Gems

- Anchoring bias is a cognitive bias describing the tendency to rely too heavily on the first piece of information received during the decision-making process. It means that when clinicians are given new information (signs, symptoms, investigation results), they interpret it through the lens of the original 'label' or diagnosis. In the case vignette above, this occurs when the senior clinician presumes the child has influenza, because most of the other patients with similar symptoms have influenza. The more junior clinician then 'anchored' to this diagnosis and did not reconsider the diagnosis considering the new information provided at the second presentation.
- To minimise diagnostic errors caused by cognitive biases, set up a system to always have a working diagnosis and a list of considered differential diagnoses. Writing these down or communicating them out loud (to a colleague and/or the parent) helps clinicians to remain more objective.
- It is also important to remember that senior clinicians can get things wrong too, so never be afraid to ask questions or challenge a diagnosis in the interest of safe and high-quality patient care.

References

1. Gangoiti, I., Gorostizaga, Z., Aranzamendi, M., Gomez, B., Benito, J., & Mintegi, S. (2021). Repeated emergency department visits among children with invasive bacterial infections. *The Pediatric Infectious Disease Journal, 40*(5), e205–e207. https://doi.org/10.1097/INF.0000000000003062. PMID: 33464016.
2. Queensland Family and Health Commission. (2024). *Queensland Paediatric sepsis mortality study*. Available from: https://www.qfcc.qld.gov.au/sites/default/files/2024-03/Paediatric%20Sepsis%20Mortality%20Study.pdf. Accessed 25 Aug 2024.
3. Harley, A., Schlapbach, L. J., Johnston, A. N. B., & Massey, D. (2022). Challenges in the recognition and management of paediatric sepsis – the journey. *Australas Emergency Care, 25*(1), 23–29. https://doi.org/10.1016/j.auec.2021.03.006. Epub 2021 Apr 15. PMID: 33865753.

4. Gangoiti, I., Fernandez, C. L., Gallego, M., Gomez, B., Benito, J., & Mintegi, S. (2021). Markers for invasive bacterial infections in previously healthy children. *The American Journal of Emergency Medicine, 48*, 83–86. https://doi.org/10.1016/j.ajem.2021.04.018. Epub 2021 Apr 13. Erratum in: Am J Emerg Med. 2021 Aug;46:806. https://doi.org/10.1016/j.ajem.2021.04.052. PMID: 33862390
5. Harley, A., Latour, J. M., & Schlapbach, L. J. (2019). The role of parental concerns in the recognition of sepsis in children: A literature review. *Frontiers in Pediatrics, 7*, 161. https://doi.org/10.3389/fped.2019.00161. PMID: 31131264; PMCID: PMC6509218.
6. Consultative Council on Obstetric and Paediatric Morbidity and Mortality. (2021). *Victoria's mothers, babies and children report*. Available from: https://www.safercare.vic.gov.au/sites/default/files/2023-11/Victoria%E2%80%99s%20mothers%20babies%20and%20children%20report%202021.pdf. Accessed 25 Aug 2024.

A Sick Child in ED Who Needs an Airway: HELP

Michael Clifford

1 Clinical Pearl

Bag and mask ventilation is lifesaving—you DO NOT HAVE TO INTUBATE if the patient is stable.

2 Clinical Case

Stephanie, a 3-year-old girl, with a past history of complex (prolonged) febrile convulsions and normal neurodevelopment has been brought to the Emergency Department with seizures. Stephanie was administered buccal midazolam at home and has had 2 doses of IM midazolam in the ambulance. On arrival she had an intravenous cannula inserted, blood cultures were taken, and antibiotics administered. Following another dose of midazolam and a load of levetiracetam her seizures continue and she is now desaturating despite oxygen supplementation via Hudson mask. The anaesthetic registrar is in theatre and unable to leave, the paediatric intensive care fellow has been contacted. The nurses ask for your assistance.

M. Clifford (✉)
Departments of Paediatric Intensive Care, Anaesthesia and Pain Management, The Royal Children's Hospital Melbourne, Parkville, VIC, Australia

C. F. Lynch et al. (eds.), *The Art of Paediatric Medicine Beyond the Evidence Base*,
https://doi.org/10.1007/978-981-96-7234-9_82

3 Discussion

Seizures are a common indication for transfer to the Emergency Department. Unfortunately, the therapy required to terminate them often results in the need for airway intervention and often transfer to PICU [1]. Simple febrile convulsions are the most common epilepsy syndrome of childhood—with a predictable natural history, a strong genetic element and a benign prognosis [2]. Many prolonged seizures present with fever, be they (by definition) atypical febrile convulsions or other epilepsies with a reduced threshold for seizures at the time of febrile illness [3]. Failure to terminate these seizures promptly is often an indication for hospital transfer. Failure to terminate them in the Emergency Department often leads to repeat doses of benzodiazepine (which begin to accumulate) and/or escalation with second agents (levetiracetam or phenytoin). The need to provide additional therapy for refractory seizures (or status epilepticus) often requires higher doses of standard therapies and/or anaesthetic agents [4–6]. Airway and breathing support will then require advanced airway management [1].

Most Paediatric (and General) Emergency Departments have considerable expertise with these patients and the decision to intubate is often sensible and reasoned [1]. Local protocols will determine which medications and doses are anticipated. They are often rapidly provided by senior nursing staff and checklists are increasingly used to provide a shared mental model. This will optimise preparation, focus the team members on roles and responses, anticipate any likely complications and clarify points of departure from a standard workflow [7, 8].

Simple things matter, such as [7]:

- preparing and checking the presence of working suction
- having an alternative oxygen or ventilation source
- attaching appropriate monitoring (and predicting the need for additional devices such as end tidal CO2)
- optimising the environment on the bed (a pillow or towel to elevate the head with or without the shoulders) and around the bed or trolley to enable access to the head end (for the airway team) and to the intravenous device (for medication administration)
- pre-cut strapping and tapes
- drawing up pre-defined doses of medications for intubation (and resuscitation)
- allocation of key roles (airway assistant, therapeutics, scribe, etc)
- age appropriate (cuffed) endotracheal tubes (ETT)
- verbalising when to STOP or CALL FOR HELP

These are all equally as important as *two working laryngoscopes, one of which is a* ***videolaryngoscope*** [9–12].

4 Positioning

Optimisation of the head (for both bag and mask ventilation or intubation) requires the so-called "neutral" position—this will vary with age. Neonates and infants have a large head (relative to the thorax) so often benefit from a small pillow (or roll) under the shoulders. Toddlers are more balanced and often require the pillow to elevate the head with (but slightly more than) the shoulders. Children and adolescents almost ALWAYS benefit from a slight head lift (towel or pillow or even multiple pillows in the obese). It is recommended for adults to have the external auditory meatus approximately level with the sternum, and this is not a bad start for most ages, so you will ALWAYS benefit from a pillow.

5 Ventilating

The head can be slightly tilted up, the mask placed over the nose and mouth and held with a C shape (thumb and first finger) and the jaw held with three fingers (middle, ring and pinky) on the bony edge of the mandible NOT the soft tissue of the floor of the mouth (the 3C technique). It helps to ensure that the mouth is open and the tongue is not stuck to the top of the mouth—this is a reason to use a Guedel airway. Gentle squeezing of the self-inflating bag (or use of a Neopuff or T-Piece) should result in movement of the chest wall—the rise and fall ensures adequate ventilation and at this point enough has been done. The child is now safe and proceeding to intubation requires adequate training in an appropriate setting.

6 Intubation

Should intubation be necessary, continue to oxygenate (and preferably ventilate) the child and administer appropriate induction agents and muscle relaxants. A video laryngoscope should ALWAYS be used (use the departmental device with an age-appropriate blade) [8–11].

The selected endotracheal tube should have a malleable stylet inside it (with the end NOT extending beyond the tip of the ETT), and this should be "bent" to reflect the "shape" of whichever video laryngoscope blade is used. This will make finding the ETT on the screen AND deployment beyond the laryngeal inlet MUCH easier.

Introduce the blade over the tongue and use the screen—stay in the midline, go forward gently, identify the epiglottis, lift it out of the way i.e. with a Macintosh blade (or squash it flat –Miller blade). The cords will now be visible and perhaps tracheal rings in the distance.

Push the endotracheal tube through the cords; often a "180-degree rotation" is required at the level of the vallecula to enable the ETT to advance into the trachea, posteriorly into the chest. Stop at the appropriate depth (there may be a "depth marker" or cm marker…or if not… ***the size of the tube (in mm) = the depth of the tube (in cm) at the larynx*** can be used—this will be correct approximately 80% of the time [13] and is THE BEST current predictor we have [14, 15].

Inflate the cuff (preferably with a manometer or confirm the pressure is safe with one, if a syringe was used) and connect and confirm the presence of end tidal CO2. The child now needs a chest x-ray to confirm that the tip of the ETT is at the body of T2 (with the head in the midline, not flexed or extended)—and it should be taped securely [16].

IT (the ETT), is not 'IN' until it is taped 'IN', and confirmed by x-ray!. Prof Frank Shann

Remember—at any time, if in doubt, STOP and GO BACK to BAG MASK VENTILATION—the child will be safe, remain oxygenated and have adequate CO2 clearance until help arrives.

7 Other Gems

- The laryngoscope is the last thing a beginner needs but the first thing they reach for.
- Airway management training is best done in the operating theatre, with an expert, without stress.
- Muscle relaxation will almost always improve the view and facilitate ventilation (but limits neurologic assessment).
- Video laryngoscopy is now the "Gold Standard" for intubation in the Paediatric Emergency Department and PICU.

References

1. Furyk, J., & Dalziel, S. (2023). Seizures and non-epileptic events. In P. Cameron, G. J. Browne, B. Mitra, S. Dalziel, & S. Craig (Eds.), *Textbook of Paediatric Emergency Medicine-E-book* (pp. 243–246). Elsevier Health Sciences.
2. Royal Children's Hospital: Clinical Practice Guidelines. Febrile Seizure. (2020). https://www.rch.org.au/clinicalguide/guideline_index/Febrile_seizure/. Accessed 13 Nov 2024.
3. Royal Children's Hospital: Clinical Practice Guidelines. Afebrile Seizures. (2020). https://www.rch.org.au/clinicalguide/guideline_index/Afebrile_Seizures/. Accessed 13 Nov 2024.
4. Tiwari, A., Meshram, R. J., & Kumar Singh, R. (2022). Febrile Seizures in Children: A Review. *Cureus, 2022*. https://doi.org/10.7759/cureus.31509
5. Messahel, S., Bracken, L., & Appleton, R. (2022). Optimal Management of Status Epilepticus in children in the emergency setting: A review of recent advances. *Open Access Emergency Medicine., 14*, 491–506. https://doi.org/10.2147/OAEM.S293258

6. Schonfeld, D., Gardner, K., Willemsen, M. A., & Ostrow, O. (2024). Reducing unnecessary investigations in paediatric seizures in the emergency department. *BMJ, 25*, 385.
7. Royal Children's Hospital: Clinical Practice Guidelines. Emergency Airway Management. (2021). https://www.rch.org.au/clinicalguide/guideline_index/Emergency_airway_management/. Accessed 13 Nov 2024.
8. Ghedina, N., Alkhouri, H., Badge, H., Fogg, T., & McCarthy, S. (2020 Jun). Paediatric intubation in Australasian emergency departments: A report from the ANZEDAR. *Emergency Medicine Australasia., 32*(3), 401–408.
9. Miller, A. G., Mallory, P., & Rotta, A. T. (2024). Video laryngoscopy as the standard of care for pediatric intubation—The time is now. *Transl Pediatr, 13*(4), 537–541. https://doi.org/10.21037/tp-23-572
10. Kaji, A. H., Shover, C., Lee, J., Yee, L., Pallin, D. J., April, M. D., Carlson, J. N., Fantegrossi, A., & Brown, C. A., III. (2020). Video versus direct and augmented direct laryngoscopy in pediatric tracheal intubations. *Academic Emergency Medicine., 27*(5), 394–402.
11. Hu, X., Jin, Y., Li, J., Xin, J., & Yang, Z. (2020). Efficacy and safety of videolaryngoscopy versus direct laryngoscopy in paediatric intubation: A meta-analysis of 27 randomized controlled trials. *Journal of Clinical Anesthesia*. https://doi.org/10.1016/j.jclinane.2020.109968
12. Serkan, Ö., Adem, D., & Nur, A. B. (2021). Comparison of direct laryngoscopy and video-assisted laryngoscopy in pediatric intensive care unit. *Archives de Pédiatrie., 28*(8), 658–662.
13. Freeman, J. A., Fredricks, B. J., & Best, C. J. (1995). Evaluation of a new method for determining tracheal tube length in children. *Anaesthesia, 50*(12), 1050–1052.
14. Clifford, M., & Butt, W. (2016). Tracheal tube insertion is an essential part of modern paediatric anaesthesia and critical care: Let us get it right. *BJA: British Journal of Anaesthesia., 116*(5), 582–584.
15. Ebenebe, C. U., Schriever, K., Apostolidou, S., Wolf, M., Herrmann, J., Singer, D., & Deindl, P. (2023). Recommendations for endotracheal tube insertion depths in children. *Emergency Medicine Journal., 40*, 583–587.
16. Shann, F., Henning, R. J., Shekerdemian, L., & Butt, W. (2008). Royal Children's hospital (Melbourne). In *Intensive Care Unit. Paediatric Intensive Care Guidelines* (3rd ed.). Collective Pty Ltd..

Critically Ill Patients: Oxygen Is Essential; an Endotracheal Tube Is Not

Richard K. Barnes

1 Clinical Pearl

When the decision is made to intubate a critically ill child, it is vital to keep in mind that ventilation and oxygenation are essential to life, whereas the placement of an endotracheal tube is not.

2 Clinical Case

An 18-month-old child, Zak, is in the Emergency Department (ED). He has a complicated past history: significant prematurity with ongoing slow growth and chronic lung disease; likely an undiagnosed syndrome. He now has an acute respiratory infection. After a period of observation in the ED, his oxygen saturation has fallen to the low 90's despite supplemental oxygen, and he has increasing work of breathing.

It is decided that Zak should be intubated and admitted to the Intensive Care Unit. He is given suitable sedation and muscle relaxant and is easy to ventilate by mask. At direct laryngoscopy, the view is poor, with perhaps just a glimpse of the epiglottis; the oxygen saturation falls rapidly into the low 80's. Bag mask ventilation has resumed, but is now more difficult. When the saturation reaches 90%, a second attempt at laryngoscopy is also unsuccessful. A second operator makes the third attempt at laryngoscopy, again without success. Bag mask ventilation is now also ineffective. Meanwhile the abdomen has become noticeably distended. The oxygen saturation is in the 60's, and not rising.

R. K. Barnes (✉)
Monash Children's Hospital, Melbourne, Australia

C. F. Lynch et al. (eds.), *The Art of Paediatric Medicine Beyond the Evidence Base*,
https://doi.org/10.1007/978-981-96-7234-9_83

At this point, the nominated "airway nurse" offers the team a size #1½ laryngeal mask airway (LMA). This is placed without difficulty and allows satisfactory ventilation. A nasogastric tube is now passed and the stomach decompressed. Zak's oxygen saturation rises to the high 90's. Everyone breathes a sigh of relief.

3 Discussion

Unsuccessful tracheal intubation does not have to become a "failure." At every intubation, all staff should have an understanding that intubation might prove to be difficult or impossible; and there should be a clear plan in place for how to proceed if that scenario arises. The clinical case illustrates several common errors, but also highlights the value of a non-intubation technique in rescuing a deteriorating situation.

Common errors include:

- continuing with an attempt despite dangerously falling oxygenation saturation. It is wise to decide in advance what oxygen saturation level would be the trigger for abandoning that attempt, and to nominate a suitable observer to advise the operator if that point is reached.
- having second and subsequent attempts without making a change that is likely to increase the likelihood of success. Changes might involve personnel, patient position and/or equipment.
- an intention to intubate "no matter what". The likelihood of success falls with each intubation attempt, while the likelihood of being unable to rescue the situation increases.

The "Vortex approach" [1] is a paradigm for approaching airway management which was developed in adult anaesthesia, but which is increasingly applied to all critical care areas and to all ages. It has the great benefit of providing a shared mental model for all staff involved in managing a patient's airway, whatever the setting.

The key premise of the Vortex approach is that there are three (non-surgical) techniques for alveolar oxygen delivery (Fig. 1):

1. face mask
2. supraglottic airway
3. endotracheal tube

This moves us away from a mental model in which intubation must be achieved. The Vortex model also emphasises:

- a "best effort" (and limited attempts) at each of the three techniques.
- a "green zone" of safety, when oxygenation is being achieved, and there is time to pause and plan the next move.
- a clear progression, if all three techniques have failed, to "neck rescue" (emergency front-of-neck access)—thankfully, an extremely rare situation in paediatric practice.

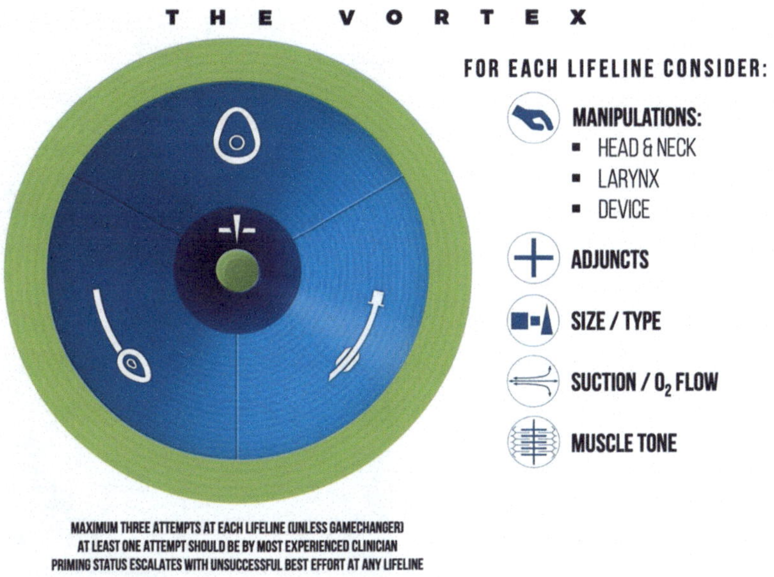

Fig. 1 A visual summary of the Vortex approach. (Vortex Approach copyright Nicholas Chrimes 2016. Used with permission)

4 Increasing the Likelihood of Successful Intubation

Several important advances in recent years have increased the likelihood of intubation success.

Apnoeic oxygenation describes the provision of oxygen to the upper airway (and thus the tracheobronchial tree) of a patient who is apnoeic. As oxygen is taken up from the alveoli into the pulmonary capillaries, it is replaced by oxygen moving down the tracheobronchial tree, thus maintaining patient oxygenation. Apnoeic oxygenation during paediatric intubation has been shown to significantly prolong the time for which safe oxygen saturation is maintained. Not surprisingly, it is associated with a higher rate of successful intubation [2].

Several techniques of apnoeic oxygenation have been described. The simplest is the use of a moderate flow of oxygen via simple nasal prongs (Fig. 2).

Videolaryngoscopy is another recent advance, increasing the success rate of intubation. As in adults, evidence is accumulating that the use of videolaryngoscopy in children results in a significantly increased rate of first-attempt and overall intubation success [3]. This is not surprising, given the strong evidence that video techniques provide a better view of the larynx. The use of a videolaryngoscope also allows for helpful input from observers. And it is a powerful means of safely teaching intubation skills.

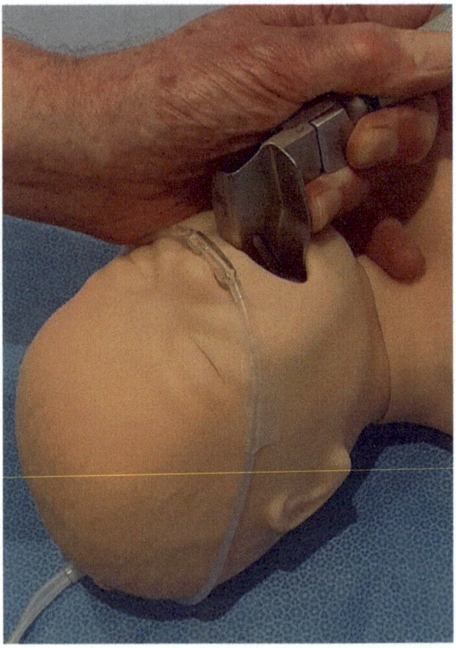

Fig. 2 Simple nasal prongs for paediatric apnoeic oxygenation (Image provided courtesy of Richard K. Barnes)

There are, however, important caveats:

- video intubation requires a different skill set, in particular hand-eye coordination; it must be learned and practised.
- the use of stylets and bougies is more important with video than with conventional laryngoscopy.
- there are several types of videolaryngoscope; familiarity with one does not necessarily translate to facility with another.
- evidence is accruing in support of videolaryngoscopy for neonates [4], however, there is less data and so the recommendations are weaker for its use.

Waveform capnography has been used in anaesthesia since the late 1980s. However, its uptake in other critical care areas has been surprisingly slow. The presence of a sustained capnography waveform is the sine qua non for confirmation of successful intubation, leading to adages such as "no trace = wrong place" [5]. Colorimetric CO_2 indicators have often substituted for waveform capnography in locations beyond the operating theatres and intensive care unit, but are not absolutely reliable, particularly when cardiac output is low. Now, however, simple portable capnographs are available which are easy to operate and give a waveform within seconds. It is difficult to justify the failure to use capnography to confirm tracheal intubation other than in very unusual places or circumstances.

Tracheal intubation is a key procedure in the management of many critically ill patients, particularly those with ventilatory failure. Nonetheless, it is important to recognise that non-invasive ventilatory support (NIV) now has a well-established role in paediatrics [6]. Although NIV is generally not appropriate for the unstable critically ill child, it should always be considered, if only as a temporising measure while awaiting the arrival of more skilled staff.

References

1. Chrimes, N. (2016). The vortex: A universal 'high-acuity implementation tool' for emergency airway management. *British Journal of Anaesthesia, 117*(S1), i20–i27. https://doi.org/10.1093/bja/aew175
2. Fuchs, A., Koepp, G., Huber, M., et al. (2024). Apnoeic oxygenation during paediatric tracheal intubation: A systematic review and meta-analysis. *British Journal of Anaesthesia, 132*(2), 392–406. https://doi.org/10.1016/j.bja.2023.10.039
3. de Carvalho, C. C., Regueira, S. L. P. A., Souza, A. B. S., et al. (2022). Videolaryngoscopes versus direct laryngoscopes in children: Ranking systematic review with network meta-analyses of randomized clinical trials. *Paediatric Anaesthesia, 32*(9), 1000–1014. https://doi.org/10.1111/pan.14521
4. Lingappan, K., Neveln, N., Arnold, J. L., et al. (2023). Videolaryngoscopy versus direct laryngoscopy for tracheal intubation in neonates. *Cochrane Database of Systematic Reviews*, (5), Art. No.: CD009975. https://doi.org/10.1002/14651858.CD009975.pub4. Accessed 09 Aug 2024.
5. Royal college of Anaesthetists, Capnography: No Trace = Wrong Place. (2018). https://www.youtube.com/watch?v=t97G65bignQ&t=17s. Accessed 18 Nov 2024.
6. Morley, S. L. (2016). Non-invasive ventilation in paediatric critical care. *Paediatric Respiratory Reviews, 20*, 24–31. https://doi.org/10.1016/j.prrv.2016.03.001

Venous Access: We Can—and Should—Do Better

Richard K. Barnes

1 Clinical Pearl

A holistic approach to IV (intravenous) insertion is essential.

2 Clinical Cases

A 3-week-old baby, Tao, is admitted with *E. coli* sepsis. The first IV lasts 24 hours, as do each of the next two. The fourth IV, placed in the foot after several attempts, lasts 2 days. The intended duration of intravenous antibiotics is 3 weeks, but after 10 days, Tao is doing well and everyone is exhausted, so he is discharged home to complete a course of oral antibiotics.

A chubby 21-month-old, Joannie, presents with acute mastoiditis. She undergoes a mastoidectomy. The anaesthetist places a cannula in the child's foot. In the post-operative recovery ward, Joannie becomes agitated and manages to kick out the IV.

A 6-year-old, Priya, with chronic suppurative lung disease is admitted with a flare-up, for treatment including ten days of intravenous antibiotics. The parents report that "she has difficult veins, and has been traumatised by previous experiences." A junior doctor has four unsuccessful attempts at cannulation, by which time Priya, the parents and the doctor are all in tears.

R. K. Barnes (✉)
Monash Children's Hospital, Melbourne, Australia

C. F. Lynch et al. (eds.), *The Art of Paediatric Medicine Beyond the Evidence Base*,
https://doi.org/10.1007/978-981-96-7234-9_84

3 Discussion

We all recognise these scenarios. In fact, we almost certainly feel the guilt of having been a party to them! Drips (IV cannulaes) can be challenging for us all [1]. They can be even more challenging for our patients—regardless of age—and for their loved ones. Unhappy drip experiences can leave serious psychological scars—and set things up for future failure.

Before any cannulation, we should pause to ask whether intravenous access is actually necessary:

1. Would oral antibiotics suffice?
2. Could oral or nasogastric rehydration be attempted first?

Apart from being challenging, time-consuming and expensive, venous access can also have serious sequelae.

Always ask "am I a suitable person for this task?"

The more the following factors apply, the greater the skill level required:

- neonate or child under 2 years (particularly if they were premature)
- serious illness
- urgency
- history of previous difficulty
- multiple cannulations already during this episode of care
- significant child and/or parent distress

There should be a clear system for escalation to a person with greater skills, usually after two unsuccessful attempts. Doctors can gain increased proficiency with didactic teaching and simulation training on venous access phantoms [2].

Age-appropriate comfort is both important and increases the likelihood of success. Techniques include swaddling and oral sucrose for infants; distraction techniques and child life therapist support for older children. Use of VR (virtual reality) headsets may be helpful.

Local anaesthetic is helpful at all ages: topical gel if there is time; a bleb of subcutaneous local anaesthetic via a 27 g or 30 g needle if in a hurry. Note that a tiny bleb of subcutaneous local anaesthetic numbs an area the size of a 5-cent piece and despite beliefs to the contrary, does not interfere with your view of the vein.

Suitable restraint of both child and cannulation site by nursing staff is important. In an infant, excellent immobilisation can be obtained by strapping the limb to a warm intravenous bag, thus leaving the proceduralist with both hands free (Fig. 1).

Sedation should be considered when there is significant patient distress. Time pressure might preclude its use. However, at the "peak distress/difficulty" age range of 12 months to 3 years, nasal midazolam 0.3 mg/kg is safe as a single agent, is effective in minutes, and will both reduce distress and increase success.

Before embarking on any cannulation, one should pause to consider whether something more than a simple peripheral intravenous cannula might be indicated. Guidelines are available which indicate the type of intravenous cannula that would

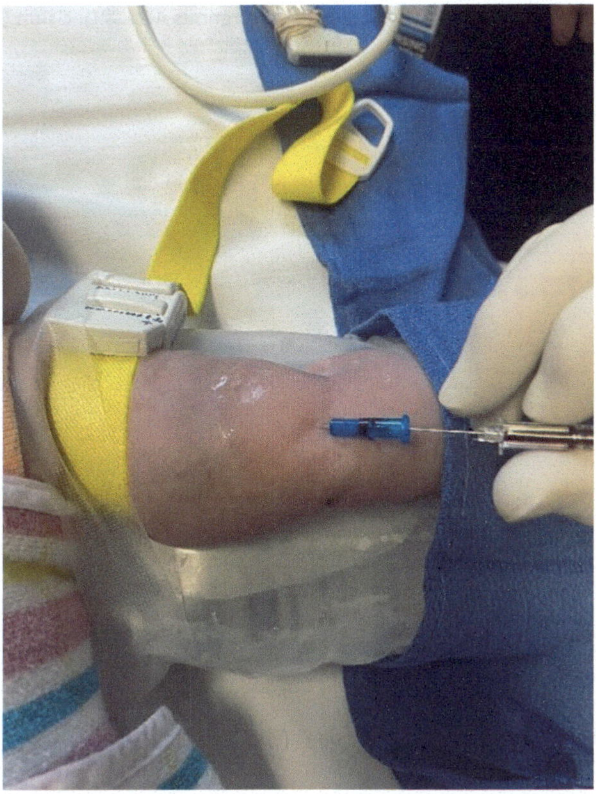

Fig. 1 Placement of a basilic vein long peripheral cannula with ultrasound guidance in an infant. The infant is sedated. The arm is secured to a warm intravenous bag. Local anaesthetic has been used. (Image provided courtesy of Richard K. Barnes)

be most appropriate in various circumstances. The most important determining factors are the intended duration of therapy, the age of the patient and whether the infusate is sclerosant, thus necessitating central access (Fig. 2).

Making the first cannulation the optimal one saves a lot of trouble and misery for everyone. Of course, this will not always be possible, particularly when what is required in the first instance is efficient cannulation to begin urgent therapy. But in almost all circumstances we should aim to make at least the second cannulation the definitive one; it is unacceptable to request expert help after five cannulations, one week into an intended 3-week course of intravenous antibiotic therapy!

If venous access will be required for more than 2–3 days, use of a long peripheral cannula (LPC) should be considered. There is strong evidence that longer cannulas last longer. 22 g × 45 mm and 64 mm cannulas are readily available, are placed by the usual technique, and will on average last twice as long as a standard 25 mm cannula [3]. In selected cases, a LPC may be suitable for Hospital-in-the-home treatment (older child, good child/parent understanding of signs of extravasation, ability to seek hospital review if required) [4].

Ultrasound and transillumination can be invaluable in the search for, and successful cannulation of, a suitable vein. Transillumination is particularly helpful in

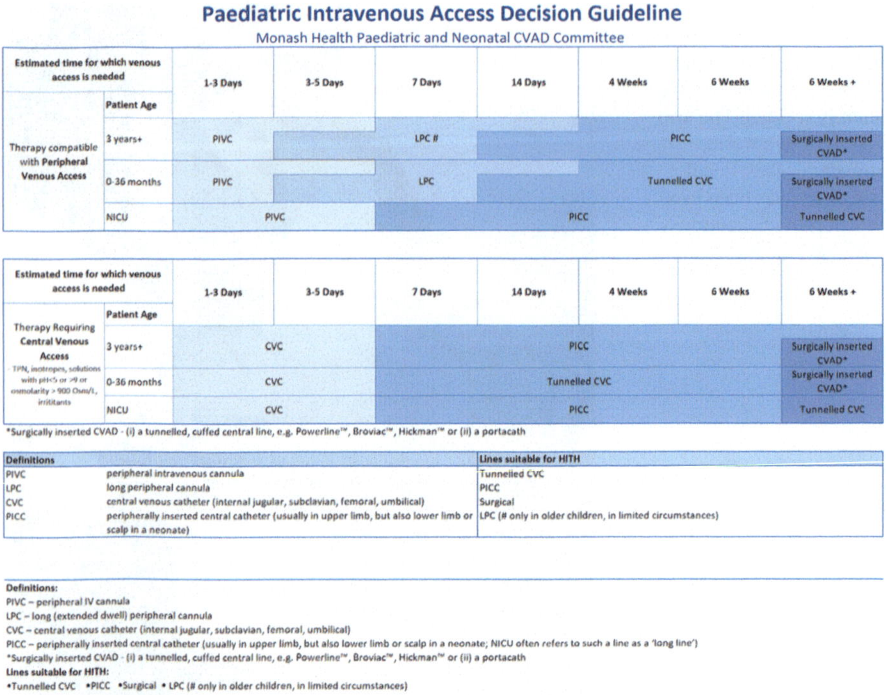

Fig. 2 Vascular access decision algorithm, courtesy of Monash Children's Hospital, Melbourne, Australia

infants: shone through the limb in a small neonate; shone from above the area of interest in older infants. The infrared light makes superficial veins more visible (Fig. 3); it also reveals when an apparent vein is actually a haematoma!

Ultrasound is a useful skill to acquire. In paediatric peripheral venous access, some key points are worth stressing:

- One needs both hands free. Assistance is required. It is important to have the skin stretched (e.g. with tape), so that it doesn't buckle as the cannula is passed (see Fig. 1).
- Ultrasound is of little use for veins which are immediately subcutaneous. The presence of some flesh between the ultrasound probe and the vein makes it possible to see the needle's journey.
- At least 2/3 of the cannula must be in the vein. This vital point is often not appreciated by novices. If a cannula of standard length is placed in a deep vein, there may be very little cannula actually within the vein, making extravasation inevitable (Fig. 4). Use of a LPC is essential.

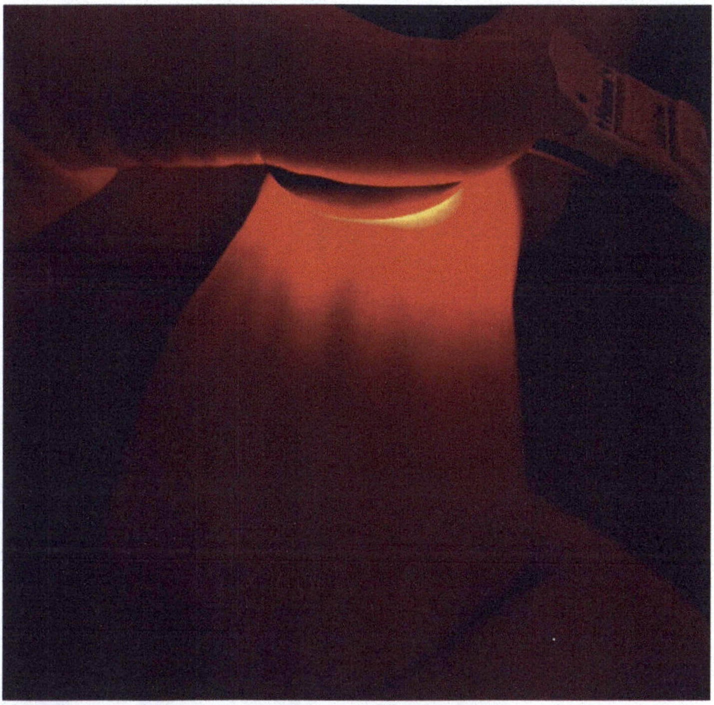

Fig. 3 Transillumination proximal to the target vein helps clarify its course. (image provided courtesy of Richard K. Barnes)

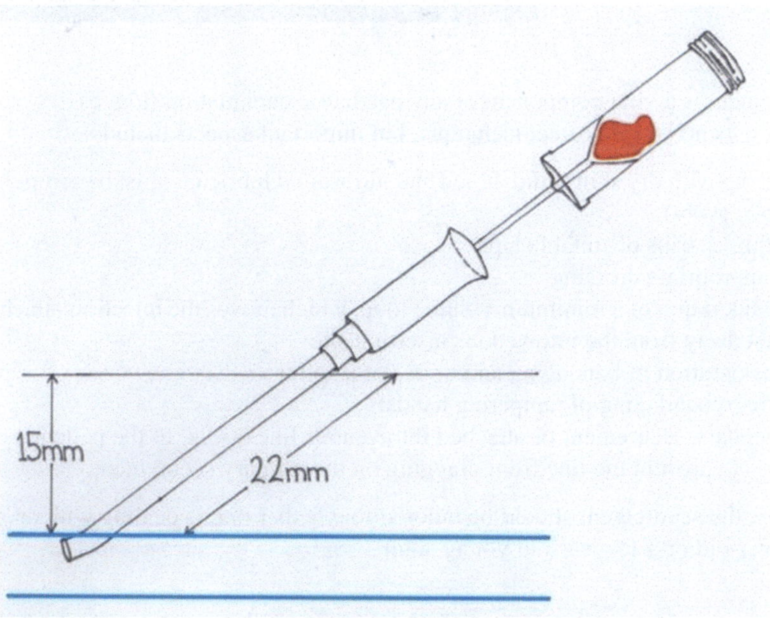

Fig. 4 Sketch to illustrate inadequate length of cannula within vein after ultrasound-guided cannulation. (image provided courtesy of Richard K. Barnes)

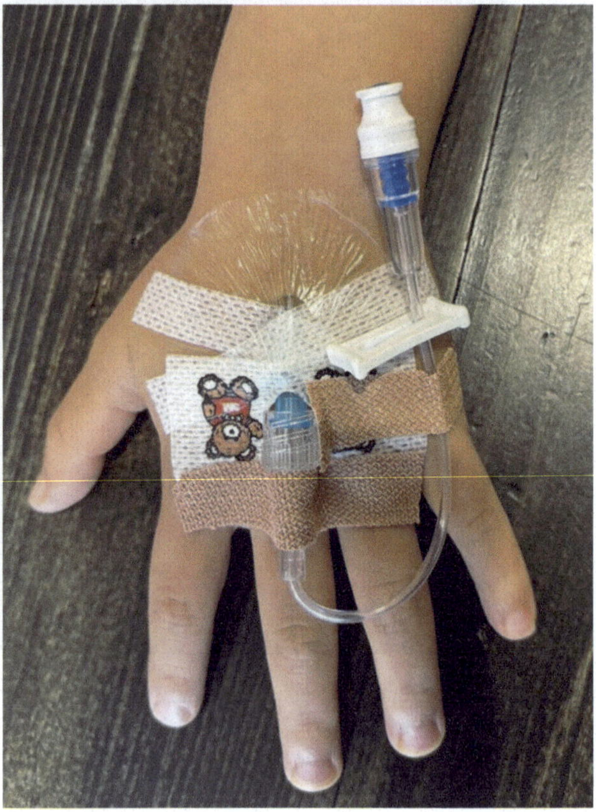

Fig. 5 Image to show a suitable securement technique. (provided courtesy of Richard K. Barnes)

Securement is a vital component of any paediatric cannulation (Fig. 5).

There is no single correct technique, but important aspects include:

- starting with dry skin (fluid, blood and ultrasound lubricant must be scrupulously wiped away)
- multiple strips of suitable tape
- an appropriate dressing
- consideration of a minimum-volume loop, which moves the injection/attachment point away from the intravenous insertion site
- consideration of bandaging and/or use of a splint
- perhaps bandaging of tampering hands!
- secondary securement of attached intravenous lines—e.g. to the patient's clothing—to prevent the line from dragging on the primary securement.

Clearly, the securement should be tailored to whether one is dealing with an angry two-year-old or a 15-year-old young adult!

4 Other Gems

- Always remember, "drips are humbling". Never hesitate to ask a colleague for help.

References

1. Paterson, R. S., Chopra, V., Brown, E., et al. (2020). Selection and insertion of vascular access devices in pediatrics: A systematic review. *Pediatrics, 145*(s3), e20193474H. https://doi.org/10.1542/peds.2019-3474H
2. Qin, K. R., Ensor, N., D'Amore, M., Barnes, R., Nataraja, R. M., & Pacilli, M. (2024). A pilot workshop for ultrasound-guided insertion of long peripheral catheters. *The Journal of Vascular Access., 25*(3), 1031–1032. https://doi.org/10.1177/11297298221125270
3. Qin, K. R., Ensor, N., Barnes, R., et al. (2021). Standard versus long peripheral catheters for multiday IV therapy: A randomized controlled trial. *Pediatrics, 147*(2), e2020000877. https://doi.org/10.1542/peds.2020-000877
4. Glazner, J., Steinfort, K., Hu, Y. J., Browne, W., Smith, I., & Brasher, C. (2023). Short midline catheters: High success rates for antibiotic therapy in children with cystic fibrosis. *The Journal of Vascular Access., 24*(3), 385–390. https://doi.org/10.1177/11297298211035310

It's Just a Needle

Dinah Humphries, Olivia Cameron, and Simon Craig

1 Clinical Pearl

Creating a positive and supportive experience for children during their first needle-stick procedure is crucial in reducing needle-phobia, procedural anxiety, and medical trauma.

2 Clinical Case

Izzy, a 4-year-old girl with cystic fibrosis, attended a regular clinic appointment with her mother. Her mother also has cystic fibrosis and has been engaged with the medical system for the duration of her life, and now presents with medical trauma and anxiety. Izzy also presents with medical anxiety and needle phobia.

Izzy requires annual blood testing to monitor her condition and has been offered a new medication that requires a 3 monthly blood test. The family are keen to try the new medication, but her mother is unsure about the requirement for regular blood tests.

Izzy and her mother presented to pathology three times before actually making it in the door for the blood test. On the third attempt, the child life therapist (CLT) met the family prior to the appointment. During a previous attempt, the CLT had discussed with the mother the advantages of numbing cream, and the patient had presented this time with cream in-situ on the left cubital fossa.

D. Humphries · O. Cameron
Monash Children's Hospital, Clayton, VIC, Australia

S. Craig (✉)
Department of Paediatrics, School of Clinical Sciences at Monash Health, Monash University, Clayton, VIC, Australia

C. F. Lynch et al. (eds.), *The Art of Paediatric Medicine Beyond the Evidence Base*,
https://doi.org/10.1007/978-981-96-7234-9_85

The CLT discussed and made a plan to support the patient with the mother, prior to the blood test. The agreed plan included comfort positioning in mum's arms, and distraction that the CLT discussed with the patient directly (patient chose fairy book and counting toy). The patient and the CLT had met previously and played prior to the procedure, to allow for rapport and trust building. The mother and the CLT spent time talking prior to the procedure during which the mother disclosed her own experience of medical trauma at the hospital. The CLT spent time validating the mother's experience and attempting to engage the mother in procedural planning to ensure a different experience for her child.

Once the patient and parent were in the procedure room, the child began to become increasingly distressed. The parent attempted to hold the child in a comfort hold that was unsuccessful due to the child's escalating behaviour. The patient was not able to engage in distraction with the CLT as planned. Although the parent was keen to continue with the blood test initially, as the procedure was taking longer than anticipated (to find the vein) she changed her mind and requested the staff stop. The parent (and CLT) needed to request this 3 times before the procedure was finally ceased. The parent and child both left the procedure visibly upset.

3 Discussion

Many children present to medical centres with pre-existing phobias and/or medical trauma, particularly relating to needle-stick procedures. Fear of needle procedures is challenging to overcome in the regular outpatient medical environment as the fear tends to be ingrained and chronic in nature.

A proactive approach to manage procedural fear is critical. *Routine* use of topical anaesthetic, comfort position and distraction are three essential ways to prevent adverse procedural experiences [1]. Just "getting on with it" to finish the procedure in the face of severe distress is likely to be very traumatic for the child and family, and may set them up for many years of medical anxiety [2].

The combination of these three methods can enhance the child and family's experience of the medical intervention, offer control and choice in a situation where the child (and family) can often feel none [3].

Sometimes, even "straightforward" procedures such as venepuncture and intravenous cannulation, may not be tolerated in the standard outpatient setting. Readily available options such as sucrose (for young infants) and topical anaesthesia are useful, however, additional sedation may be necessary, and can occur either as a planned day procedure, or within some outpatient settings.

Sedation options include inhaled nitrous oxide, or medications including midazolam, clonidine, dexmedetomidine or ketamine. The choice of sedation will depend on the age of the child, duration of the procedure, the likelihood of "successful" sedation, the anticipated onset and recovery time, and the level of monitoring available. Any sedation should be provided in a safe environment with appropriate monitoring. Resuscitation equipment and medication should be readily available.

4 Other Gems

- Some parents enter the medical space with their own history of negative medical interventions. This can have a detrimental effect on the child, often despite the parent's best efforts to maintain control over their own feelings of distress. In order to meet the needs of children and families who have a propensity towards needle-phobia, basic standard care (as discussed above) should be offered to avoid negative medical experiences and build health literacy, competence and confidence.
- Sedation often lasts longer than the procedure. Ensure the child has appropriate monitoring until they have recovered.
- Falls can occur if a sedated child is inadequately supervised. Ensure that cot sides are up and that the parent (or an appropriate staff member) is able to provide supervision until the child has recovered.

References

1. Kids Health Info: Vaccination and Needle Phobia [Online resource, last updated June 2024, accessed 19/9/2024. Available from www.rch.org.au/kidsinfo/fact_sheets/Vaccination_and_needle_phobia] The Royal Children's Hospital Melbourne.
2. Claridge, A., Hajec, L., Montgomery, L., & Knapp, B. (2020). Child and parent psychosocial experiences of hospitalization: An examination of the role of child life specialists. *The Journal of Child Life: Psychosocial Theory and Practice, 1*(1).
3. Postier, A. C., Eull, D., Schulz, C., et al. (2018). Pain experience in a US children's hospital: A point prevalence survey undertaken after the implementation of a system-wide protocol to eliminate or decrease pain caused by needles. *Hospital Pediatrics, 8*(9), 515–523. (In eng). https://doi.org/10.1542/hpeds.2018-0039

Knowledge is Power

Olivia Cameron, Dinah Humphries, and Simon Craig

1 Clinical Pearl

Empowering children with knowledge and agency in their healthcare can improve their ability to cope with medical treatment.

2 Clinical Case

A 14-year-old boy, Shane, presented to the emergency department with a foreign body in his ear. He had a history of a moderate intellectual disability. Medical staff engaged a child life therapist (CLT) to assess the teenager's ability to cope, to assist with procedure planning. Shane was assessed as having a good ability to cope.

The CLT clarified the procedure steps with medical staff, and subsequently provided medical education using real equipment to ensure the patient understood the steps involved in the procedure. The education session included information about how each step would feel and sound like for the patient. Shane was then given opportunities to ask questions to clarify his understanding. During the education session, the CLT was able to further assess the teenager's coping ability based on his reaction to the medical education provided.

The child responded well to education, and the CLT communicated this to medical staff and articulated that she felt he would manage the procedure without pharmacological support. Shane was given the choice of sitting upright or lying down

O. Cameron · D. Humphries
Monash Children's Hospital, Clayton, VIC, Australia

S. Craig (✉)
Department of Paediatrics, School of Clinical Sciences at Monash Health,
Monash University, Clayton, VIC, Australia

C. F. Lynch et al. (eds.), *The Art of Paediatric Medicine Beyond the Evidence Base*,
https://doi.org/10.1007/978-981-96-7234-9_86

for the procedure. Medical staff attended to Shane and began to undertake the steps in the procedure. The CLT reminded Shane throughout, of the procedural plan and what each step would feel/sound like. Shane managed the steps with ease, the foreign body was removed, and Shane was subsequently discharged.

3 Discussion

Most children experience medical procedures during their childhood. While many children undergoing medical procedures and interactions with healthcare professionals have positive experiences, others do not. Increasing evidence shows the harm which can be caused to children when they are not informed or involved in their care [1].

Effective procedural pain management encompasses both pharmacological and non-pharmacological interventions. Non-pharmacological interventions aim to minimise anxiety and pain, therefore promoting coping for current procedures, and building a better capacity for coping with future interventions.

4 Procedural Preparation and Planning

Children often experience anxiety and uncertainty when facing unfamiliar medical procedures. These procedures can be frightening and overwhelming for young patients, leading to negative feelings and a reluctance to return to the healthcare setting.

Provision of clear and developmentally appropriate information, including the sensory aspects of the procedure, is crucial for preparing children. For some children verbal information will be sufficient, and other children will require use of visual tools and medical equipment. They should have the opportunity to ask questions to clarify their understanding. This can help reduce their anxiety, increase their sense of agency, and improve their coping ability. During the procedure, some children may benefit from step-by-step instructions [1].

The level of detail and intervention provided will depend on the child's age, developmental stage, and coping style. Younger children or those with a reduced capacity to cope may benefit from simpler explanations [2].

During procedural planning, children should be supported to share their views, feelings and procedural preferences. They should be involved in decision making where possible, which can enhance their agency and sense of control, leading to improved procedural coping and positive outcomes.

5 Coping strategies

Coping strategies can be effective tools for children during medical procedures and hospitalisation. Coping strategies involve conscious efforts to manage emotions, thoughts, behaviours, and physical reactions to stress. This helps individuals maintain control over their responses during stressful situations. Effective coping strategies include but are not limited to: play as an alternate activity, deep breathing, mindful activities like counting, visual blocking of the procedure site and non-procedural talk. Choosing a coping strategy will depend on the child's age and stage, preference and coping style [3, 4].

6 Procedural positioning

Children often experience fear, uncertainty, and anxiety during medical procedures, which can lead to resistance. Some healthcare professionals may resort to holding children when they become uncooperative, which can undermine their rights [5].

Alternatives to restraining a child for a procedure, include taking a clinical pause to consider children's preferences and explore alternative approaches to holding, or developing a Plan B at the start and pivoting to an approach that is better tolerated [6]. By choosing alternatives to holding, healthcare professionals can make more informed decisions that respect the child's rights and promote a positive procedural experience. Positive childhood experiences with healthcare can lead to improved access to and a positive relationship with healthcare in adulthood [7].

Comfort positioning (a secure, "hugging" hold by a trusted caregiver) is optimal as it helps children feel safe and secure while facilitating access for the medical procedure [8].

7 Other Gems

- High parental anxiety can have a significant negative impact on a child's ability to cope. Supporting parents can enhance the psychosocial outcomes of the child [2].
- Child life therapists and experienced paediatric nurses can improve the patient experience, reducing the risk of distress, and can potentially reduce the need for procedural sedation.

References

1. Bray, L., Appleton, V., & Sharpe, A. (2019). The information needs of children having clinical procedures in hospital: Will it hurt? Will I feel scared? What can I do to stay calm? *Child Care Health Dev, 45*(5), 737–743. https://doi.org/10.1111/cch.12692. (In eng).
2. Koller, D. (2008). *Child Life Council Evidence-Based Practice Statement: Child Life Assessment: Variables Associated with a Child's Ability to Cope with Hospitalization*. Association of Child Life Professionals.
3. Thompson, R. (2018). *The Handbook of Child Life: A Guide for Pediatric Psychosocial Care*: Charles C Thomas Pub Ltd.
4. Kuttner, L. (2010). *Child in Pain: What Health Professionals Can Do to Help*. Crown House Publishing.
5. Bray, L., Carter, B., Kiernan, J., et al. (2023). Developing rights-based standards for children having tests, treatments, examinations and interventions: using a collaborative, multi-phased, multi-method and multi-stakeholder approach to build consensus. *Eur J Pediatr, 182*(10), 4707–4721. https://doi.org/10.1007/s00431-023-05131-9. (In eng).
6. The Royal Children's Hospital, Melbourne, Australia, Clinical Practice Guideline on Procedural Sedation, [last updated December 2021; cited 5 Sept 2024], Available from: https://wwww.rch.org.au/clinicalguide/
7. Mackenzie, A. (2014). *Everybody Stay Calm: How to support your young child through medical tests and procedures*. Global Publishing Group.
8. Children's Hopsital of Philadelphia. Comfort Positioning During Procedures. Available at https://www.chop.edu/centers-programs/child-life-education-and-creative-arts-therapy/prepare-your-child-visit-doctor/comfort-positioning-during-procedures. Accessed 6 Sep 2024.

Improving Medication Safety During Resuscitation

Simon Craig

1 Clinical Pearl

Maths is hard when you are stressed! Ensure that systems are in place to enable reliable medication dosing during resuscitation.

2 Clinical Case

Sunith is a three-year-old boy who was admitted to the paediatric ward for observation after a possible seizure at home. At 2 am, he is noted to have a prolonged seizure, and an emergency response is activated.

Sunith receives two intravenous doses of midazolam and the seizure stops. However, he has severe respiratory depression and requires bag-mask ventilation and eventually intubation prior to transfer to the intensive care unit.

Shortly after transfer, it is apparent that Sunith received a five-fold dosing error of midazolam, on both occasions. The treating team had requested 2.2 mL of midazolam, and the nursing staff had administered the 15 mg/3 mL solution (11 mg) rather than the 5 mg in 5 mL solution (2.2 mg).

S. Craig (✉)
Department of Paediatrics, School of Clinical Sciences at Monash Health,
Monash University, Clayton, VIC, Australia

C. F. Lynch et al. (eds.), *The Art of Paediatric Medicine Beyond the Evidence Base*,
https://doi.org/10.1007/978-981-96-7234-9_87

3 Discussion

Fortunately, in most high-income countries, paediatric resuscitation is a rare event. However, the rarity of the event leads to resuscitation of a child being emotionally charged, technically challenging, and potentially error prone [1].

One significant challenge relates to the rapid and accurate preparation of resuscitation medications, often in response to verbal orders given in a high-stress situation. This requires knowledge of the child's weight, the recommended dose (in mg/kg), the concentration of the available preparation (in mg/mL), the appropriate dilution, and rapid administration of the correct volume. Medication errors during paediatric resuscitation have been demonstrated in the pre-hospital [1, 2], emergency department [3, 4] and intensive care setting [5].

The Broselow Tape was developed to rapidly assist in determining a child's weight, based on their length (height). Although it provides a rough guide to medication dosing, the tape tends to overestimate weight in low- and middle-income countries, and does not provide sufficient information on medication administration, thereby requiring additional resources [6]. The PAWPER tape, developed in South Africa, provides a more accurate weight estimate which accounts for body habitus as well as length [6, 7].

Determining an accurate weight, although very important, is only the first step. Clinical staff must be able to confidently and rapidly prepare and administer the correct dose of medication at the correct time. This relies on a series of calculations to determine dose, dilution and volume. These calculations were previously done "in the moment" at the bedside, often on a whiteboard, mirroring teaching in Advanced Paediatric Life Support courses. Dosing errors are a significant risk during time-pressured, stressful resuscitations [3, 8].

In recent years, the use of pre-calculated resources such as medication books (often stored in medication rooms or resuscitation trolleys), electronic medical record modules or smartphone apps [2, 9] has increased the reliability of medication dosing during paediatric resuscitation. Other resources which may be helpful include pre-filled medication syringes [10] and standardised formularies [11].

Medications are usually drawn up and administered by nursing staff, although the presence of a pharmacist (if available) may improve safety in this setting [12]. It is worth remembering that paediatric resuscitation requires contributions from a multidisciplinary team, who usually work in different parts of the hospital environment (e.g. anaesthetics, intensive care, emergency, inpatient wards). It is important to **ensure that a single resource is endorsed and used throughout the hospital/healthcare organisation** to increase efficiency and make sure that everyone is "on the same page."

4 Other Gems

- If a patient is anticipated to be at significant risk of deterioration, ensure that the likely medications (e.g. to treat seizures, manage cardiac arrest or facilitate emergency intubation) are anticipated, pre-calculated and readily available at the bedside.
- Nursing staff are most likely to be drawing up and diluting medications and will require ready access to any bedside medication resources. Physical resources (such as a book or printout) have some advantages over smartphone apps in that they do not time out, do not require passwords or logins, and are visible to multiple people at once, which facilitates medication checking. A smartphone app in a doctor's pocket may not be readily available and accessible to all team members during a resuscitation.

References

1. Woods, B., Lang, B., Blayney, C., et al. (2019). Medic one pediatric (MOPed) cards: Standardising paramedic paediatric resuscitation. *BMJ Open Quality, 8*(3), e000534. (In eng). https://doi.org/10.1136/bmjoq-2018-000534
2. Siebert, J. N., Bloudeau, L., Ehrler, F., et al. (2019). A mobile device app to reduce prehospital medication errors and time to drug preparation and delivery by emergency medical services during simulated pediatric cardiopulmonary resuscitation: Study protocol of a multicenter, prospective, randomized controlled trial. *Trials, 20*(1), 634. (In eng). https://doi.org/10.1186/s13063-019-3726-4
3. Kaufmann, J., Laschat, M., & Wappler, F. (2012). Medication errors in pediatric emergencies: A systematic analysis. *Deutsches Ärzteblatt International, 109*(38), 609–616. (In eng). https://doi.org/10.3238/arztebl.2012.0609
4. Foster, M., & Tagg, A. (2019). A systems-centred approach to reducing medication error: Should pre-hospital providers and emergency departments dose children by age during resuscitation? *Journal of Paediatrics and Child Health, 55*(11), 1299–1303. (In eng). https://doi.org/10.1111/jpc.14626
5. Cimino, M. A., Kirschbaum, M. S., Brodsky, L., & Shaha, S. H. (2004). Assessing medication prescribing errors in pediatric intensive care units. *Pediatric Critical Care Medicine, 5*(2), 124–132. (In eng). https://doi.org/10.1097/01.Pcc.0000112371.26138.E8
6. Wells, M., Goldstein, L. N., Bentley, A., Basnett, S., & Monteith, I. (2017). The accuracy of the Broselow tape as a weight estimation tool and a drug-dosing guide—A systematic review and meta-analysis. *Resuscitation, 121*, 9–33. (In eng). https://doi.org/10.1016/j.resuscitation.2017.09.026
7. Wells, M., & Goldstein, L. N. (2018). An algorithm to improve the accuracy of emergency weight estimation in obese children. *The Pan African Medical Journal, 31*, 90. (In eng). https://doi.org/10.11604/pamj.2018.31.90.13821
8. Luten, R. (2002). Error and time delay in pediatric trauma resuscitation: Addressing the problem with color-coded resuscitation aids. *The Surgical Clinics of North America, 82*(2), 303–14, vi. (In eng). https://doi.org/10.1016/s0039-6109(02)00007-5

9. Ehrler, F., & Siebert, J. N. (2020). PedAMINES: A disruptive mHealth app to tackle paediatric medication errors. *Swiss Medical Weekly, 150*, w20335. (In eng). https://doi.org/10.4414/smw.2020.20335
10. Moreira, M. E., Hernandez, C., Stevens, A. D., et al. (2015). Color-coded prefilled medication syringes decrease time to delivery and dosing error in simulated emergency department pediatric resuscitations. *Annals of Emergency Medicine, 66*(2), 97–106.e3. (In eng). https://doi.org/10.1016/j.annemergmed.2014.12.035
11. Bosson, N., Kaji, A. H., & Gausche-Hill, M. (2022). A standardized formulary to reduce pediatric medication dosing errors: A mixed methods study. *Prehospital Emergency Care, 26*(4), 492–502. (In eng). https://doi.org/10.1080/10903127.2021.1955058
12. Porter, E., Barcega, B., & Kim, T. Y. (2014). Analysis of medication errors in simulated pediatric resuscitation by residents. West. *The Journal of Emergency Medicine, 15*(4), 486–490. (In eng). https://doi.org/10.5811/westjem.2014.2.17922

The Other Side of the Bed

Milin Vasudevan, Sarah Arachchi, Clementine Binks, and Catherine F Lynch

1 Clinical Pearl

The "doctor-parent" is an unenviable dual role but deepens our connections both personal and professional.

2 Clinical Cases

Case 1

An 8-year-old boy had been unwell with fever and cough for two days after returning from an overseas holiday. His paediatrician parent noted his cough started whilst overseas but deemed it a postviral cough. After returning home he developed a fever and began vomiting. She noted this symptom was unusual for him and was concerned given their recent travel history. She took him to her own hospital for review. After initial blood tests, he was commenced on high dose oral antibiotics for a confirmed pneumonia and discharged home. However, upon discharge, he began vomiting profusely. He was subsequently admitted to hospital. Multiple medical teams were involved due to the persistent vomiting, being a returned traveller, the unusual nature of his presentation and the requirement for both intravenous fluids and antibiotics. After a stormy few days, he was discharged home.

M. Vasudevan · C. Binks
Melbourne, VIC, Australia

S. Arachchi (✉)
Department of Paediatric Emergency Medicine, Monash Health, Melbourne, VIC, Australia

C. F. Lynch
Alfred Health, Melbourne, VIC, Australia

C. F. Lynch et al. (eds.), *The Art of Paediatric Medicine Beyond the Evidence Base*,
https://doi.org/10.1007/978-981-96-7234-9_88

2.1 The Patient's Reflection

As I walked into the hospital, I could hear people talking, trolleys clattering and children crying. I clutched my mother's hand tightly and tried not to vomit. However, I could not help from hurtling down my stomach contents into a long, white plastic vomit bag, handed to me by a friendly nurse dressed in dark blue scrubs.

My mother told me not to be afraid because she was a paediatrician, but I could see the pain in her eyes and so I tried my best to be brave for her.

When Dr. Sally told me that I needed to have a blood test, I could feel my heart beating rapidly like a drum and my palms were sweating. Dr. Sally said, "You might like to try the VR (virtual reality) headset."

As I slid the VR headset onto my head, I felt my body begin to relax. I could glimpse a blue and white whale in the ocean. I did not feel the sharp needle going into my arm.

Becoming a patient even for a few days meant that I missed my family, friends, dogs and school. However, my family was by my side always and my friends came to visit me in the hospital which made the days seem less grey.

I was wheeled around for imaging, had numerous blood tests (always with the VR headset) and lots of medication to make me feel better. My mother told me I had pneumonia but to me it was a long word for the horrible cough that I could not shake.

When I was finally discharged home, I felt glad to smell the fresh air, the wind blowing against my skin and the blue sky reminded me that I was no longer a patient. I smiled because I could not wait to get home and play with my younger brother and sleep in my own bed.

2.2 The Paediatrician Parent's Reflection

I vividly recall the challenge of advocating for my child's needs while striving to maintain my professional composure, particularly when his illness strayed from the typical course of pneumonia.

The extra care required during that time weighed heavily on me, as I navigated the dual role of being a 'doctor-parent.'

I felt immense gratitude when my colleagues showed compassion toward my child, and I was especially thankful to those who took the time to truly listen to my concerns as a parent.

I was deeply touched by the colleagues who reached out to offer support—whether it was through phone calls, delivering coffee while they were at work, or simply popping in to check on us. The visits from family and friends were also a source of comfort.

As a paediatrician, I found myself in the vulnerable position of being a mother first, while my child fought a serious illness. The pain and worry of knowing too much, coupled with the constant need to be present for medical updates, were emotionally and physically draining. Yet, this experience also taught me the profound importance of listening to parents, who spend the most time with their children and truly know them best.

Case 2
An 11-yr old girl had been limping for several months. Her paediatrician parent finally takes her to the local doctor and imaging is undertaken. The results are frightening, with a lesion noted in the bone requiring urgent hospital admission. Surgery reveals a benign but rare lesion. After several days, she is discharged home in a wheelchair and advised to remain on crutches for 4 weeks.

2.3 The Patient's Perspective

I remember the doctor with the Superman T-shirt. I remember a doctor telling me a silly golf joke (that I didn't get). I remember being desperate to see my friends from school and disoriented by the way time works in hospitals. I remember giggling at my dad, who had "four eyes, two noses", as the morphine kicked in. What I remember best is watching my parents push for my well-being, advocating for me in a scary hospital setting. My 'doctor-parent' had extra tools to navigate through the stress, and to explain what was happening in plain language.

2.4 The Paediatrician Parent Reflection

I remember a challenging time with the burden of being the 'expert parent.'

I remember being so grateful for kindness; the nurse who gently brushed my daughter's hair, the cleaner who greeted her in Spanish every day knowing she was learning the language, the junior doctor who sat alongside me and said, "This must be hard" and gave my hand a squeeze.

I remember suppressing the outrage I felt at being called 'an anxious little mother' by the anaesthetic consultant, and being appalled at the clinician's failure to prescribe postoperative pain relief. I remember running down the corridor demanding to see the person in charge simultaneously anxious not to make a scene yet determined to help my child. The mixture of emotional parent and rational doctor was challenging!

3 Discussion

As a parent, our role is to care for, provide for, and look after *our* children. As a paediatrician, our role is to care for, provide for, and look after *other people's* children. We bring a different lens and different emotions to these roles. Whether your child is a 6-month babe, a 6-year-old primary schooler or a 16-year-old adolescent, the first inpatient hospital stay for your own child is a particular challenge. You may be an expert in caring for sick children and you are an expert in your own child's health and well-being but you are 'first timers' as a parent of a sick child. Your workplace and home life now collide.

Our dual identity, as a doctor and parent, brings benefits and challenges. Our roles can sometimes blur the picture in front of us. The best practice is to always seek medical help when one has an unwell child. But what if one is the doctor? This role reversal is challenging and requires us to assume a 'dual citizenship' [1]. When parenting and professional worlds collide, the question is this: who will you be during your own family's medical situation?

As doctors, we are used to being in control of medical decision making, shared care, communication within a team, offering explanations, reassurance, ordering investigations, and prescribing medication. Doctor-parents are usually very conscious of the needs of the treating team and strive not to be "difficult" or be treated as "special", but the therapeutic relationship does change on both sides of the bed when treating a colleague's child. Sometimes it can be better for everyone if the staff do not know the parent's occupation. Advocacy is hard even when as a doctor you may be familiar with escalation pathways and systems. Relinquishing your level of control, to a hospital, a different team, can be challenging. It does, at times, come with a heavy emotional cost, especially if your child is not receiving appropriate care or their illness trajectory is unusual.

Internally, there is a conflict of being emotionally attached to your child, whilst also trying to keep a clinical perspective. The experience may become an internal battleground for the doctor-parent, seesawing between the calm, collected professional and a parent struggling to push away the fears swirling within their own mind; the 'what ifs.'

Perhaps, we want to be seen a certain way and may dismiss concerns or provide too much clinical information to our child, about certain procedures or investigations, whilst trying to allay their concerns. "Don't worry you will be fine. Mummy does this all the time", or "The X-ray is a quick burst of photos that does not produce too much radiation."

Nights in the hospital are long but in a different way from being a busy night doctor. As a parent, you are woken late at night whilst intravenous antibiotics are administered, or by the noises of the nurses' footsteps. These things become a frequent irritation in the early hours of the night. The exhaustion, lack of sleep and poor food are also a very different experience. When the morning team arrives to commence their ward round and review your child, this may become a source of turmoil as we struggle to take in the information provided. The effects can linger even after discharge.

It is important to always advocate for our children. But the care of sick children is a shared responsibility. Whilst acknowledging the challenge of losing control, it is also important to refine our role—as a doctor and as a parent. Both roles are equally important, and we must ensure that we do not allow one role to blur the role of the other. We must never forget that medical care is a team effort that involves all members of the team, including the parent. When we are the doctor-parent we are a unique team member!

4 Other Gems

- When treating a child of a doctor-parent (or parents), there are positives and pitfalls. The parent will usually be a good historian and observer, and the treating clinician will have a shared language with them. But beware the additional struggles of their dual roles. Also, the doctor-parent's field of expertise may be in areas other than childhood illness.
- Beware creating a "special" patient. "Special status" can lead to boundary crossing, unnecessary investigations and does not always ensure better outcomes.
- A non-medical parent can be a great asset but is easily marginalised during the medical conversations.
- If as a clinician you find yourself treating any patient as special, reflect on what it is about the situation that has meaning for you.

Reference

1. Stone, L. (2022). Being a doctor -parent of a sick child. In *Don't forget the Bubbles*. https://doi.org/10.31440/DFTB.50189. Accessed 25 Jan 25.

To Heal the Body, We Also Must Comfort the Soul

Dinesh Bandara Palipana

1 Clinical Pearl

If we are to best support our patients to heal physically, we must make sure that the soul is comforted.

2 Clinical Case

The handover happens on a late shift in a paediatric short stay unit, where a 14-year-old girl, Yasmin, who is undergoing some investigations for an undifferentiated abdominal pain, is on the handover list to be discussed. The handover describes a difficult course of interactions with the teenager, who is now about 15 h into admission. Yasmin is frustrated. She is refusing an ultrasound, which is indicated. She wants to leave the department. Her mother is under pressure, furthering the rift between family and staff. The therapeutic relationship is broken. There have been 5 hours of difficult conversations to progress to the next step.

The doctor takes a deep breath. It is the start of the shift. They are beginning with yet another difficult patient. The hospital environment has been challenging of late. The doctor has their own personal problems at home, topped off with a malfunctioning parking permit on arrival causing tardiness to work.

The doctor pauses on the way to reviewing the patient. They take a moment to remember that they were once a patient in a hospital, with a lengthy admission for

D. B. Palipana (✉)
Gold Coast University Hospital, Southport, QLD, Australia

Griffith University, Nathan, QLD, Australia

Bond University, Robina, QLD, Australia

C. F. Lynch et al. (eds.), *The Art of Paediatric Medicine Beyond the Evidence Base*,
https://doi.org/10.1007/978-981-96-7234-9_89

a critical illness. They remember the disempowering scary environment of a hospital, with their own frustrations. They decide to start again with this patient.

The doctor wanders in, introduces themselves, and asks Yasmin how she is. The doctor spends 10 min just listening to her frustrations. "No one has explained to me what's happening or why the plan is changing", she says in near tears. The mother expresses her own frustrations. She is a single parent. She is meant to be at work but has taken another sick day. The rent has been late many times recently. The doctor spends five minutes talking about the course of care, then why the ultrasound is necessary. Yasmin agrees to do the ultrasound, thanking the doctor for listening.

An hour later, the ultrasound is done. It is the last negative test needed to reassure the team of a safe discharge. The family goes home. The bed is cleared for another outlier.

3 Discussion

Plato is said to have taught that, "The greatest mistake in the treatment of diseases is that there are physicians for the body and physicians for the soul, although the two cannot be separated" [1]. This principle has for a long time been a foundational, though sometimes forgotten, tenet of medicine. Empathy is a part of being a physician for the soul.

Since he said it, Plato's principle has been supported by evidence. A 2023 meta-analysis revealed that empathy may be associated with better outcomes in clinical outcomes; provider performance; patient experiences and states; provider well-being; subsequent empathy; patient behaviour; and non-clinical behaviour or attitude [2]. In considering this, it is worth pondering how much human and financial resources we expend in healthcare to improve these outcomes with various interventions, when empathy as a single intervention may make an impact. Studies have even explored a reduction in the duration of the common cold [3], and better diabetes control [4], with an empathetic doctor.

It is also worth considering the time we spend, and compromises we make, practising defensive medicine to mitigate medicolegal risk. Positive communication skills have been linked with patient perceptions of doctor competence, as well as decreased medicolegal claim intentions [5, 6].

There are several simple steps to address empathy, facilitate communication, and aid in comforting the patient. These include:

- *sitting down* to talk to the patient, which has been associated by patients with listening carefully and explaining things clearly [7]—a natural advantage for a doctor with a spinal cord injury like this author.
- *listening*, which is associated with better outcomes, but it is also associated with a reduction in 'late-arising' concerns [8] - this cannot be taken for granted, with one study suggesting that patients experience a median time to interruption of 11 seconds [9].

- considering *non-verbal communication* including body language such as posture, gesture, facial expression and spatial distance [10].
- thinking of *digital tools* as an aid, rather than a barrier, for it was said by the cardiologist Dr. Eric Topol that technology is an opportunity "to restore the precious and time-honoured connection and trust - the human touch - between patients and doctors" [11].
- as *components of empathy*, spend time to understand what patients feel, express interest, and demonstrate concern. This has been shown to improve interactions between the doctor and patient [12].

The literature and tools available on empathy and communication are broad. The goal of this chapter is to reinforce the importance of it, the utility of it, and to encourage exploring it to better clinical practice.

In the pressures of practising medicine, it is easy to see the patient as an interruption to our work. With relation to customer service, Mahatma Gandhi said that "A customer is the most important visitor on our premises. He is not dependent on us. We are dependent on him. He is the purpose of our doing business" [13]. Similarly, the patient is the purpose of our work. Without a patient, there is no doctor.

As we go on serving our purpose, then, it is important to remember, as Hippocrates said to, "cure sometimes, treat often and comfort always" [14].

References

1. Brooks, A. T., Silverman, L., & Wallen, G. R. (2013). Shared decision making: A fundamental tenet in a conceptual framework of integrative healthcare delivery. *Integrative Medicine Insights, 8*, IMI-S12783.
2. Nembhard, I. M., David, G., Ezzeddine, I., Betts, D., & Radin, J. (2023). A systematic review of research on empathy in health care. *Health Services Research, 58*(2), 250–263.
3. Rakel, D. P., Hoeft, T. J., Barrett, B. P., Chewning, B. A., Craig, B. M., & Niu, M. (2009). Practitioner empathy and the duration of the common cold. *Family Medicine, 41*(7), 494.
4. Hojat, M., Louis, D. Z., Markham, F. W., Wender, R., Rabinowitz, C., & Gonnella, J. S. (2011). Physicians' empathy and clinical outcomes for diabetic patients. *Academic Medicine, 86*(3), 359–364.
5. Trumble, S. C., O'Brien, M. L., O'Brien, M., & Hartwig, B. (2006). Communication skills training for doctors increases patient satisfaction. *Clinical Governance: An International Journal, 11*(4), 299–307.
6. Huntington, B., & Kuhn, N. (2003). Communication gaffes: A root cause of malpractice claims. *Baylor University Medical Center Proceedings, 16*(2), 157–161. Taylor & Francis.
7. Merel, S. E., McKinney, C. M., Ufkes, P., Kwan, A. C., & White, A. A. (2016). Sitting at patients' bedsides may improve patients' perceptions of physician communication skills. *Journal of Hospital Medicine, 11*(12), 865–868.
8. Jagosh, J., Boudreau, J. D., Steinert, Y., MacDonald, M. E., & Ingram, L. (2011). The importance of physician listening from the patients' perspective: Enhancing diagnosis, healing, and the doctor–patient relationship. *Patient Education and Counseling, 85*(3), 369–374.
9. Singh Ospina, N., Phillips, K. A., Rodriguez-Gutierrez, R., Castaneda-Guarderas, A., Gionfriddo, M. R., Branda, M. E., & Montori, V. M. (2019). Eliciting the patient's agenda-secondary analysis of recorded clinical encounters. *Journal of General Internal Medicine, 34*, 36–40.

10. Ranjan, P., Kumari, A., & Chakrawarty, A. (2015). How can doctors improve their communication skills? *Journal of Clinical and Diagnostic Research: JCDR, 9*(3), JE01.
11. Topol, E. (2019). *Deep medicine: How artificial intelligence can make healthcare human again*. Hachette UK.
12. Decety, J. (2020). Empathy in medicine: What it is, and how much we really need it. *The American Journal of Medicine, 133*(5), 561–566.
13. Dadwal, S., Agarwal, D. D., Tanwar, D., & Sahu, A. (2022). Gandhian CRM-Mahatma Gandhi's philosophy on managing relationship with customers. *Journal of Positive School Psychology, 26*, 2968–2975.
14. Chan, Y. (2024). "Cure sometimes, treat often and comfort always"—Hippocrates. *American Journal of Rhinology & Allergy, 38*(4), 200–202.

The manufacturer's authorised representative in the EU is Springer Nature Customer Service Centre GmbH, Europaplatz 3, 69115 Heidelberg, Germany. If you have any concerns regarding our products, please contact ProductSafety@springernature.com

Printed and bound by CPI Group (UK) Ltd, Croydon, CR0 4YY
01/10/2026
02225921-0014